Neuron Signaling in Metabolic Regulation

Methods in Signal Transduction

Series Editors: Joseph Eichberg, Jr. and Michael X. Zhu

The overall theme of this series continues to be the presentation of the wealth of up to date research methods applied to the many facets of signal transduction. Each volume is assembled by one or more editors who are pre-eminent in their specialty. In turn, the guiding principle for editors is to recruit chapter authors who will describe procedures and protocols with which they are intimately familiar in a reader-friendly format. The intent is to assure that each volume will be of maximum practical value to a broad audience, including students and researchers just entering an area, as well as seasoned investigators.

Calcium Entry Channels in Non-Excitable Cells
Juliusz Ashot Kozak and James W. Putney, Jr.

Autophagy and Signaling
Esther Wong

Signal Transduction and Smooth Muscle
Mohamed Trebak and Scott Earley

Polycystic Kidney Disease
Jinghua Hu and Yong Yu

New Techniques for Studying Biomembranes
Qiu-Xing Jiang

Ion and Molecule Transport in Lysosomes
Bruno Gasnier and Michael X. Zhu

Neuron Signaling in Metabolic Regulation
Qingchun Tong

Non-Classical Ion Channels in the Nervous System
Tian-Le Xu, Long-Ju Wu

For more information about this series, please visit: https://www.crcpress.com/Methods-in-Signal-Transduction-Series/book-series/CRCMETSIGTRA?page=&order=pubdate&size=12&view=list&status=published,forthcoming

Neuron Signaling in Metabolic Regulation

Edited by
Qingchun Tong

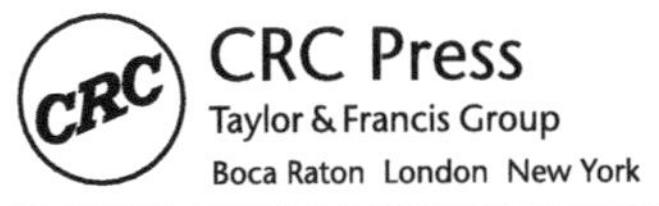
CRC Press
Taylor & Francis Group
Boca Raton London New York

CRC Press is an imprint of the
Taylor & Francis Group, an **informa** business

CRC Press
Boca Raton and London

First edition published 2021
by CRC Press
6000 Broken Sound Parkway NW, Suite 300, Boca Raton, FL 33487-2742

and by CRC Press
2 Park Square, Milton Park, Abingdon, Oxon, OX14 4RN

ISBN: 978-0-367-42029-1 (hbk)
ISBN: 978-0-367-74466-3 (pbk)
ISBN: 978-0-367-82326-9 (ebk)

Typeset in Times
by SPi Global, India

Contents

Preface

In recent years, obesity has become an epidemic and currently more than one-third of the American population develop it. Importantly, obesity is a significant contributor to a series of other diseases including, but not limited to, diabetes, cardiovascular dysfunction, and cancer. It is therefore imperative to gain mechanistic insights on the cause of obesity development. Body weight homeostasis is achieved by balanced energy homeostasis between energy intake and expenditure. More energy intake in the form of feeding than energy expenditure in the form of metabolism results in obesity. As both feeding and metabolism are ultimately controlled by the brain, understanding how brain dysfunction causes obesity development has become a major research focus in the field of metabolism.

The research on brain function in metabolism has been spurred by the discovery of leptin, an adipose-tissue-derived hormone that acts on the brain neurons to control feeding and metabolism. With the development of Cre-LoxP technology, animal models with neuron-specific gene manipulations have greatly enabled identifications of neurons, signaling pathways within neurons, and neural pathways that play an important role in feeding, energy expenditure, and obesity development. Importantly, recent technical advances in achieving acute manipulation of neuron activity with optogenetics and chemogenetics have revolutionized the approach to examining the brain function and led to important findings on key brain neurons in feeding and metabolism. In addition, recent success in adapting Ca2+ imaging to monitor *in vivo* neuron activity has allowed monitoring the activity of selective brain neurons during specific episodes of animal behaviors associated with feeding, providing important insights on the function of these neurons in normal physiology. As a result, exciting discoveries have been gained in the field during recent decades.

This volume of the CRC series on Neuron Signaling in Metabolic Regulation is dedicated to the discussion of the concept and methodology used to study brain neurons in feeding and metabolism related to obesity development. The 13 chapters cover a broad range of topics including the current state-of-the-art experimental approaches to manipulating and monitoring neuron activity, and importantly their usage in animal models to reveal the function of specific neurons, neural pathways, and neurotransmitters in the regulation of feeding, energy expenditure, and obesity development. Important insights on the role of key neurons, neural pathways, neuropeptides, hormones, as well as the interactions between brain and peripheral tissues, including nodose ganglia and adipose tissues, are also covered in this series. The chapters are intended for both accomplished investigators who want to broaden their views on this important subject and young investigators and trainees who need to acquire comprehensive knowledge and technical skills for working with brain neurons and metabolism. We anticipate this book will be a valuable menu for both basic and clinical scientists.

Qingchun Tong

Notes on the Editor

Qingchun Tong received his B.S. in Biology from Anhui Normal University in China in 1996, and his M.S. in Physiology from Shanghai Institute of Physiology, Chinese Academy of Sciences in 1999. He then moved to the USA and obtained his PhD in Neural and Behavioral Sciences from SUNY Downstate Medical Center in 2003. He expanded his PhD studies during his postdoctoral training at Beth Israel Deaconess Medical Center and Harvard Medical School during 2003–2009, where he used mouse genetics to study hypothalamic neurocircuits in metabolism and feeding behaviors related to obesity and diabetes. In 2009, he was recruited to the Institute of Molecular Medicine (IMM) of the University of Texas Health Science Center at Houston (UTHealth) and has remained a faculty member ever since. Tong is currently Professor and Cullen Chair in Molecular Medicine at IMM of the McGovern Medical School of UTHealth. He is also an adjunct faculty member of the Department of Neurobiology and Anatomy of McGovern Medical School and the Endocrine Division of the Department of Medicine at Baylor College of Medicine.

Tong's research focuses on brain control of feeding behaviors and metabolism. The current obesity epidemic and its associated metabolic syndrome have imposed unprecedented challenges to society and medicine, but with no apparent effective therapeutics. His research goal is to understand the fundamental mechanistic insights on key driving causes for defective feeding and body weight regulation, therefore providing conceptual and effective targets for the prevention and treatment of eating disorders, obesity, and its associated diabetes. Toward this goal, he employs animal models in combination with state-of-the-art techniques, including electrophysiology, optogenetics, chemogenetics, neuronal tracing, and *in vivo* live imaging to dissect key functional neurocircuits in the regulation of feeding, body weight, and glucose homeostasis.

Tong has published over 70 peer-reviewed research articles and is frequently invited as a speaker at national and international conferences. He currently serves as active manuscript reviewer for numerous academic journals and is an editorial board member of *Molecular Metabolism* and *Obesity Medicine*.

List of Contributors

Alan de Araujo, University of Florida, Gainesville, FL, USA
Arashdeep Singh, University of Florida, Gainesville, FL, USA
Calyn B. Maske, PhD, Florida State University, Tallahassee, FL, USA and University of Florida, Gainesville, FL, USA
Carlos Ramos, Baylor College of Medicine, Houston, TX, USA
Cristian Coarfa, Baylor College of Medicine, Houston, TX, USA
Danielle N. Tapp, Miami University, Oxford, Ohio, USA
Dean P. Edwards, PhD, Baylor College of Medicine, Houston, TX, USA
Diana L. Williams, PhD, Florida State University, Tallahassee, FL, USA
Dimuthu Nuwan Perera, Baylor College of Medicine, Houston, TX, USA
Guillaume de Lartigue, PhD, University of Florida, Gainesville, FL, USA
Haifei Shi, PhD, Miami University, Oxford, Ohio, USA
Hao Ying, PhD, Shanghai Institutes for Biological Sciences, University of Chinese Academy of Sciences, Chinese Academy of Sciences, Shanghai 200031, China
Hsin-Yi Lu, PhD, Baylor College of Medicine, Houston, TX, USA
Isabel I. Coiduras, Florida State University, Tallahassee, FL, USA
Jennifer W. Hill, PhD, The University of Toledo, Toledo, OH 43606, USA
Jessie Morrill, University of Texas Health Science Center at Houston, Houston, TX, USA
Jian Xiong, PhD, University of Texas Health Science Center at Houston, Houston, TX, USA
Jianqiao Zhang, Johns Hopkins University School of Medicine, Baltimore, MD, USA
Jing Cai, University of Texas Health Science Center at Houston, Houston, TX, USA
Jingjing Jiang, PhD, Zhongshan Hospital, Fudan University, Shanghai 200031, China
Julia Wulfkuhle, PhD, George Mason University, Manassas, VA, USA
Kapil Suchal, Johns Hopkins University School of Medicine, Baltimore, MD, USA
Kimal Rajapakshe, Baylor College of Medicine, Houston, TX, USA
Kimberly R. Holloway, PhD, Baylor College of Medicine, Houston, TX, USA
Ki Woo Kim, PhD, Yonsei University College of Dentistry, Seoul, 03722, Korea
Kristen N. Krolick, Miami University, Oxford, Ohio, USA
Le Trung Tran, Yonsei University College of Dentistry, Seoul, 03722, Korea
Lisa R. Anderson, Florida State University, Tallahassee, FL, USA
Macarena Vergara, University of Florida, Gainesville, FL, USA
Makoto Fukuda, PhD, Baylor College of Medicine, Houston, TX, USA
Matthew S. McMurray, Miami University, Oxford, Ohio, USA
Michael X. Zhu, PhD, University of Texas Health Science Center at Houston, Houston, TX, USA
Mitchell T. Harberson, The University of Toledo, Toledo, OH 43606, USA
Myra Costello, Baylor College of Medicine, Houston, TX, USA
Ni Zhang, Johns Hopkins University School of Medicine, Baltimore, MD, USA

Qingchun Tong, PhD, University of Texas Health Science Center at Houston, Houston, TX, USA
Ryan M. Cassidy, MD, PhD, University of Texas Health Science Center at Houston, Houston, TX, USA
Sandra L. Grimm, PhD, Baylor College of Medicine,Houston, TX, USA
Sheng Bi, MD, Johns Hopkins University School of Medicine, Baltimore, MD, USA
Shengnan Liu, Shanghai Institutes for Biological Sciences, University of Chinese Academy of Sciences, Chinese Academy of Sciences, Shanghai 200031, China
Shixia Huang, PhD, Baylor College of Medicine, Houston, TX, USA
Siyi Shen, Shanghai Institutes for Biological Sciences, University of Chinese Academy of Sciences, Chinese Academy of Sciences, Shanghai 200031, China
Tooru M. Mizuno, PhD, University of Manitoba, Winnipeg, Manitoba, Canada
Wenwen Zeng, PhD, Tsinghua University, Beijing, China
Xinmin Qian, Tsinghua University, Beijing, China
Xuan Wang, PhD, Baylor College of Medicine, Houston, TX, USA
Yan Li, Jiangnan University, Wuxi 214122, China
Ying Yan, Shanghai Institutes for Biological Sciences, University of Chinese Academy of Sciences, Chinese Academy of Sciences, Shanghai 200031, China
Yong Xu, MD, PhD, Baylor College of Medicine, Houston, TX, USA
Yongjie Yang, PhD, Baylor College of Medicine, Houston, TX, USA

1 Regulation of Energy Balance by Hypothalamic cAMP-Related Signaling

Makoto Fukuda

Baylor College of Medicine, USA

CONTENTS

1.1 CYCLIC AMP AND DOWNSTREAM SIGNALING

Cyclic adenosine monophosphate (cAMP) is a ubiquitous second messenger that plays a critical role in coupling extracellular signals to intracellular responses in virtually all cell types (Patra et al. 2020, Rall and Sutherland 1958). cAMP is produced in response to various extracellular signals that bind to and activate G-protein-coupled receptors (GPCRs) which are coupled with their associated heterotrimeric GTP-binding protein (G protein) alpha subunits (Gαs) (Kroeze, Sheffler, and Roth 2003, Dessauer et al. 2017) (Figure 1.1). The Gαs stimulate adenylyl cyclases that catalyze the cyclization of adenosine triphosphate (ATP), thereby producing cAMP, which then directly binds intracellular effector proteins to initiate cellular processes.

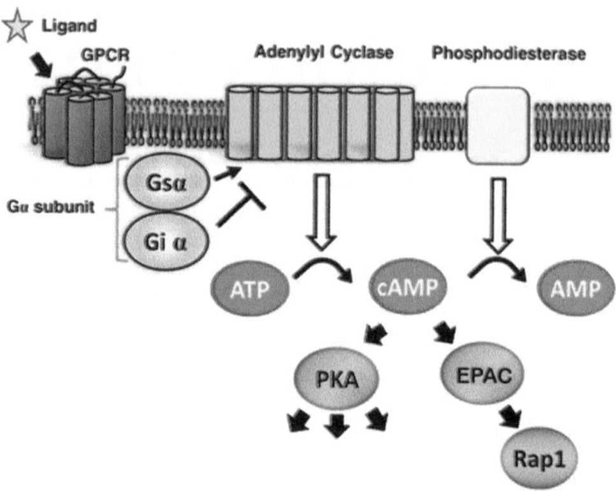

FIGURE 1.1 Schematic illustration of cAMP-related signaling. cAMP is produced from the cyclization of adenosine triphosphate (ATP), which is catalyzed by adenylyl cyclase (AC, encoded by ADCYs). The enzymatic activity of adenylyl cyclase is stimulated or inhibited by the stimulatory or inhibitory alpha subunits (Gsα or Giα) of G proteins linked to G protein-coupled receptors (GPCRs). Increased intracellular levels of cAMP induce the activation of effector proteins containing cyclic nucleotide-binding domains, such as protein kinase A (PKA), and exchange proteins directly activated by cAMP (EPAC), mediating specific downstream effects. cAMP is degraded, and its signal is terminated by phosphodiesterases (PDEs) that hydrolyze cAMP into AMP. Additional details and abbreviations are described in the text.

Termination of cAMP signaling is achieved by the degradation of cAMP by phosphodiesterases, enzymes that catalyze the hydrolysis of cAMP to AMP (Conti and Beavo 2007), and also by inhibition of adenyl cyclase by Gα subunits of the Gi family (Dessauer et al. 2017) (Figure 1.1).

cAMP exerts its pleiotropic effects by directly binding to its effector proteins containing the cyclic nucleotide-binding domain (CNBD) (Berman et al. 2005), a small and evolutionarily conserved regulatory module comprising ~120 amino acids that directly binds to cAMP and cGMP. The binding of cAMP to CNBDs elicits an allosteric reversible change in the conformation of proteins, which ultimately alters the activities of cAMP effector proteins. Eukaryotic cAMP effector proteins identified to date commonly contain CNBDs and include cAMP-dependent protein kinase (PKA) (Walsh, Perkins, and Krebs 1968), exchange protein directly activated by cAMP (EPAC, the guanine nucleotide-exchange factor for the small GTPase Rap1) (de Rooij et al. 1998), cyclic nucleotide-regulated channels (Kaupp and Seifert 2002), popeye domain-containing proteins (Brand and Schindler 2017), and cyclic nucleotide receptors involved in sperm function (CRIS) (Krähling et al. 2013).

Protein kinase A (PKA), also commonly known as cAMP-dependent protein kinase, is the first identified and the most extensively studied cAMP effector (Walsh, Perkins, and Krebs 1968, Taylor et al. 2012). PKA is a tetrameric holoenzyme consisting of two regulatory and two catalytic subunits. When cAMP levels are low, the catalytic subunits are associated with an inhibitory regulatory subunit dimer, which inactivates the kinase activity of the catalytic domain. As cAMP levels increase, two cAMP molecules directly bind to each regulatory subunit, eliciting an allosteric reversible change in conformation, which dissociates the inhibitory regulatory subunits from the catalytic subunits. The free catalytic subunits interact with target proteins and the phosphorylate amino acid residues of serine or threonine.

Subsequently, cAMP was discovered to directly bind to EPAC1 and EPAC2 (exchange proteins activated by cAMP), which are guanine nucleotide exchange factors (GEFs) that catalyze the exchange of guanosine diphosphate (GDP) for guanosine-5'-triphosphate (GTP) on the small GTPase Rap1 (de Rooij et al. 1998). cAMP-bound and active EPACs promote the exchange of GDP for GTP on Rap1, thereby leading to the activation of the latter. In addition, cyclic nucleotide-regulated (CNG) channels were found to be activated by cAMP and to contain the CNBDs (Kaupp and Seifert 2002). The binding of cAMP to CNG channels induces their conformational change which stabilizes the open channel state. CNG channels are known to mediate visual and olfactory signal transduction. More recently, the cyclic AMP binding motif was identified in two novel classes of proteins, the popeye domain-containing (POPDC) proteins (Brand and Schindler 2017) and cyclic nucleotide receptors involved in sperm function (CRIS) (Krähling et al. 2013). The physiological roles of POPDC and CRIS in metabolic controls are unclear.

Increasing the number of cAMP effector proteins suggests that cAMP plays a broader range of roles in various biological contexts. While the broad topics of cAMP signaling and its cellular responses have been extensively reviewed elsewhere (e.g. Kroeze, Sheffler, and Roth 2003, Patra et al. 2020, Gold, Gonen, and Scott 2013, Zaccolo 2009, Perera and Nikolaev 2013), this chapter will primarily focus on the roles of cAMP-related signaling in the hypothalamus which is a key brain region involved in the central control of feeding and body weight.

1.2 HYPOTHALAMIC CONTROL OF ENERGY BALANCE

The hypothalamus is a crucial regulator of feeding and energy metabolism (Barsh, Farooqi, and O'Rahilly 2000, Cone 2005, van der Klaauw and Farooqi 2015, Myers and Olson 2012, Schwartz and Porte 2005, Gautron, Elmquist, and Williams 2015). Hypothalamic neurons receive a number of neural and hormonal inputs and integrate the diverse signals into the coordinated endocrine, autonomic, and behavioral responses to maintain whole-body energy homeostasis. Among the peripheral mediators acting through the hypothalamus, leptin is one of the most powerful anorectic hormones for maintaining normal body weight. Leptin is an adipocyte hormone that is produced and secreted by fat cells in proportion to fat mass (Zhang et al. 1994, Friedman 2019) and it acts through the central nervous system, in particular the hypothalamus, to modulate food intake and energy metabolism (Elmquist, Elias, and Saper 1999). The functional leptin receptor, ObRb, is highly expressed in the hypothalamus and other neuronal populations in the midbrain and hindbrain (Elmquist et al. 1998). Neural deficiency of this receptor significantly increases body weight and adiposity (Cohen et al. 2001). Decades of extensive studies of leptin have uncovered hypothalamic neural circuits of energy balance that include two sets of prototypical cell types: one expressing proopiomelanocortin (POMC) and another expressing neuropeptide Y and agouti-related peptide (AgRP/NPY) (Figure 1.2) (Barsh, Farooqi, and O'Rahilly 2000, Cone 2005, van der Klaauw and Farooqi 2015, Myers and Olson 2012, Schwartz and Porte 2005, Gautron, Elmquist, and Williams 2015). POMC and

AgRP/NPY neurons are neural populations that exist in the arcuate nucleus (ARC), a hypothalamic nucleus anatomically located at the base of the hypothalamus in close proximity to the median eminence, which contains leaky fenestrated capillaries (Schwartz and Porte 2005, Toda et al. 2017, Cowley et al. 2001, Atasoy et al. 2012, Varela and Horvath 2012). Both neurons express the leptin receptor. Selective deletion of the receptor in these neurons reproduces some (Balthasar et al. 2004, van de Wall et al. 2008) or all (Xu et al. 2018) of the obesity phenotypes observed in ob/ob or db/db mice. Thus, POMC and AgRP neurons are the target cells of leptin that mediate at least some aspects of the metabolic effects of leptin. Both neurons directly innervate neurons expressing melanocortin 4 receptor (MC4R) in the paraventricular nucleus of the hypothalamus (PVH) to mediate leptin's action (Cone 2005). Upon leptin stimulation, POMC neurons are activated and increase the release of the MC4R agonist α-MSH that promotes negative energy balance, whereas AgRP/NPY neurons are inhibited and decrease the release of the MC4R antagonist AgRP peptide that promotes positive energy balance, thereby promoting negative energy balance as a whole (Cowley et al. 2001, Elias et al. 1999, Schwartz et al. 1997, Cone 2005). Furthermore, mutations in ligands and receptors of the leptin–melanocortin pathway result in obesity in humans (Farooqi and O'Rahilly 2008). Thus, the leptin–melanocortin pathway embedded in the hypothalamus serves as the central regulator of whole-body metabolism.

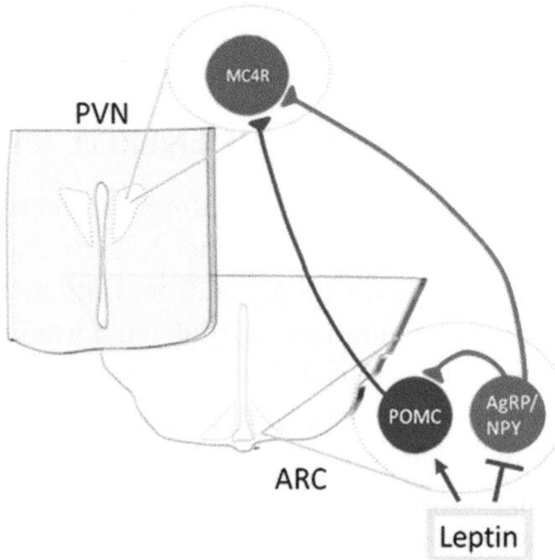

FIGURE 1.2 The hypothalamic melanocortin system. Two primary neurons of the melanocortin system, POMC and AgRP/NPY neurons, are located in the arcuate nucleus of the hypothalamus, a nucleus morphologically located at the base of the hypothalamus. POMC neurons produce and release an anorexigenic hormone, α-melanocyte-stimulating hormone (α-MSH), that directly binds and activates the melanocortin 4 receptor (MC4R). AgRP/NPY neurons secrete the AgRP peptide that is a potent antagonist of MC4R. These neurons project to neurons in the PVN that express MC4R. Leptin stimulates POMC neurons, but inhibits AgRP/NPY neurons, thereby negatively regulating MC4R, suppressing food intake, and reducing body weight. AgRP/NPY neurons send inhibitory projections onto neighboring POMC cells. The leptin–melanocortin pathway is a critical neural circuit mediating the hypothalamic control of energy balance.

1.3 OREXIGENIC EFFECT OF CAMP SIGNALING IN THE HYPOTHALAMUS

The potential role of cAMP in feeding behavior was documented as early as the 1960s. For example, Breckenridge et al. reported that implanted dibutyryl cAMP in various hypothalamic sites resulted in hyperphagia and increased locomotor activity (Breckenridge and Lisk 1969). However, this conclusion in early studies remained controversial because subsequent studies failed to reproduce the effect of intrahypothalamic injection of cAMP or its mimetics on food intake (Booth 1972, Sciorelli, Poloni, and Rindi 1972, Rindi et al. 1972, Poloni, Sciorelli, and Rindi 1974, Herberg and Stephens 1976). In the 1990s, Stanley's group reported a series of elegant works demonstrating that cAMP promotes feeding behavior when directly infused into hypothalamic areas (Gillard et al. 1997). They demonstrated that direct infusion of the membrane-permeant cAMP analog 8-bromo-cAMP (8-BrcAMP) into the perifornical (PFH) and lateral hypothalamus (LH) stimulated food intake in a dose-dependent manner. This effect is specific to the lateral and adjacent nucleus PFH because 8-BrcAMP did not elicit an anorectic effect when injected into other areas, such as the anterior and posterior LH, paraventricular nucleus of the hypothalamus, thalamus, and amygdala.

Consistent with the orexigenic role of hypothalamic cAMP, cAMP signaling is stimulated during fasting that is known to increase the expression of a most potent orexigenic neuropeptide NPY in the ARC. Using a cAMP-inducible reporter mouse that produces LacZ that faithfully reflects cAMP response element (CRE)-dependent gene expression, Shimizu-Albergine et al. showed that fasting markedly induced LacZ expression in a subset of neurons within the ARC (Shimizu-Albergine, Ippolito, and Beavo 2001). Phosphorylation of endogenous CREB in the ARC was also detected in response to fasting (Shimizu-Albergine, Ippolito, and Beavo 2001). ARC neurons, positive for LacZ or pCREB, were colocalized with NPY but not with POMC (Shimizu-Albergine, Ippolito, and Beavo 2001), suggesting that fasting increases cAMP signaling in NPY neurons. Furthermore, fasting-induced pCREB in AgRP neurons was also confirmed using AgRP-Cre-dependent reporter mice (Podyma et al. 2020, Nakajima et al. 2016). In addition, the cAMP analogue was reported to promote the orexigenic NPY peptide in the ARC (Akabayashi et al. 1994). A recent study using chemogenetics with a Gs-coupled designer GPCR (Gs-DREADD) showed that selective activation of cAMP signaling in AgRP neurons triggers a rapid and long-lasting increase in food intake and causes body weight gain (Nakajima et al. 2016).

1.4 PROTEIN KINASE A

Classically, cAMP is known to act through PKA. The evidence for the role of PKA in energy homeostasis was clearly demonstrated by powerful mouse genetic studies of each PKA subunit. PKA consists of four regulatory subunits (RIα, RIβ, RIIα, and RIIβ) and three C subunits (Cα, Cβ, and Cγ), and they are all expressed by the hypothalamus, except the catalytic subunit Cγ in humans and mice (the Human Protein Atlas resource; Uhlen et al. 2015). RIIβ is the best-studied regulatory subunit of PKA

(Cummings et al. 1996, London, Bloyd, and Stratakis 2020, Schreyer et al. 2001). Genetic deletion of the RIIβ gene leads to a lean phenotype and protects mice against high fat diet-induced obesity and subsequent metabolic consequences such as insulin resistance (Cummings et al. 1996). While RIIβ is highly expressed in brain and white-and-brown adipose tissue, the lean phenotype was reversed by re-expression of RIIβ only in the brain but not in adipocytes (Zheng et al. 2013). Furthermore, hypothalamic re-expression of RIIβ was sufficient to restore the lean phenotype (Zheng et al. 2013). Thus, the lean phenotype of RIIβ knockout mice appears to stem from its deletion in the brain, more specifically in the hypothalamus. Collectively, these studies indicate that the PKA regulatory subunit RIIβ is a critical regulator of energy balance via the hypothalamic metabolic pathways. Genetic deletion of the PKA regulatory subunit RIIα also protects mice from diet-induced obesity, a fatty liver, and glucose intolerance (London et al. 2014). In contrast to RIIβ KO mice, which exhibit marked hyperphagia, food intake was not changed in mice lacking RIIα (London et al. 2014). Similar resistance to diet-induced obesity was also observed in mice with a deficiency of PKA catalytic subunit β (Cβ) (Enns et al. 2009, London et al. 2019).

While the knockout mice of PKA subunits exhibit the common phenotypes: leanness and resistance to diet-induced obesity, the detailed phenotypes vary among RIIα KO, RIIβ KO, and Cβ KO mice, indicating specific roles of the PKA subunits in the control of energy and glucose homeostasis. Interestingly, sexual dimorphism exists in terms of the degree of phenotypic manifestations caused by genetic perturbations of the PKA pathway (London et al. 2019). The underlying causes of the differences in metabolic phenotypes of each subunit and/or between sexes are still unknown. To advance our understanding of the relevance of PKA signaling in the hypothalamic control of metabolism, future studies, particulary studies employing a powerful genetic approach enabling the genetic dissection of the pathway in a cell-type-specific manner are warranted.

1.5 EPAC-RAP1 SIGNALING

1.5.1 EPAC1/2

In addition to PKA, cAMP signaling is mediated by a relatively new cAMP target protein, EPAC (Exchange protein directly activated by cAMP), the guanine nucleotide-exchange factor for the small GTPase Rap1 (de Rooij et al. 1998).

EPAC is directly activated by cAMP, which in turn activates the small GTPase Rap1 by virtue of its ability to stimulate GTP/GDP exchange activity. There are two mammalian EPAC isoforms, EPAC1 and EPAC2, which are encoded by Rapgef3 and Rapgef4, respectively. EPAC1 is ubiquitously expressed throughout the body in humans and rodents (Kawasaki et al. 1998).

Mouse genetic studies have implicated both EPAC1 and EPAC2 in the control of energy and glucose metabolism. Yan et al. produced mice with systemic deletion of EPAC1 and demonstrated that EPAC1 null mice had lower body weight and adiposity. Under overnutrition conditions, the mutant mice gained less body weight and were protected from diet-induced glucose intolerance (Yan et al. 2013). In contrast to the lean phenotype of EPAC1 KO mice, another report demonstrated that the global deletion of EPAC1 augmented diet-induced obesity and glucose imbalance (Kai et al. 2013). While the reason for the discrepancy in the metabolic phenotypes in the two studies is still unclear, it could be due to different methods of generating EPAC1-deficient mice (the deletion of the region flanking exons 3–5 (Yan et al. 2013) vs. deletion of exons 8-21; Kai et al. 2013), the different genetic backgrounds, or the different types and durations of HFD feeding.

Another layer of evidence supporting the link between EPAC1 and obesity came from a recent study that searched for rare and low-frequency coding variants associated with body mass index (BMI) in humans. Meta-analysis of exome-targeted genotyping data from 718,734 individuals successfully identified several variants associated with BMI, including a coding variant in RAPGEF3 which encodes EPAC1 (Turcot et al. 2018). Coding variants generally change amino acids, which influences protein structure, stability, and biochemical actions, thereby likely modifying protein function. Indeed, the obesity-associated variant of RAPGEF3 results in a change in an amino acid residue at 300 from leucine to proline, suggesting a potential link between the EPAC1 function and obesity in humans.

In contrast to the ubiquitously expressed EPAC1, EPAC2 is relatively selectively expressed in a limited number of tissues, such as heart, beta-cell, adrenal gland, liver, and brain, including the hypothalamus (Kawasaki et al. 1998). One study showed that EPAC2a-null mice are prone to diet-induced obesity (Hwang et al. 2017). Under chronic high-fat diet feeding, EPAC2a KO mice had higher food intake and lower energy expenditure than control mice (Hwang et al. 2017). While the brain is one of the major tissues expressing EPAC2, however, again the direct role of EPAC2 in the hypothalamus remains to be established. Clearly, more studies are needed to understand the role of EPAC2 in the hypothalamus in body weight control.

1.5.2 Rap1

The small GTPase Rap1 is the direct target of EPAC1 and 2 (de Rooij et al. 1998). Rap1 is a small GTPase of the Ras superfamily, which acts as a binary molecular switch: the GTP-bound active form is ON, and the GDP-bound inactive form is OFF (Caron 2003). EPAC is a GTP/GDP exchange factor (GEF) for Rap1, which catalyzes the exchange from the Rap1-bound GDP with GTP, thereby activating Rap1 signaling. EPAC directly binds to cAMP and increases its GEF activity towards Rap1. cAMP strongly promotes the GEF activity of EPAC towards Rap1. Thus, EPAC mediates the activation of Rap1 in response to stimuli that increase cAMP levels. Neural Rap1 has recently emerged as a critical mediator of diet-induced obesity and its associated disorders. The GTP-bound active Rap1 protein is increased following acute and chronic HFD feeding, which promotes obesity (Fukuda et al. 2011, Kaneko et al. 2016). Mice with forebrain-specific deletion of Rap1a and Rap1b (brain Rap1 KO mice) were protected from the metabolic consequences of high-fat diet feeding (Kaneko et al. 2016). Brain Rap1 KO mice gained lower body weight and adiposity, maintained normoglycemia, and had better glucose and insulin tolerance under HFD conditions, than control mice (Kaneko et al. 2016). While HFD-fed control mice lost their ability to respond to exogenously administered leptin, HFD-fed brain Rap1 KO mice still maintained cellular and anorectic responses to administered leptin (Kaneko et al. 2016). These data collectively suggest that Rap1 plays an important role in the hypothalamic control of leptin action and energy balance.

1.6 GSα

Gsα is an α-subunit of the heterotrimeric G protein that couples cell surface receptors for hormones and other extracellular signals to adenylyl cyclase and stimulates intracellular cyclic AMP production. The Gs alpha subunit (Gsα) is ubiquitously expressed in many tissues including the hypothalamus. Recent genetic studies have uncovered the metabolic roles of Gsα expressed in distinct hypothalamic neural populations.

Heterozygous inactivating mutations of Gsα cause Albright hereditary osteodystrophy (AHO), a rare genetic disorder characterized by phenotypic abnormalities, including short stature, bone and tooth abnormalities, and developmental problems (Weinstein et al. 2001). Interestingly, AHO patients who inherit the mutation from their mother also develop early onset severe obesity and insulin resistance. This is because the Gsα gene is selectively expressed from the maternal allele in some tissues, such as the hypothalamus (Spiegel and Weinstein 2004). A mouse model of AHO recapitulated the key metabolic features of AHO by demonstrating that loss of the maternal (but not paternal) Gsα allele induced severe obesity, insulin resistance, and diabetes in mice (Chen et al. 2005, Germain-Lee et al. 2005, Xie et al. 2008). Using AHO mouse models, Weinstein's group narrowed down the site mediating the obese phenotype of the maternal deficiency of the Gsα allele. Mice with whole-brain deficiency of the maternal allele of Gsα develop obesity, probably due to reduced energy expenditure (Chen et al. 2009). This obesity phenotype seems to be mediated via a defect in Gsα signaling in the dorsomedial nucleus of the hypothalamus (DMH) (Chen et al. 2019) because AAV-mediated deletion of the maternal allele of Gsα in the DMH causes obesity (Chen et al. 2019). Maternal Gsα deletion-induced obesity was not detected when the allele was deleted in the ventromedial hypothalamus (VMH) (Berger et al. 2016), the paraventricular nucleus of the hypothalamus (PVN) (Chen et al. 2012), or Agrp neurons (Chen et al. 2017). Thus, the metabolic effect of AHO likely arises from defects in Gsα signaling in the hypothalamus.

Using mice with a loss of the Gsα alleles in distinct neural populations, Weinstein's group determined the metabolic roles of Gsα in distinct hypothalamic neurons. DMH-specific deletion of Gsα resulted in hyperphagia, reduced energy expenditure and locomotor activity, and impaired brown adipose tissue thermogenesis (Chen et al. 2019), thereby causing severe, early onset obesity. The mice also developed insulin resistance, hyperglycemia, and hyperlipidemia (Chen et al. 2019). DMH Gsα deficient mice had an increased level of the protein tyrosine phosphatase 1B, an inhibitor of leptin signaling, and decreased cellular leptin action within the DMH. While VMH-specific deficiency of Gsα had no effect on body weight on either a regular or high-fat diet (Berger et al. 2016), glucose metabolism was significantly improved in male knockout mice (Berger et al. 2016), and the effects were enhanced under high-fat diet conditions. Loss of VMH Gsα enhanced the leptin response, demonstrating a greater leptin-induced anorexigenic effect and increased STAT3 phosphorylation (Berger et al. 2016). Thus, Gsα in the VMH negatively controls cellular leptin actions and mediates whole-body glycemic control under overnutrition conditions. While loss of Gsα in the PVH was embryonically lethal in mice, haploinsufficiency of Gsα in PVN caused obesity with reductions in energy expenditure; the mice subsequently exhibited impaired glucose tolerance and insulin resistance (Chen et al. 2012). These mouse genetic studies clearly point to the critical role of Gsα in controlling energy and glucose balance in a neuron-specific manner.

The direct effect of Gsα on AgRP neurons was recently demonstrated by using a Gsα-coupled designer GPCR (Gs-DREADD) which is activated by a physiologically inert designer synthetic ligand and which initiates the Gsα-cAMP signaling cascade (Nakajima et al. 2016). By expressing Gsα-DREADD selectively in AgRP neurons, Nakajima et al. demonstrated that activation of cAMP signaling in AgRP neurons increased food intake and caused adiposity. As expected, stimulation with Gsα-DREADD increased the phosphorylation of CREB, a direct target of PKA, suggesting the activation of the cAMP–PKA pathway. cAMP signaling increased AgRP expression, and this process is required for cAMP-induced increased food intake and body weight gain. Interestingly, this manipulation did not cause neuronal excitability of AgRP neurons in brain slices or c-fos induction, a cellular marker for neural activation, suggesting that cAMP signaling induces AgRP expression, hyperplasia, and weight gain without changing AgRP neural activity. In contrast, Palmiter's group reported that chronic neural activation of AgRP neurons by Gq-DREADD was not sufficient to cause obesity (Ewbank et al. 2020). Thus, Gsα-cAMP signaling has physiological relevance in controlling cellular AgRP action and energy balance.

1.7 ADENYLYL CYCLASES

cAMP is produced solely by adenylate cyclases that catalyze the intramolecular transfer of the adenylyl group of ATP from pyrophosphate to the 3' hydroxyl group (Hanoune and Defer 2001, Cooper 2003). There are ten isoforms of mammalian adenylate cyclases, nine of which are membrane-bound forms encoded by ADCY1-9 and ADCY10 encoding soluble adenylyl cyclase.

Multiple lines of evidence suggest that ADCY3 is likely to play a role in controlling energy balance and contribute to the development of obesity in humans and animals. The first evidence linking ADCY3 to human obesity appeared in a genetic association study of ADCY3 in the Swedish population ($n = 630$) with type 2 diabetes and obesity (Nordman et al. 2008). Three single nucleotide polymorphisms (SNPs) in the ADCY3 gene were found to be associated with BMI, providing the first evidence that ADCY3 polymorphisms confer susceptibility to obesity. A subsequent genetic association study with a cohort of obese and lean Chinese subjects ($n=3{,}396$) also confirmed that ADCY3 genetic polymorphisms are associated with obesity (Wang et al. 2010).

Storm's group developed a mouse model of ADCY3 deficiency to further explore the potential link between ADCY3 and body weight control. Whole body ADCY3 knockout mice showed remarkable obesity (Wang et al. 2009). The obesity phenotype is likely due to decreased physical activity and hyperphagia because weight-matched young knockout mice exhibit reduced locomotor activity and increased food intake, even before the onset of obesity (Wang et al. 2009). These metabolic phenotypes, such as altered food intake/energy expenditure, could imply the central effect of ADCY3. Supporting this view, ADCY3 is expressed in several regions of the brain, including multiple hypothalamic nuclei responsible for the control of energy metabolism. Indeed, Cao et al. produced ADCY3-floxed mice and selectively deleted ADCY3 from the hypothalamus by a virus-mediated hypothalamic expression of Cre recombinase (Cao et al. 2016). Similar to the obese phenotype of ADCY3 deficiency, hypothalamic deletion of ADCY3 also resulted in increased body weight and adiposity. They also showed that mice with VMH-specific ablation of the ADCY3 gene had increased food intake and body weight (Cao et al. 2016). Thus, ADCY3 in the hypothalamus regulates energy balance, and its deficiency sufficiently promotes hyperphagia and obesity. In contrast, mice with a constitutively hyperactive ADCY3 mutation demonstrated a lean phenotype and were protected from diet-induced obesity (Pitman et al. 2014). The mutant mouse was found during the course of random N-ethyl-N-nitrosourea mutagenesis screening aimed at identifying genes that confer resistance to HFD-induced obesity. The mice had a single coding mutation yielding a methionine-to-isoleucine substitution at position 279 of the ADCY3 protein, which increases ADCY3 activity.

Consistent with earlier human genetic studies and animal studies, two recent studies have found homozygous variants of ADCY3 associated with severe obesity (Grarup et al. 2018, Saeed et al. 2018). One study identified obesity-causal homozygous and compound heterozygous mutations in ADCY3 in children with severe obesity (Saeed et al. 2018). Another study found novel loss-of-function variants of ADCY3-associated obesity in the Greenlandic cohort (Grarup et al. 2018). Thus, ADCY3 is recognized as a gene whose homozygous variants cause monogenic obesity in humans.

In addition, recent studies have started to provide mechanistic insight into the cellular action of ADCY3 in the hypothalamus by demonstrating a link between ADCY3, the cilia, and the hypothalamus. ADCY3 localizes to primary cilia throughout many regions of the adult mouse brain (Bishop et al. 2007). The primary cilium is a hair-like solitary structure emanating from the cell surface of most eukaryotic organisms (Goetz and Anderson 2010, Davis and Katsanis 2012, Singla and Reiter 2006) and acts as a hub for cellular signaling. Defects in many cilia-associated proteins have been linked to obesity. Wang and colleagues pointed out a remarkable similarity between ADCY3 knockout mice (Wang et al. 2009) and a mouse model of Bardel-Biedl syndrome (BBS) (Davis et al. 2007), a rare disease caused by dysfunctional cilia. Both mutant mice showed obesity, increased food intake, decreased locomotor activity, and diminished responsiveness to leptin (Davis et al. 2007, Wang et al. 2009). Furthermore, anosmia and loss of olfactory responses were also described in both mice (Wong et al. 2000, Wang et al. 2006, Kulaga et al. 2004). Siljee et al. suggested that ADCY3 is colocalized in hypothalamic neurons with MC4R, a central gene of the melanocortin system accounting for ~5% of all severe human obesity (Siljee et al. 2018). Selective inhibition of adenylyl cyclase at the primary cilia of hypothalamic neurons expressing MC4R sufficiently drives obesity in mice (Siljee et al. 2018). These results demonstrate that cAMP signaling generated by ADCY3 is a crucial regulator of energy balance by acting through cilia.

1.8 PHOSPHODIESTERASE

Intracellular levels of cAMP are tightly controlled, not only by adenylyl cyclase that stimulates the production of cAMP, but also by phosphodiesterase (PDE) that degrades cAMP, thereby terminating cAMP signaling. Currently, there are 12 structurally related but functionally distinct PDEs that catalyze the hydrolysis of the 3′-phosphoester bonds of cAMP and/or cyclic GMP to form 5'-AMP and/or 5'-GMP. Among them, PDE3B is the best-studied PDE in terms of hypothalamic metabolic functions.

The Sahuh laboratory demonstrated that leptin activated PDE3B in the hypothalamus and that the PDE3 inhibitor cilostamide blocked leptin-induced anorexia and body weight reduction as well as leptin-stimulated phosphorylation of STAT3 (Zhao et al. 2002), suggesting the existence of the leptin–PDE3b–cAMP pathway. They further generated PDE3B flox mice to produce hypothalamic-specific PDE3b deletion by crossing them to Nkx2.1-Cre mice (Sahu, Anamthathmakula, and Sahu 2018). The female mice showed increased body weight under both low- and high-fat diet feeding conditions. As the study did not assess the effect of PDE3b deficiency on leptin action, it remains to be determined whether hypothalamic PDE3B is required for leptin actions. In addition to PDE3B, Zhang and colleagues reported that whole-body deletion of PDE4B in mice reduced adiposity and high-fat diet-induced adipose inflammation (Zhang, Maratos-Flier, and Flier 2009). Another PDE that affects metabolism is PDE10A. Mice with PDE10A deficiency were protected from diet-induced obesity and associated metabolic disorders. PDE10A deficiency caused hypophagia but did not affect locomotor activity (Nawrocki et al. 2014). Pharmacological inhibition of PDE10A-induced weight loss, reduced food intake, and increased energy expenditure (Nawrocki et al. 2014). Interestingly, both PDE4B (Cherry and Davis 1999) and PDE10A (Coskran et al. 2006) are known to be expressed by multiple brain areas, including the hypothalamus, and it is of interest to determine whether the hypothalamus is the site mediating the metabolic effects of their deletion.

1.9 CAMP AND LEPTIN ACTION IN THE HYPOTHALAMUS

Leptin activates JAK-STAT3 signaling in leptin receptor-expressing neurons within the central nervous system to decrease food intake and maintain normal body weight (Bjorbaek and Kahn 2004, Spiegelman and Flier 2001, Flier 2006, Coll, Farooqi, and O'Rahilly 2007, Elmquist, Elias, and Saper 1999, Friedman 2004, Morton et al. 2006, Simerly 2008, Pan and Myers 2018). Genetic studies suggest that forebrain-specific STAT3 knockout mice display similar to those of leptin- or receptor-deficient mice (Gao et al. 2004). Bates and colleagues generated a mutant leptin receptor that selectively loses its ability to activate the STAT3 pathway by introducing a substitution mutation of tyrosine for serine at amino acid residue 1138 of the leptin receptor long-form (LRb) (Bates et al. 2003). While the mutant mice failed to modulate STAT3 signaling in response to leptin, other signaling pathways, such as MAPK signaling, remained intact in terms of leptin-dependent modulation (Bates et al. 2003). While leptin receptor mutant mice did not produce some of the phenotypes of leptin receptor-deficient mice which include infertility, severe hyperglycemia, and a shortened snout-anus length, LepR mutant mice were hyperphagic and obese, almost comparable to leptin receptor-deficient mice (Bates et al. 2003). These results collectively suggest that STAT3 signaling is a major pathway that mediates the leptin control of energy balance.

Evidence suggests that cAMP suppresses STAT3 signaling. Early studies demonstrated that cAMP plays a role as a downregulator of interleukin (IL)-6 signaling that uses JAK-STAT3 signaling (Park et al. 2000, Delgado and Ganea 2000, Bousquet et al. 2001, Gasperini et al. 2002, Fasshauer et al. 2002, Sands et al. 2006). For example, a cAMP analog inhibited IL-6-induced STAT3 activation in mononuclear cells (Sengupta, Schmitt, and Ivashkiv 1996) and in vascular endothelial cells (Sands et al. 2006). IL-6-STAT3 signaling is also inhibited by activation of Gαs-coupled receptors that lead to cAMP production (Bousquet et al. 2001, Sands et al. 2006). In several cell lines, cAMP-elevating agents were reported to induce SOCS-3 (Delgado and Ganea 2000, Bousquet et al. 2001, Gasperini et al. 2002, Fasshauer et al. 2002, Sands et al. 2006), which is a potent inhibitor of cytokine-STAT signaling. Consistent with the fact that the leptin receptor belongs to the IL-6 receptor subfamily and that cAMP promotes SOCS3 induction, cAMP was similarly shown to block leptin-STAT3 signaling. The first experimental evidence supporting the link between cAMP and leptin action came from Zhao's study demonstrating that central administration of a PDE3B inhibitor blunted the leptin-induced anorectic effect and hypothalamic STAT3 phosphorylation (Zhao et al. 2002). Additionally elevated cAMP induces the production of a potent inhibitor of cellular leptin signaling, SOCS3, in the hypothalamus, which is a primary site of action of leptin (Fukuda et al. 2011, Cordonier et al. 2019). Thus, cAMP signaling negatively controls hypothalamic leptin actions.

Recent studies further revealed the downstream signaling mechanisms underlying the inhibitory effects of cAMP on leptin action. An EPAC-selective cAMP analog sufficiently promotes SOCS-3 induction and inhibits leptin-induced STAT3 phosphorylation in vascular endothelial cells and in hypothalamic explants (Sands et al. 2006, Fukuda et al. 2011). The EPAC agonist impaired leptin-dependent neural activation of POMC neurons, a key neural population mediating the biological action of leptin (Fukuda et al. 2011). The pharmacological activation of EPAC negatively regulates the anorectic effect of leptin *in vivo* (Fukuda et al. 2011). In contrast, treatment with specific inhibitors of EPAC, such as ESI-05 or ESI-09 enhanced leptin sensitivity in hypothalamic slices or in the brain (Fukuda et al. 2011, Yan et al. 2013). Further, the genetic deletion of EPAC1 also improves leptin sensitivity (Yan et al. 2013). However, a recent study demonstrated that systemic EPAC2a knockout mice were characterized by impaired hypothalamic leptin action (Hwang et al. 2017), suggesting EPAC2a might be involved in the process of promoting leptin sensitivity. It is important to note that EPAC2a is enriched not only in the brain, including the hypothalamus, but also in peripheral endocrine organs. Thus, how EPAC2 contributes cell-autonomously to the control of leptin actions remains to be established, and further studies especially studies employing tissue-specific EPAC2 knockout mouse models, are needed to clarify this point.

In support of the role of EPAC signaling in controlling leptin sensitivity, Rap1, the direct target of EPAC1/2, was also reported to negatively control leptin sensitivity in the hypothalamus. Cellular leptin sensitivity is commonly enhanced in multiple mouse models lacking Rap1 in the brain (Kaneko et al. 2016) or distinct hypothalamic neural populations, such as VMH neurons, POMC neurons, and leptin-responsive neurons (unpublished data). In addition to the EPAC–Rap1 axis, Yang and colleagues demonstrated that mice lacking the RIIβ regulatory subunit of PKA had an enhanced response to exogenously administered leptin (Yang and McKnight 2015), suggesting that PKA contributes to determining leptin sensitivity.

1.10 POTENTIAL UPSTREAM MEDIATORS OF HYPOTHALAMIC CAMP SIGNALING

cAMP-related signaling in the hypothalamus is accordingly modulated in response to metabolic conditions. For example, in AgRP/NPY neurons, fasting leads to activation of the cAMP-related pathway and induction of AgRP expression (Shimizu-Albergine, Ippolito, and Beavo 2001, Ollmann et al. 1997). Nakajima and colleagues have shown that AgRP-specific activation of Gsα sufficiently promotes AgRP expression, food intake, and weight gain (Nakajima et al. 2016). They further showed that activation of the PAC1 receptor, one of the Gsα-coupled receptors endogenously expressed by AgRP neurons, sufficiently induced AgRP expression and subsequently promoted food intake, providing a proof of concept for the idea that Gsα-coupled receptor(s) endogenously expressed by AgRP neurons could mediate fasting-induced food intake (Nakajima et al. 2016). While physiologically relevant factors are unclear, recent progress has been made to identify potential upstream factors linking fasting and cAMP signaling.

Duerrschmid and colleagues have shown that the fasting-induced hormone, asprosin, likely mediates the fasting-induced activation of AgRP neurons (Duerrschmid et al. 2017). Asprosin is a ~30 kDa fasting-induced hormone that is highly expressed in adipose tissue and promotes hepatic glucose production (Romere et al. 2016). They found that asprosin in the circulation reached the hypothalamus, directly activated AgRP neurons, and promoted food intake via the cAMP signaling pathway (Duerrschmid et al. 2017). Exposure to asprosin acutely increased the firing frequency and the resting membrane potential of AgRP neurons, thereby inducing AgRP neural activation (Duerrschmid et al. 2017). Asprosin-induced neural activation was blocked by the pharmacological inhibition of Gαs, adenylate cyclase, and PKA (Duerrschmid et al. 2017), suggesting that asprosin activates AgRP neurons via the Gαs–cAMP–PKA pathway.

In the context of diet-induced obesity, the cAMP-related pathway was documented to be involved in leptin resistance in diet-induced obesity. The hypothalamic EPAC–Rap1 pathway is activated upon acute and chronic HFD feeding and negatively controls leptin actions (Kaneko et al. 2016, Fukuda et al. 2011). Kaneko et al. screened for circulating factors that potentially drive the activation of the EPAC–Rap1 pathway and leptin resistance using cultured brain slices, and found that the gut-derived hormone GIP blocked cellular leptin signaling in hypothalamic explants (Kaneko et al. 2019). Furthermore, centrally administered GIP diminished hypothalamic sensitivity to leptin and increased hypothalamic levels of SOCS3 (Kaneko et al. 2019). In contrast, inhibition of the GIP receptor, a GPCR coupled to Gαs, by GIPR deficiency or a GIPR-neutralizing antibody reduced body weight and adiposity and decreased the hypothalamic level of SOCS3 (Kaneko et al. 2019). We also demonstrated that activation of brain GIPR resulted in the induction of hypothalamic inflammation and insulin resistance within the hypothalamus (Fu et al. 2020). Considering that GIP levels in the blood are increased in obese humans and animals, GIP is likely a factor linking obesity and hypothalamic pathological alterations such as inflammation, leptin, and insulin resistance.

1.11 CONCLUSION

cAMP is a fundamental second messenger across many biological processes. In the hypothalamus, which comprises a complex array of distinct neural populations and non-neural cells, cAMP signaling plays different roles in different contexts. These facts underscore the need to elucidate the precise mode of action of cAMP in specific cell groups under physiological and pathological conditions. Delineating cell-specific cAMP signaling networks in the hypothalamus may result in a better understanding of the metabolic role of cAMP signaling and further create opportunities for therapeutic interventions for metabolic diseases.

REFERENCES

Akabayashi, A., C. T. Zaia, S. M. Gabriel, I. Silva, W. K. Cheung, and S. F. Leibowitz. 1994. “Intracerebroventricular injection of dibutyryl cyclic adenosine 3’,5’-monophosphate increases hypothalamic levels of neuropeptide Y.” *Brain Res* 660 (2): 323–328. doi: 10.1016/0006-8993(94)91306-4.

Atasoy, D., J. N. Betley, H. H. Su, and S. M. Sternson. 2012. “Deconstruction of a neural circuit for hunger.” *Nature* 488 (7410): 172–177. doi: 10.1038/nature11270.

Balthasar, N., R. Coppari, J. McMinn, S. M. Liu, C. E. Lee, V. Tang, C. D. Kenny, R. A. McGovern, S. C. Chua, Jr., J. K. Elmquist, et al. 2004. “Leptin receptor signaling in POMC neurons is required for normal body weight homeostasis.” *Neuron* 42 (6):983–991. doi: 10.1016/j.neuron.2004.06.004.

Barsh, G. S., I. S. Farooqi, and S. O’Rahilly. 2000. “Genetics of body-weight regulation.” *Nature* 404 (6778):644–651. doi: 10.1038/35007519.

Bates, S. H., W. H. Stearns, T. A. Dundon, M. Schubert, A. W. Tso, Y. Wang, A. S. Banks, H. J. Lavery, A. K. Haq, E. Maratos-Flier, et al. 2003. “STAT3 signalling is required for leptin regulation of energy balance but not reproduction.” *Nature* 421 (6925):856–859. doi: 10.1038/nature01388.

Berger, A., A. Kablan, C. Yao, T. Ho, B. Podyma, L. S. Weinstein, and M. Chen. 2016. “Gsalpha Deficiency in the Ventromedial Hypothalamus Enhances Leptin Sensitivity and Improves Glucose Homeostasis in Mice on a High-Fat Diet.” *Endocrinology* 157 (2):600–610. doi: 10.1210/en.2015-1700.

Berman, H. M., L. F. Ten Eyck, D. S. Goodsell, N. M. Haste, A. Kornev, and S. S. Taylor. 2005. “The cAMP binding domain: an ancient signaling module.” *Proc Natl Acad Sci U S A* 102 (1):45–50. doi: 10.1073/pnas.0408579102.

Bishop, G. A., N. F. Berbari, J. Lewis, and K. Mykytyn. 2007. “Type III adenylyl cyclase localizes to primary cilia throughout the adult mouse brain.” *J Comp Neurol* 505 (5):562–571. doi: 10.1002/cne.21510.

Bjorbaek, C., and B. B. Kahn. 2004. “Leptin signaling in the central nervous system and the periphery.” *Recent Prog Horm Res* 59:305–331.

Booth, D. A. 1972. "Unlearned and learned effects of intrahypothalamic cyclic AMP injection on feeding." *Nat New Biol* 237 (76):222–224. doi: 10.1038/newbio237222a0.

Bousquet, C., V. Chesnokova, A. Kariagina, A. Ferrand, and S. Melmed. 2001. "cAMP neuropeptide agonists induce pituitary suppressor of cytokine signaling-3: novel negative feedback mechanism for corticotroph cytokine action." *Mol Endocrinol* 15 (11):1880–1890. doi: 10.1210/mend.15.11.0733.

Brand, T., and R. Schindler. 2017. "New kids on the block: The Popeye domain containing (POPDC) protein family acting as a novel class of cAMP effector proteins in striated muscle." *Cell Signal* 40:156–165. doi: 10.1016/j.cellsig.2017.09.015.

Breckenridge, B. M., and R. D. Lisk. 1969. "Cyclic adenylate and hypothalamic regulatory functions." *Proc Soc Exp Biol Med* 131 (3):934–935. doi: 10.3181/00379727-131-34012.

Cao, H., X. Chen, Y. Yang, and D. R. Storm. 2016. "Disruption of type 3 adenylyl cyclase expression in the hypothalamus leads to obesity." *Integr Obes Diabetes* 2 (2):225–228. doi: 10.15761/iod.1000149.

Caron, E. 2003. "Cellular functions of the Rap1 GTP-binding protein: a pattern emerges." *J Cell Sci* 116 (Pt 3):435–440. doi: 10.1242/jcs.00238.

Chen, M., A. Berger, A. Kablan, J. Zhang, O. Gavrilova, and L. S. Weinstein. 2012. "Gsα deficiency in the paraventricular nucleus of the hypothalamus partially contributes to obesity associated with Gsα mutations." *Endocrinology* 153 (9):4256–4265. doi: 10.1210/en.2012-1113.

Chen, M., O. Gavrilova, J. Liu, T. Xie, C. Deng, A. T. Nguyen, L. M. Nackers, J. Lorenzo, L. Shen, and L. S. Weinstein. 2005. "Alternative Gnas gene products have opposite effects on glucose and lipid metabolism." *Proc Natl Acad Sci U S A* 102 (20):7386–7391. doi: 10.1073/pnas.0408268102.

Chen, M., Y. B. Shrestha, B. Podyma, Z. Cui, B. Naglieri, H. Sun, T. Ho, E. A. Wilson, Y. Q. Li, O. Gavrilova, et al. 2017. "Gsα deficiency in the dorsomedial hypothalamus underlies obesity associated with Gsα mutations." *J Clin Invest* 127 (2):500–510. doi: 10.1172/jci88622.

Chen, M., J. Wang, K. E. Dickerson, J. Kelleher, T. Xie, D. Gupta, E. W. Lai, K. Pacak, O. Gavrilova, and L. S. Weinstein. 2009. "Central nervous system imprinting of the G protein G(s)alpha and its role in metabolic regulation." *Cell Metab* 9 (6):548–555. doi: 10.1016/j.cmet.2009.05.004.

Chen, M., E. A. Wilson, Z. Cui, H. Sun, Y. B. Shrestha, B. Podyma, C. H. Le, B. Naglieri, K. Pacak, O. Gavrilova, et al. 2019. "G(s)α deficiency in the dorsomedial hypothalamus leads to obesity, hyperphagia, and reduced thermogenesis associated with impaired leptin signaling." *Mol Metab* 25:142–153. doi: 10.1016/j.molmet.2019.04.005.

Cherry, J. A., and R. L. Davis. 1999. "Cyclic AMP phosphodiesterases are localized in regions of the mouse brain associated with reinforcement, movement, and affect." *J Comp Neurol* 407 (2):287–301.

Cohen, P., C. Zhao, X. Cai, J. M. Montez, S. C. Rohani, P. Feinstein, P. Mombaerts, and J. M. Friedman. 2001. "Selective deletion of leptin receptor in neurons leads to obesity." *J Clin Invest* 108 (8):1113–1121. doi: 10.1172/JCI13914.

Coll, A. P., I. S. Farooqi, and S. O'Rahilly. 2007. "The hormonal control of food intake." *Cell* 129 (2):251–262. doi: 10.1016/j.cell.2007.04.001.

Cone, R. D. 2005. "Anatomy and regulation of the central melanocortin system." *Nat Neurosci* 8 (5):571–578. doi: 10.1038/nn1455.

Conti, M., and J. Beavo. 2007. "Biochemistry and physiology of cyclic nucleotide phosphodiesterases: essential components in cyclic nucleotide signaling." *Annu Rev Biochem* 76:481–511. doi: 10.1146/annurev.biochem.76.060305.150444.

Cooper, D. M. 2003. "Regulation and organization of adenylyl cyclases and cAMP." *Biochem J* 375 (Pt 3):517–529. doi: 10.1042/bj20031061.

Cordonier, E. L., T. Liu, K. Saito, S. S. Chen, Y. Xu, and M. Fukuda. 2019. "Luciferase Reporter Mice for In Vivo Monitoring and Ex Vivo Assessment of Hypothalamic Signaling of Socs3 Expression." *J Endocr Soc* 3 (7):1246–1260. doi: 10.1210/js.2019-00077.

Coskran, T. M., D. Morton, F. S. Menniti, W. O. Adamowicz, R. J. Kleiman, A. M. Ryan, C. A. Strick, C. J. Schmidt, and D. T. Stephenson. 2006. "Immunohistochemical localization of phosphodiesterase 10A in multiple mammalian species." *J Histochem Cytochem* 54 (11):1205–1213. doi: 10.1369/jhc.6A6930.2006.

Cowley, M. A., J. L. Smart, M. Rubinstein, M. G. Cerdan, S. Diano, T. L. Horvath, R. D. Cone, and M. J. Low. 2001. "Leptin activates anorexigenic POMC neurons through a neural network in the arcuate nucleus." *Nature* 411 (6836):480–484.

Cummings, D. E., E. P. Brandon, J. V. Planas, K. Motamed, R. L. Idzerda, and G. S. McKnight. 1996. "Genetically lean mice result from targeted disruption of the RII beta subunit of protein kinase A." *Nature* 382 (6592):622–626. doi: 10.1038/382622a0.

Davis, E. E., and N. Katsanis. 2012. "The ciliopathies: a transitional model into systems biology of human genetic disease." *Curr Opin Genet Dev* 22 (3):290–303. doi: 10.1016/j.gde.2012.04.006.

Davis, R. E., R. E. Swiderski, K. Rahmouni, D. Y. Nishimura, R. F. Mullins, K. Agassandian, A. R. Philp, C. C. Searby, M. P. Andrews, S. Thompson, et al. 2007. "A knockin mouse model of the Bardet-Biedl syndrome 1 M390R mutation has cilia defects, ventriculomegaly, retinopathy, and obesity." *Proc Natl Acad Sci U S A* 104 (49):19422–19427. doi: 10.1073/pnas.0708571104.

de Rooij, J., F. J. Zwartkruis, M. H. Verheijen, R. H. Cool, S. M. Nijman, A. Wittinghofer, and J. L. Bos. 1998. "Epac is a Rap1 guanine-nucleotide-exchange factor directly activated by cyclic AMP." *Nature* 396 (6710):474–477. doi: 10.1038/24884.

Delgado, M., and D. Ganea. 2000. "Inhibition of IFN-gamma-induced janus kinase-1-STAT1 activation in macrophages by vasoactive intestinal peptide and pituitary adenylate cyclase-activating polypeptide." *J Immunol* 165 (6):3051–3057. doi: 10.4049/jimmunol.165.6.3051.

Dessauer, Carmen W., Val J. Watts, Rennolds S. Ostrom, Marco Conti, Stefan Dove, and Roland Seifert. 2017. "International Union of Basic and Clinical Pharmacology. CI. Structures and Small Molecule Modulators of Mammalian Adenylyl Cyclases." *Pharmacol Rev* 69 (2):93–139. doi: 10.1124/pr.116.013078.

Duerrschmid, C., Y. He, C. Wang, C. Li, J. C. Bournat, C. Romere, P. K. Saha, M. E. Lee, K. J. Phillips, M. Jain, et al. 2017. "Asprosin is a centrally acting orexigenic hormone." *Nat Med* 23 (12):1444–1453. doi: 10.1038/nm.4432.

Elias, C. F., C. Aschkenasi, C. Lee, J. Kelly, R. S. Ahima, C. Bjorbaek, J. S. Flier, C. B. Saper, and J. K. Elmquist. 1999. "Leptin differentially regulates NPY and POMC neurons projecting to the lateral hypothalamic area." *Neuron* 23 (4):775–786.

Elmquist, J. K., C. Bjørbaek, R. S. Ahima, J. S. Flier, and C. B. Saper. 1998. "Distributions of leptin receptor mRNA isoforms in the rat brain." *J Comp Neurol* 395 (4):535–547.

Elmquist, J. K., C. F. Elias, and C. B. Saper. 1999. "From lesions to leptin: hypothalamic control of food intake and body weight." *Neuron* 22 (2):221–232.

Enns, L. C., J. F. Morton, R. S. Mangalindan, G. S. McKnight, M. W. Schwartz, M. R. Kaeberlein, B. K. Kennedy, P. S. Rabinovitch, and W. C. Ladiges. 2009. "Attenuation of age-related metabolic dysfunction in mice with a targeted disruption of the Cbeta subunit of protein kinase A." *J Gerontol A Biol Sci Med Sci* 64 (12):1221–1231. doi: 10.1093/gerona/glp133.

Ewbank, S. N., C. A. Campos, J. Y. Chen, A. J. Bowen, S. L. Padilla, J. L. Dempsey, J. Y. Cui, and R. D. Palmiter. 2020. "Chronic G(q) signaling in AgRP neurons does not cause obesity." *Proc Natl Acad Sci U S A* 117 (34):20874–20880. doi: 10.1073/pnas.2004941117.

Farooqi, I. S., and S. O'Rahilly. 2008. "Mutations in ligands and receptors of the leptin-melanocortin pathway that lead to obesity." *Nat Clin Pract Endocrinol Metab* 4 (10):569–577. doi: 10.1038/ncpendmet0966.

Fasshauer, M., J. Klein, U. Lossner, and R. Paschke. 2002. "Isoproterenol is a positive regulator of the suppressor of cytokine signaling-3 gene expression in 3T3-L1 adipocytes." *J Endocrinol* 175 (3):727–733.

Flier, J. S. 2006. "Neuroscience. Regulating energy balance: the substrate strikes back." *Science* 312 (5775):861–864. doi: 10.1126/science.1127971.

Friedman, J. M. 2004. "Modern science versus the stigma of obesity." *Nat Med* 10 (6):563–569. doi: 10.1038/nm0604-563.

Friedman, J. M. 2019. "Leptin and the endocrine control of energy balance." *Nat Metab* 1 (8):754–764. doi: 10.1038/s42255-019-0095-y.

Fu, Y., K. Kaneko, H. Y. Lin, Q. Mo, Y. Xu, T. Suganami, P. Ravn, and M. Fukuda. 2020. "Gut Hormone GIP Induces Inflammation and Insulin Resistance in the Hypothalamus." *Endocrinology* 161 (9). doi: 10.1210/endocr/bqaa102.

Fukuda, M., K. W. Williams, L. Gautron, and J. K. Elmquist. 2011. "Induction of leptin resistance by activation of cAMP-Epac signaling." *Cell Metab* 13 (3):331–339. doi: 10.1016/j.cmet.2011.01.016.

Gao, Q., M. J. Wolfgang, S. Neschen, K. Morino, T. L. Horvath, G. I. Shulman, and X. Y. Fu. 2004. "Disruption of neural signal transducer and activator of transcription 3 causes obesity, diabetes, infertility, and thermal dysregulation." *Proc Natl Acad Sci U S A* 101 (13):4661–4666. doi: 10.1073/pnas.0303992101.

Gasperini, S., L. Crepaldi, F. Calzetti, L. Gatto, C. Berlato, F. Bazzoni, A. Yoshimura, and M. A. Cassatella. 2002. "Interleukin-10 and cAMP-elevating agents cooperate to induce suppressor of cytokine signaling-3 via a protein kinase A-independent signal." *Eur Cytokine Netw* 13 (1):47–53.

Gautron, L., J. K. Elmquist, and K. W. Williams. 2015. "Neural control of energy balance: translating circuits to therapies." *Cell* 161 (1):133–145. doi: 10.1016/j.cell.2015.02.023.

Germain-Lee, E. L., W. Schwindinger, J. L. Crane, R. Zewdu, L. S. Zweifel, G. Wand, D. L. Huso, M. Saji, M. D. Ringel, and M. A. Levine. 2005. "A mouse model of albright hereditary osteodystrophy generated by targeted disruption of exon 1 of the Gnas gene." *Endocrinology* 146 (11):4697–4709. doi: 10.1210/en.2005-0681.

Gillard, E. R., A. M. Khan, Haq Ahsan ul, R. S. Grewal, B. Mouradi, and B. G. Stanley. 1997. "Stimulation of eating by the second messenger cAMP in the perifornical and lateral hypothalamus." *Am J Phys* 273 (1 Pt 2):R107–R112. doi: 10.1152/ajpregu.1997.273.1.R107.

Goetz, S. C., and K. V. Anderson. 2010. "The primary cilium: a signalling centre during vertebrate development." *Nat Rev Genet* 11 (5):331–344. doi: 10.1038/nrg2774.

Gold, M. G., T. Gonen, and J. D. Scott. 2013. "Local cAMP signaling in disease at a glance." *J Cell Sci* 126 (Pt 20):4537–4543. doi: 10.1242/jcs.133751.

Grarup, N., I. Moltke, M. K. Andersen, M. Dalby, K. Vitting-Seerup, T. Kern, Y. Mahendran, E. Jørsboe, C. V. L. Larsen, I. K. Dahl-Petersen, et al. 2018. "Loss-of-function variants in ADCY3 increase risk of obesity and type 2 diabetes." *Nat Genet* 50 (2):172–174. doi: 10.1038/s41588-017-0022-7.

Hanoune, J., and N. Defer. 2001. "Regulation and role of adenylyl cyclase isoforms." *Annu Rev Pharmacol Toxicol* 41:145–174. doi: 10.1146/annurev.pharmtox.41.1.145.

Herberg, L. J., and D. N. Stephens. 1976. "Cyclic AMP and central noradrenaline receptors: failure to activate diencephalic adrenergic feeding pathways." *Pharmacol Biochem Behav* 4 (1):107–110. doi: 10.1016/0091-3057(76)90183-0.

Hwang, M., Y. Go, J. H. Park, S. K. Shin, S. E. Song, B. C. Oh, S. S. Im, I. Hwang, Y. H. Jeon, I. K. Lee, et al. 2017. "Epac2a-null mice exhibit obesity-prone nature more susceptible to leptin resistance." *Int J Obes* 41 (2):279–288. doi: 10.1038/ijo.2016.208.

Kai, A. K., A. K. Lam, Y. Chen, A. C. Tai, X. Zhang, A. K. Lai, P. K. Yeung, S. Tam, J. Wang, K. S. Lam, et al. 2013. "Exchange protein activated by cAMP 1 (Epac1)-deficient mice develop beta-cell dysfunction and metabolic syndrome." *FASEB J* 27 (10):4122–4135. doi: 10.1096/fj.13-230433.

Kaneko, K., Y. Fu, H. Y. Lin, E. L. Cordonier, Q. Mo, Y. Gao, T. Yao, J. Naylor, V. Howard, K. Saito, et al. 2019. "Gut-derived GIP activates central Rap1 to impair neural leptin sensitivity during overnutrition." *J Clin Invest* 130:3786–3791. doi: 10.1172/JCI126107.

Kaneko, K., P. Xu, E. L. Cordonier, S. S. Chen, A. Ng, Y. Xu, A. Morozov, and M. Fukuda. 2016. "Neuronal Rap1 Regulates Energy Balance, Glucose Homeostasis, and Leptin Actions." *Cell Rep* 16 (11):3003–3015. doi: 10.1016/j.celrep.2016.08.039.

Kaupp, U. B., and R. Seifert. 2002. "Cyclic nucleotide-gated ion channels." *Physiol Rev* 82 (3):769–824. doi: 10.1152/physrev.00008.2002.

Kawasaki, H., G. M. Springett, N. Mochizuki, S. Toki, M. Nakaya, M. Matsuda, D. E. Housman, and A. M. Graybiel. 1998. "A family of cAMP-binding proteins that directly activate Rap1." *Science* 282 (5397):2275–2279.

Krähling, A. M., L. Alvarez, K. Debowski, Q. Van, M. Gunkel, S. Irsen, A. Al-Amoudi, T. Strünker, E. Kremmer, E. Krause, et al. 2013. "CRIS-a novel cAMP-binding protein controlling spermiogenesis and the development of flagellar bending." *PLoS Genet* 9 (12):e1003960. doi: 10.1371/journal.pgen.1003960.

Kroeze, W. K., D. J. Sheffler, and B. L. Roth. 2003. "G-protein-coupled receptors at a glance." *J Cell Sci* 116 (Pt 24):4867–4869. doi: 10.1242/jcs.00902.

Kulaga, H. M., C. C. Leitch, E. R. Eichers, J. L. Badano, A. Lesemann, B. E. Hoskins, J. R. Lupski, P. L. Beales, R. R. Reed, and N. Katsanis. 2004. "Loss of BBS proteins causes anosmia in humans and defects in olfactory cilia structure and function in the mouse." *Nat Genet* 36 (9):994–998. doi: 10.1038/ng1418.

London, E., M. Bloyd, and C. A. Stratakis. 2020. "PKA functions in metabolism and resistance to obesity: lessons from mouse and human studies." *J Endocrinol* 246 (3):R51–r64. doi: 10.1530/joe-20-0035.

London, E., M. Nesterova, N. Sinaii, E. Szarek, T. Chanturiya, S. A. Mastroyannis, O. Gavrilova, and C. A. Stratakis. 2014. "Differentially regulated protein kinase A (PKA) activity in adipose tissue and liver is associated with resistance to diet-induced obesity and glucose intolerance in mice that lack PKA regulatory subunit type IIα." *Endocrinology* 155 (9):3397–3408. doi: 10.1210/en.2014-1122.

London, E., A. Noguchi, D. Springer, M. Faidas, O. Gavrilova, G. Eisenhofer, and C. A. Stratakis. 2019. "The Catalytic Subunit β of PKA Affects Energy Balance and Catecholaminergic Activity." *J Endocr Soc* 3 (5):1062–1078. doi: 10.1210/js.2019-00029.

Morton, G. J., D. E. Cummings, D. G. Baskin, G. S. Barsh, and M. W. Schwartz. 2006. "Central nervous system control of food intake and body weight." *Nature* 443 (7109):289–295. doi: 10.1038/nature05026.

Myers, M. G., Jr., and D. P. Olson. 2012. "Central nervous system control of metabolism." *Nature* 491 (7424):357–363. doi: 10.1038/nature11705.

Nakajima, K., Z. Cui, C. Li, J. Meister, Y. Cui, O. Fu, A. S. Smith, S. Jain, B. B. Lowell, M. J. Krashes, and J. Wess. 2016. "Gs-coupled GPCR signalling in AgRP neurons triggers sustained increase in food intake." *Nat Commun* 7:10268. doi: 10.1038/ncomms10268.

Nawrocki, A. R., C. G. Rodriguez, D. M. Toolan, O. Price, M. Henry, G. Forrest, D. Szeto, C. A. Keohane, Y. Pan, K. M. Smith, et al. 2014. "Genetic deletion and pharmacological inhibition of phosphodiesterase 10A protects mice from diet-induced obesity and insulin resistance." *Diabetes* 63 (1):300–311. doi: 10.2337/db13-0247.

Nordman, S., A. Abulaiti, A. Hilding, E. C. Långberg, K. Humphreys, C. G. Ostenson, S. Efendic, and H. F. Gu. 2008. "Genetic variation of the adenylyl cyclase 3 (AC3) locus and its influence on type 2 diabetes and obesity susceptibility in Swedish men." *Int J Obes* 32 (3):407–412. doi: 10.1038/sj.ijo.0803742.

Ollmann, M. M., B. D. Wilson, Y. K. Yang, J. A. Kerns, Y. Chen, I. Gantz, and G. S. Barsh. 1997. "Antagonism of central melanocortin receptors in vitro and in vivo by agouti-related protein." *Science* 278 (5335):135–138. doi: 10.1126/science.278.5335.135.

Pan, W. W., and M. G. Myers, Jr. 2018. "Leptin and the maintenance of elevated body weight." *Nat Rev Neurosci* 19 (2):95-105. doi: 10.1038/nrn.2017.168.

Park, E. S., H. Kim, J. M. Suh, S. J. Park, O. Y. Kwon, Y. K. Kim, H. K. Ro, B. Y. Cho, J. Chung, and M. Shong. 2000. "Thyrotropin induces SOCS-1 (suppressor of cytokine signaling-1) and SOCS-3 in FRTL-5 thyroid cells." *Mol Endocrinol* 14 (3):440–448. doi: 10.1210/mend.14.3.0433.

Patra, C., K. Foster, J. E. Corley, M. Dimri, and M. F. Brady. 2020. "Biochemistry, cAMP." In *StatPearls*. Treasure Island (FL): StatPearls Publishing Copyright © 2020, StatPearls Publishing LLC.

Perera, R. K., and V. O. Nikolaev. 2013. "Compartmentation of cAMP signalling in cardiomyocytes in health and disease." *Acta Physiol (Oxford)* 207 (4):650–662. doi: 10.1111/apha.12077.

Pitman, J. L., M. C. Wheeler, D. J. Lloyd, J. R. Walker, R. J. Glynne, and N. Gekakis. 2014. "A gain-of-function mutation in adenylate cyclase 3 protects mice from diet-induced obesity." *PLoS One* 9 (10):e110226. doi: 10.1371/journal.pone.0110226.

Podyma, B., D. A. Johnson, L. Sipe, T. P. Remcho, K. Battin, Y. Liu, S. O. Yoon, C. D. Deppmann, and A. D. Güler. 2020. "The p75 neurotrophin receptor in AgRP neurons is necessary for homeostatic feeding and food anticipation." *elife* 9. doi: 10.7554/eLife.52623.

Poloni, M., G. Sciorelli, and G. Rindi. 1974. "[Ingestive responses to cyclic amp administration to the lateral rat hypothalamus and their nature]." *Arch Sci Biol (Bologna)* 58 (1-4):57–69.

Rall, T. W., and E. W. Sutherland. 1958. "Formation of a cyclic adenine ribonucleotide by tissue particles." *J Biol Chem* 232 (2):1065–1076.

Rindi, G., G. Sciorelli, M. Poloni, and F. Acanfora. 1972. "Induction of ingestive responses by cAMP applied into the rat hypothalamus." *Experientia* 28 (9):1047–1049. doi: 10.1007/bf01918664.

Romere, C., C. Duerrschmid, J. Bournat, P. Constable, M. Jain, F. Xia, P. K. Saha, M. Del Solar, B. Zhu, B. York, et al. 2016. "Asprosin, a Fasting-Induced Glucogenic Protein Hormone." *Cell* 165 (3):566–579. doi: 10.1016/j.cell.2016.02.063.

Saeed, S., A. Bonnefond, F. Tamanini, M. U. Mirza, J. Manzoor, Q. M. Janjua, S. M. Din, J. Gaitan, A. Milochau, E. Durand, et al. 2018. "Loss-of-function mutations in ADCY3 cause monogenic severe obesity." *Nat Genet* 50 (2):175–179. doi: 10.1038/s41588-017-0023-6.

Sahu, M., P. Anamthathmakula, and A. Sahu. 2018. "Hypothalamic PDE3B deficiency alters body weight and glucose homeostasis in mouse." *J Endocrinol* 239 (1):93–105. doi: 10.1530/joe-18-0304.

Sands, W. A., H. D. Woolson, G. R. Milne, C. Rutherford, and T. M. Palmer. 2006. "Exchange protein activated by cyclic AMP (Epac)-mediated induction of suppressor of cytokine signaling 3 (SOCS-3) in vascular endothelial cells." *Mol Cell Biol* 26 (17):6333–6346. doi: 10.1128/MCB.00207-06.

Schreyer, S. A., D. E. Cummings, G. S. McKnight, and R. C. LeBoeuf. 2001. "Mutation of the RIIbeta subunit of protein kinase A prevents diet-induced insulin resistance and dyslipidemia in mice." *Diabetes* 50 (11):2555–2562. doi: 10.2337/diabetes.50.11.2555.

Schwartz, M. W., and D. Porte, Jr. 2005. "Diabetes, obesity, and the brain." *Science* 307 (5708):375–379. doi: 10.1126/science.1104344.

Schwartz, M. W., R. J. Seeley, S. C. Woods, D. S. Weigle, L. A. Campfield, P. Burn, and D. G. Baskin. 1997. "Leptin increases hypothalamic pro-opiomelanocortin mRNA expression in the rostral arcuate nucleus." *Diabetes* 46 (12):2119–2123. doi: 10.2337/diab.46.12.2119.

Sciorelli, G., M. Poloni, and G. Rindi. 1972. "Evidence of cholinergic mediation of ingestive responses elicited by dibutyryladenosine-3',5'-monophosphate in rat hypothalamus." *Brain Res* 48:427–431. doi: 10.1016/0006-8993(72)90205-3.

Sengupta, T. K., E. M. Schmitt, and L. B. Ivashkiv. 1996. "Inhibition of cytokines and JAK-STAT activation by distinct signaling pathways." *Proc Natl Acad Sci U S A* 93 (18):9499–9504. doi: 10.1073/pnas.93.18.9499.

Shimizu-Albergine, M., D. L. Ippolito, and J. A. Beavo. 2001. "Downregulation of fasting-induced cAMP response element-mediated gene induction by leptin in neuropeptide Y neurons of the arcuate nucleus." *J Neurosci* 21 (4):1238–1246. doi: 10.1523/jneurosci.21-04-01238.2001.

Siljee, J. E., Y. Wang, A. A. Bernard, B. A. Ersoy, S. Zhang, A. Marley, M. Von Zastrow, J. F. Reiter, and C. Vaisse. 2018. "Subcellular localization of MC4R with ADCY3 at neuronal primary cilia underlies a common pathway for genetic predisposition to obesity." *Nat Genet* 50 (2):180–185. doi: 10.1038/s41588-017-0020-9.

Simerly, R. B. 2008. "Hypothalamic substrates of metabolic imprinting." *Physiol Behav* 94 (1):79–89. doi: 10.1016/j.physbeh.2007.11.023.

Singla, V., and J. F. Reiter. 2006. "The primary cilium as the cell's antenna: signaling at a sensory organelle." *Science* 313 (5787):629–633. doi: 10.1126/science.1124534.

Spiegel, A. M., and L. S. Weinstein. 2004. "Inherited diseases involving g proteins and g protein-coupled receptors." *Annu Rev Med* 55:27–39. doi: 10.1146/annurev.med.55.091902.103843.

Spiegelman, B. M., and J. S. Flier. 2001. "Obesity and the regulation of energy balance." *Cell* 104 (4):531–543.

Taylor, S. S., R. Ilouz, P. Zhang, and A. P. Kornev. 2012. "Assembly of allosteric macromolecular switches: lessons from PKA." *Nat Rev Mol Cell Biol* 13 (10):646–658. doi: 10.1038/nrm3432.

Toda, C., A. Santoro, J. D. Kim, and S. Diano. 2017. "POMC neurons: from birth to death." *Annu Rev Physiol* 79:209–236. doi: 10.1146/annurev-physiol-022516-034110.

Turcot, V., Y. Lu, H. M. Highland, C. Schurmann, A. E. Justice, R. S. Fine, J. P. Bradfield, T. Esko, A. Giri, M. Graff, et al. C. H. D. Exome+ Consortium, Epic-Cvd Consortium, B. P. Consortium Exome, Consortium Global Lipids Genetic, T. D. Genes Consortium Go, Epic InterAct Consortium, Interval Study, Consortium ReproGen, T. D-Genes Consortium, Magic Investigators, and Group Understanding Society Scientific. 2018. "Protein-altering variants associated with body mass index implicate pathways that control energy intake and expenditure in obesity." *Nat Genet* 50 (1):26–41. doi: 10.1038/s41588-017-0011-x.

Uhlen, M., L. Fagerberg, B. M. Hallstrom, C. Lindskog, P. Oksvold, A. Mardinoglu, A. Sivertsson, C. Kampf, E. Sjostedt, A. Asplund, et al. 2015. "Proteomics. Tissue-based map of the human proteome." *Science* 347 (6220):1260419. doi: 10.1126/science.1260419.

van de Wall, E., R. Leshan, A. W. Xu, N. Balthasar, R. Coppari, S. M. Liu, Y. H. Jo, R. G. MacKenzie, D. B. Allison, N. J. Dun, et al. 2008. "Collective and individual functions of leptin receptor modulated neurons controlling metabolism and ingestion." *Endocrinology* 149 (4):1773–1785. doi: 10.1210/en.2007-1132.

van der Klaauw, A. A., and I. S. Farooqi. 2015. "The hunger genes: pathways to obesity." *Cell* 161 (1):119–132. doi: 10.1016/j.cell.2015.03.008.

Varela, L., and T. L. Horvath. 2012. "Leptin and insulin pathways in POMC and AgRP neurons that modulate energy balance and glucose homeostasis." *EMBO Rep* 13 (12):1079–1086. doi: 10.1038/embor.2012.174.

Walsh, D. A., J. P. Perkins, and E. G. Krebs. 1968. "An adenosine 3',5'–monophosphate-dependant protein kinase from rabbit skeletal muscle." *J Biol Chem* 243 (13):3763–3765.

Wang, H., M. Wu, W. Zhu, J. Shen, X. Shi, J. Yang, Q. Zhao, C. Ni, Y. Xu, H. Shen, et al.. 2010. "Evaluation of the association between the AC3 genetic polymorphisms and obesity in a Chinese Han population." *PLoS One* 5 (11):e13851. doi: 10.1371/journal.pone.0013851.

Wang, Z., C. Balet Sindreu, V. Li, A. Nudelman, G. C. Chan, and D. R. Storm. 2006. "Pheromone detection in male mice depends on signaling through the type 3 adenylyl cyclase in the main olfactory epithelium." *J Neurosci* 26 (28):7375–7379. doi: 10.1523/jneurosci.1967-06.2006.

Wang, Z., V. Li, G. C. Chan, T. Phan, A. S. Nudelman, Z. Xia, and D. R. Storm. 2009. "Adult type 3 adenylyl cyclase-deficient mice are obese." *PLoS One* 4 (9):e6979. doi: 10.1371/journal.pone.0006979.

Weinstein, L. S., S. Yu, D. R. Warner, and J. Liu. 2001. "Endocrine manifestations of stimulatory G protein alpha-subunit mutations and the role of genomic imprinting." *Endocr Rev* 22 (5):675–705. doi: 10.1210/edrv.22.5.0439.

Wong, S. T., K. Trinh, B. Hacker, G. C. Chan, G. Lowe, A. Gaggar, Z. Xia, G. H. Gold, and D. R. Storm. 2000. "Disruption of the type III adenylyl cyclase gene leads to peripheral and behavioral anosmia in transgenic mice." *Neuron* 27 (3):487–497. doi: 10.1016/s0896-6273(00)00060-x.

Xie, T., M. Chen, O. Gavrilova, E. W. Lai, J. Liu, and L. S. Weinstein. 2008. "Severe obesity and insulin resistance due to deletion of the maternal Gsalpha allele is reversed by paternal deletion of the Gsalpha imprint control region." *Endocrinology* 149 (5):2443–2450. doi: 10.1210/en.2007-1458.

Xu, J., C. L. Bartolome, C. S. Low, X. Yi, C. H. Chien, P. Wang, and D. Kong. 2018. "Genetic identification of leptin neural circuits in energy and glucose homeostases." *Nature* 556 (7702):505–509. doi: 10.1038/s41586-018-0049-7.

Yan, J., F. C. Mei, H. Cheng, D. H. Lao, Y. Hu, J. Wei, I. Patrikeev, D. Hao, S. J. Stutz, K. T. Dineley, et al. 2013. "Enhanced leptin sensitivity, reduced adiposity, and improved glucose homeostasis in mice lacking exchange protein directly activated by cyclic AMP isoform 1." *Mol Cell Biol* 33 (5):918–926. doi: 10.1128/MCB.01227-12.

Yang, L., and G. S. McKnight. 2015. "Hypothalamic PKA regulates leptin sensitivity and adiposity." *Nat Commun* 6:8237. doi: 10.1038/ncomms9237.

Zaccolo, M. 2009. "cAMP signal transduction in the heart: understanding spatial control for the development of novel therapeutic strategies." *Br J Pharmacol* 158 (1):50–60. doi: 10.1111/j.1476-5381.2009.00185.x.

Zhang, R., E. Maratos-Flier, and J. S. Flier. 2009. "Reduced adiposity and high-fat diet-induced adipose inflammation in mice deficient for phosphodiesterase 4B." *Endocrinology* 150 (7):3076–3082. doi: 10.1210/en.2009-0108.

Zhang, Y., R. Proenca, M. Maffei, M. Barone, L. Leopold, and J. M. Friedman. 1994. "Positional cloning of the mouse obese gene and its human homologue." *Nature* 372 (6505):425–432. doi: 10.1038/372425a0.

Zhao, A. Z., J. N. Huan, S. Gupta, R. Pal, and A. Sahu. 2002. "A phosphatidylinositol 3-kinase phosphodiesterase 3B-cyclic AMP pathway in hypothalamic action of leptin on feeding." *Nat Neurosci* 5 (8):727–728. doi: 10.1038/nn885.

Zheng, R., L. Yang, M. A. Sikorski, L. C. Enns, T. A. Czyzyk, W. C. Ladiges, and G. S. McKnight. 2013. "Deficiency of the RIIβ subunit of PKA affects locomotor activity and energy homeostasis in distinct neuronal populations." *Proc Natl Acad Sci U S A* 110 (17):E1631–E1640. doi: 10.1073/pnas.1219542110.

2 Brain Melanocortins Regulate Weight in Animals and Humans

Yongjie Yang and Yong Xu
Baylor College of Medicine, USA

CONTENTS

2.1 INTRODUCTION

Obesity is a serious global health problem due to its increasing prevalence and comorbidities. According to the World Health Organization, more than 650 million adults worldwide are obese and 40 million children are overweight or obese. The Centers for Disease Control and Prevention reported that 42.4% of adults in the United States were obese in 2017–2018. Through decades of research using cells and/or experimental animals as model systems, a great deal of knowledge has been obtained regarding the molecular, cellular, and systemic mechanisms for the regulation of body weight balance in the studied models. However, a major question in the field still remains unsolved: what causes human obesity?

Recent studies revealed genetic and epigenetic bases for variations in human body mass index (BMI) (Farooqi and O'Rahilly, 2000; Locke et al., 2015; Wahl et al., 2017); strikingly the majority of BMI-associated genetic variants affect genes that are enriched in the brain (Locke et al., 2015). Thus, the dysfunctions of the central nervous system have been implicated in the susceptibility of obesity development in humans. However, due to the limited access to human brain tissues for research purposes, data are rare regarding the anatomical, neurochemical, neurocircuitry, and synaptic alterations in the brains of obese humans, which represents a major challenge in the study of human obesity. In addition, the etiology of human obesity is expected to be highly heterogeneous. In other words, patients may develop similar obesity syndromes due to different pathophysiological processes, which makes human population study alone less powerful to reveal the complicated causes and mechanisms of the disease. Notably, an emerging strategy to reveal the causes of human obesity and the underlying mechanisms is to combine human genetic and metabolic research and basic animal neuroendocrinology studies. Through these efforts, an increasing number of genetic variants have been identified as causes of weight dysregulations in at least subpopulations of obese patients, and the underlying mechanisms have been revealed. In particular, many of these genetic variants directly or indirectly affect the melanocortin system in the brain. This chapter discusses a number of key components of the brain melanocortin system that have been shown to be dysregulated and cause human obesity.

2.2 THE MELANOCORTIN SYSTEM

The melanocortin system in the brain consists of neurons that release endogenous melanocortin ligands and neurons that express the melanocortin receptors (MCRs) (Dores et al., 2016; Shen et al., 2017; Toda et al., 2017). One group of neurons located within the arcuate nucleus of the hypothalamus (ARH) releases orexigenic neuropeptide agouti-related protein (AGRP) and neuropeptide Y (NPY), as well as a neurotransmitter γ-aminobutyric acid (GABA) (Broberger et al., 1998). In this chapter, these neurons are referred to as AGRP neurons. Importantly, AGRP is an endogenous melanocortin inverse agonist which can inhibit MCRs (Cone, 2006; Pritchard et al., 2002; Toda et al., 2017). Interestingly, another distinct group of neurons within the ARH express pro-opiomelanocortin (POMC) (Elias et al., 1998), which are referred to as POMC neurons. While a small population of POMC neurons are also present in the nucleus of the solitary tract (NTS) of the brain stem, these NTS POMC neurons do not appear to affect food intake and body weight (Appleyard et al., 2005; Bronstein et al., 1992; Fan et al., 2004; Grill et al., 1998; Zhan et al., 2013). The POMC gene transcript can be processed post-translationally to produce multiple melanocortin ligands, including α-, β-, or γ-melanocyte stimulating hormones (α-, β-, or γ-MSH) which are endogenous agonists of MCRs (Cone, 2006; Pritchard et al., 2002; Toda et al., 2017). While there are five subtypes of MCRs (MC1R, MC2R, MC3R, MC4R, and MC5R), only the MC3R and MC4R are abundantly expressed in the brain. Through binding with the endogenous melanocortin ligands, these receptors, especially the MC4R, play a key role in the regulation of energy homeostasis (Andermann and Lowell, 2017; Cowley et al., 2001; Dores et al., 2016; Gautron et al., 2015; Toda et al., 2017). For example, in the fasted condition, AGRP neurons are activated by the orexigenic hormones, e.g. ghrelin and asprosin, and POMC neurons are inhibited, which in turn promotes feeding behavior and decreases energy expenditure (Atasoy et al., 2012; Duerrschmid et al., 2017; Heisler et al., 2006; Ollmann et al., 1997; Romere et al., 2016; Zhan et al., 2013). On the other hand, in the satiated condition, anorexigenic hormones or neurotransmitters such as leptin, insulin, and serotonin can activate POMC neurons and inhibit AGRP neurons, which leads to activation of the MC4R to prevent overeating. Readers are referred to the various excellent reviews (Baldini and Phelan, 2019; Kuhnen et al., 2019; Morton et al., 2006; Shen et al., 2017; Xu et al., 2011) for more detailed discussions about the functions of the melanocortin system on energy homeostasis. This chapter will discuss the melanocortin ligands, the MC4R, and the signals/molecules that module these ligands and receptor, with a focus on their pathophysiological relevance in the development of human obesity.

2.3 POMC

In experimental animals, activation of POMC neurons causes decreases in food intake and increases in energy expenditure (Dores et al., 2016; Gautron et al., 2015; Mercer et al., 2013; Toda et al., 2017; Zhan et al., 2013), whereas ablation of POMC neurons results in hyperphagia, decreased energy expenditure, and obesity (Greenman et al., 2013; Zhan et al., 2013). Mice with POMC gene deficiency also display hyperphagia and obesity (Challis et al., 2004; Smart et al., 2006; Yaswen et al., 1999), further confirming the anorexigenic functions of the POMC gene. In humans, multiple POMC gene mutations have been identified since the first case was reported in 1998 (Farooqi et al., 2006; Krude et al., 1998). Although the number of identified human cases is extremely low, all these patients with the deficiency of POMC gene-derived peptides developed severe, early onset obesity associated with hyperphagia (Farooqi and O'Rahilly, 2008). In addition, even the loss of one copy of the POMC gene predisposes to obesity in humans (Farooqi and O'Rahilly, 2008). Moreover, multiple heterozygous point mutations in the POMC gene can cause loss of function of α-MSH or β-MSH, and increase the risk of obesity. For example, the Tyr221Cys variant is located within the β-MSH-encoding region which impairs its ability to activate the MC4R. Importantly, children carrying this variant are hyperphagic and obese (Farooqi and O'Rahilly, 2008; Lee et al., 2006).

In addition to the POMC gene itself, other genetic variants can also result in human obesity via decreasing the expression levels of POMC. For instance, steroid receptor co-activator-1 (SRC-1), encoded by the NCOA1 gene, is a nuclear receptor co-activator which can enhance POMC gene expression in the hypothalamus (Yang et al., 2019). A group of SRC-1 variants were recently identified from early onset, severely obese children (Yang et al., 2019). In cultured cells, these mutated SRC-1 proteins compete and disrupt the normal functions of wild type SRC-1 protein *and* impair POMC expression. Importantly, a knockin mouse model mimicking one of these human variants (SRC-$1^{L1376P/+}$) developed hyperphagia and obesity associated with decreased POMC gene expression (Yang et al., 2019). These data indicate that the loss-of-function SRC-1 variants result in obesity in humans, likely due to impaired regulations on POMC gene expression.

POMC neurons project to various other brain regions, including the MC4R-expressing neurons in the paraventricular nucleus of the hypothalamus (PVH) (Wang et al., 2015). Through these projections, POMC neurons can activate MC4R neurons to decrease food intake and increase energy expenditure by modulating the sympathetic outputs to the periphery (Cone, 2006; Gautron et al., 2015; Ghamari-Langroudi et al., 2015; Ollmann et al., 1997; Zhang et al., 1994). Recent studies demonstrated that the POMC-originated projections to the PVH require normal functions of the class 3 semaphorin ligands (SEMA3) and their receptors. In animals, the loss of one SEMA3 receptor, namely neuropilin-2 receptor (NRP2), in POMC neurons disrupts their projections to the PVH, which causes reduced energy expenditure and weight gain (van der Klaauw et al., 2019). Interestingly, multiple missense mutations have been identified in genes encoding SEMA3 ligands and their receptors in patients with severe early onset obesity, which likely cause weight gain in these individuals due to impaired formation of POMC projections (van der Klaauw et al., 2019).

2.4 AGRP

AGRP neurons are orexigenic in nature and they are essential for triggering feeding behavior. Transgenic mice with overexpression of AGRP develop obesity (Graham et al., 1997; Ollmann et al., 1997), and central administration of AGRP increases food intake and body weight gain in animals (Fekete et al., 2002). Notably, animals with germline deletion of the AGRP gene do not show changes in food intake and body weight (Qian et al., 2002). However, ablation of AGRP neurons during adulthood leads to hypophagia and weight loss that can cause death due to starvation (Bewick et al., 2005; Gropp et al., 2005; Luquet et al., 2005). Food deprivation increases levels of NPY and AGRP mRNAs in AGRP neurons (Swart et al., 2002), increases the firing activity of AGRP neurons (Takahashi and Cone, 2005), and inhibits downstream MC4R neurons in the PVH (Atasoy et al., 2012; Cowley et al., 1999; Cowley et al., 2001), which facilitates the conservation of energy storage and also promotes animals to eat when food becomes available again.

Mutation screening in human genes has revealed some single nucleotide polymorphisms (SNPs) in the AGRP gene that show potential linkage to body weight dysregulations (Ilnytska and Argyropoulos, 2008). The SNP −38C>T (rs5030981) has been associated with lower promoter activity, low body fatness, and resistance to the developing of type 2 diabetes in the black population (Argyropoulos et al., 2003; Bai et al., 2004; Bonilla et al., 2006; Mayfield et al., 2001). The SNP +79G>A (rs34018897) was identified in two individuals of European descent. One carrier had a reduced resting metabolic rate and was obese, which suggests a potential predisposition for a decreased resting metabolic rate and increased fat mass (Sözen et al., 2007). The SNP 131-42C>T (rs11575892) is located in the second intron of the human AGRP gene, and heterozygotes at this position are associated with severe obesity in the Latvian population (Kalnina et al., 2009). One most investigated SNP, rs5030980, 199G>A, is located in the coding region of AGRP and leads to amino acid substitution, Ala67Thr (Argyropoulos et al., 2002). Individuals homozygous for Ala67Ala have a higher BMI and increased body fat in an age-dependent fashion (Argyropoulos et al., 2002; Li et al., 2014), whereas those homozygous for Thr67Thr have a lower BMI and body fat (Marks et al., 2004). Interestingly, in the Dutch, Ala67Ala is associated with lower BMI, but only in men (van Rossum et al., 2006), suggesting a possible sexual dimorphism in the functions of this SNP.

While no SNPs located within the *in vivo* active form of AGRP (aa 83–132) have been associated with altered metabolism in humans, some SNPs have been deposited in the NIH Variation Viewer database (Ericson and Haskell-Luevano, 2018). Most recently, these SNPs have been tested *in vitro* for potential impacts on cellular signaling and functions of MC4R. All the SNPs tested result in at least a ten-fold decreased potency in inhibiting MC4R, indicating that SNPs may impact AGRP functions (Koerperich et al., 2020).

2.5 MC4R

The MC4R neurons receive excitatory inputs from POMC neurons and inhibitory inputs from AGRP neurons (Cowley et al., 1999). Genetic and pharmacological evidence obtained from animal studies demonstrates the key role of MC4R in regulating energy homeostasis. For example, MC4R null mice display massive obesity associated with hyperphagia (Huszar et al., 1997). Central administration of the agonist of MC4R decreases food intake and body weight, which can be blocked by the MC4R antagonist (Fan et al., 1997). MC4R is widely expressed in various brain regions, including the PVH (Kishi et al., 2003; Liu et al., 2003). Importantly, PVH MC4R neurons play an essential role in suppressing appetite and reducing body weight (Seeley et al., 1997). Restoration of MC4R in the PVH at the MC4R null background can prevent about 60% of weight gain and completely normalize the hyperphagia, while reduced energy expenditure is unaffected (Balthasar et al., 2005).

Consistent with observations from animal studies, MC4R mutations are often associated with severe, early onset obesity in humans (Vaisse et al., 1998; Yeo et al., 1998). Indeed, MC4R mutations account for approximately 5% of obese patients, representing the most common cause of human monogenic obesity (Farooqi et al., 2003; Farooqi and O'Rahilly, 2008; Larsen et al., 2005). Further, 636 single-nucleotide variants (SNVs), 239 copy number variants and 10 deletion variants have been reported in the MC4R gene region. These mutations may affect various aspects of MC4R functions, including ligand binding, intracellular trafficking, and downstream signaling (Farooqi and O'Rahilly, 2008; Kuhnen et al., 2019). For example, a nonsense p.Tyr35Ter MC4R SNV (rs13447324) is present in about 1 in 5,000 individuals and results in a ~7 kg higher body weight for a 1.7 m tall person (Turcot et al., 2018). Interestingly, not all MC4R variants are detrimental. For example, those MC4R variants with enhanced β-arrestin-biased signaling are associated with a lower BMI, lower risk of obesity, and cardio-metabolic complications (Lotta et al., 2019).

Factors that are required for normal development and functions of MC4R neurons also regulate body weight balance. For example, a basic helix-loop-helix-PAS transcription factor, namely single-minded 1 (SIM1), has been shown to regulate development of PVH neurons, including those expressing MC4R (Kublaoui et al., 2008; Ramachandrappa et al., 2013). Loss of SIM1 impairs the development of secretory neurons (such as oxytocin neurons) in the PVH and the supraoptic nucleus; mice with germline deletion of SIM1 die shortly after birth (Michaud et al., 1998). The heterozygous SIM1 knockout mice are viable, but develop early onset obesity associated with hypocellular PVH (average 24% fewer cells) (Michaud et al., 2001). In addition, SIM1 deletion during adulthood, which does not affect the development of

PVH neurons, also results in hyperphagic obesity in mice (Tolson et al., 2010). The reduced expression of oxytocin and MC4R in the PVH may mediate the hyperphagic phenotype (Kublaoui et al., 2008; Tolson et al., 2010). Collectively, in animals, SIM1 is required to mediate normal development and functions of PVH MC4R neurons, and therefore loss of SIM1 causes obesity in animals at least partly due to impaired melanocortin signaling (Michaud et al., 2001; Michaud et al., 1998; Tolson et al., 2010). Consistent with findings from animal studies, in humans, chromosomal deletions involving 6q16.2 result in SIM1 gene deficiency and are associated with early onset obesity (Faivre et al., 2002; Villa et al., 1995; Wang et al., 2008). In addition, a patient with severe early onset obesity is reported to have the balanced 1p22.1 and 6q16.2 chromosome translocation, which disrupts one allele of the SIM1 gene (Holder et al., 2000). Further, in the Pima Indian population, common variations in SIM1 are associated with an increased BMI (Traurig et al., 2009). Moreover, 13 heterozygous variants in the SIM1 coding region were identified from patients with severe, early onset obesity (Ramachandrappa et al., 2013). Collectively, these human genetic observations are in line with evidence obtained from animal studies which supports SIM1 as having a key role in regulating body weight balance.

MC4R is coupled to the Gsα protein and induces activation of adenylate cyclase and the production of cAMP (Gantz et al., 1993; Sarkar et al., 2002); this MC4R-initiated signaling requires the accessory protein, melanocortin receptor accessory protein (MRAP). In particular, MRAP2 can directly interact with MC4R and enhance its signaling (Asai et al., 2013). Abundant MRAP2 is expressed by PVH MC4R neurons (Asai et al., 2013; Liang et al., 2018; Novoselova et al., 2016; Schonnop et al., 2016). Mice deficient in the MRAP2 gene are severely obese (Asai et al., 2013). More importantly, the selective deletion of MRAP2 only in PVH neurons causes similar obese phenotypes. These animal studies indicate that MRAP2 is required for normal MC4R functions and therefore contributes to the regulation of energy homeostasis. Consistently, MRAP2 variants were found in obese individuals. Four rare heterozygous variants (N88Y, L115V, R125C, E24X) were identified, and one of the variants (E24X) was shown to impair MC4R signaling (Asai et al., 2013). Similarly, other variants, such as N88Y and R125C, impair α-MSH-induced MC4R or MC3R activation (Liang et al., 2018). In addition, two novel MRAP2 variants (A137T and Q174R) were found to be associated with extreme obesity; in particular, the Q174R mutant cannot potentiate an effect on MC4R (Schonnop et al., 2016). Most recently, 23 rare heterozygous MRAP2 variants were found to be associated with increased obesity risk (Baron et al., 2019). The functional assessment of each variant shows that loss-of-function MRAP2 variants are pathogenic for monogenic hyperphagic obesity (Baron et al., 2019). Collectively, these findings suggest that the loss-of-function mutations in the MRAP2 gene can cause human obesity through disrupting MC4R signaling.

2.6 LEPTIN

ARH neurons, including POMC and AGRP neurons, can be regulated by a broad range of circulating hormones (Shen et al., 2017). One such hormone is leptin. Leptin is an adipocyte-derived hormone that functions to reduce food intake and body weight.

Leptin deficient (ob/ob) mice are massively hyperphagic and obese (Zhang et al., 1994). Most of leptin's actions on energy balance are mediated by leptin receptor (LEPR) expressed in the brain (Friedman, 2016). In particular, both POMC and AGRP neurons express LEPRs and are considered to be the first-order leptin-responsive neurons. Interestingly, leptin can inhibit AGRP neuron activity and suppress AGRP gene expression; on the other hand, leptin activates a portion of POMC neurons and increases POMC gene expression. Both these actions of leptin contribute to energy homeostasis by decreasing feeding and/or increasing energy expenditure (Cowley et al., 2001; Friedman, 2016; Mizuno and Mobbs, 1999; Schwartz et al., 1997; Shen et al., 2017). Leptin can trigger multiple intracellular signals within AGRP and POMC neurons. In particular, upon binding to leptin, LEPR is phosphorylated at Tyr^{1138} by Janus kinase 2 (JAK2), which further leads to phosphorylation of the signal transducer and activator of transcription 3 (STAT3). Phosphorylated STAT3 (pSTAT3) translocates to the nucleus and functions as a transcription factor to regulate gene expression (Baldini and Phelan, 2019), including increasing POMC gene expression and decreasing AGRP gene expression (Kitamura et al., 2006). Importantly, mice carrying the point mutation with the substitution of Tyr^{1138} to Ser develop severe obesity and hyperphagia, phenotypes similar to those observed in db/db mice that are deficient in the LEPR gene. Thus, these results indicate that JAK2-STAT3 signaling mediates the majority of leptin's actions to reduce appetite and body weight (Bates et al., 2003).

In humans, multiple forms of leptin gene mutations have been identified, including homozygous frameshift, and nonsense and missense mutations, which lead to an inability to produce the leptin protein. Consistent with animals deficient in the leptin gene, humans with leptin gene deficiency are obese and diabetic (Farooqi and O'Rahilly, 2008; Montague et al., 1997). Imporatntly, administration of leptin to leptin-deficient mice can rescue the hyperphagia and obesity. Similarly, leptin treatment can also correct obesity in patients with leptin gene deficiency, which is largely attributed to decreases in food intake (Farooqi et al., 1999; Halaas et al., 1995; Pelleymounter et al., 1995). The therapeutic response to leptin in leptin-deficient humans provides compelling evidence that leptin is essential for body weight control.

Mice carrying loss-of-function mutations of LEPR are severely obese (Chen et al., 1996; Chua et al., 1996; Hummel et al., 1966; Lee et al., 1996). Notably, in humans, up to 3% of patients with severe obesity are found to carry mutations in the LEPR gene that are associated with a loss of function in the protein (Farooqi and O'Rahilly 2008). For example, a homozygous mutation of the LEPR gene causes a truncated leptin receptor without both the transmembrane and the intracellular domains, and patients carrying this mutation show early onset morbid obesity (Clement et al., 1998). In addition, a LEPR SNP (rs8179183) has been reported to be significantly associated with obesity in Chinese Han and European adolescents (Labayen et al., 2011; Ren et al., 2019).

Leptin actions are also regulated by multiple intracellular molecules, including the Src homology 2B adaptor protein 1 (SH2B1). SH2B1 can interact with numerous protein tyrosine kinases, including JAK2, and this SH2B1–JAK2 interaction can enhance leptin sensitivity (Ahmed and Pillay, 2003; Duan et al., 2004; Ren et al., 2005; Ren et al., 2007). Mice lacking SH2B1 develop severe obesity (Ren et al., 2005; Ren et al., 2007). Re-expression of SH2B1 only in the brain can improve leptin actions and correct obesity in SH2B1 null mice (Ren et al., 2007). These results highlight an important role of brain SH2B1 in leptin signaling and body weight regulation. In humans, 16p11.2 deletions are associated with highly penetrant, familial, severe, early onset obesity, hyperphagia, and severe insulin resistance (Bochukova et al., 2010). Notably, the 16p11.2 deletions encompass several genes including SH2B1 (Bochukova et al., 2010). Although the contribution of other genes or non-coding genetic material cannot be excluded, the phenotype is consistent with the role of SH2B1 in human energy homeostasis.

2.7 ASPROSIN

A novel hunger hormone, asprosin, was discovered through studies in patients with a genetic disorder called neonatal progeroid syndrome (NPS) (Romere et al., 2016). The clinical characteristics of NPS patients include extreme leanness and hypophagia (Duerrschmid et al., 2017; Romere et al., 2016). Through the whole exome sequencing, similar mutations on the fibrillin 1 (FBN1) gene were found from seven NPS patients, which are all clustered around the cleavage site of the pro-fibrillin protein, which leads to truncated mutations and the loss of a 140-amino-acid long, C-terminal cleavage product (Romere et al., 2016). This C-terminal cleavage product was later found to be able to enter the circulation and function as a hormone, and was named asprosin (Romere et al., 2016). Asprosin levels in the circulation increase upon fasting and one major function of asprosin is to act in the liver to promote rapid glucose release during food deprivation (Romere et al., 2016). In addition, asprosin can also cross the blood–brain barrier and directly activate AGRP neurons and indirectly inhibit POMC neurons, which leads to increased feeding (Duerrschmid et al., 2017). Importantly, neutralizing asprosin with an antibody reduces food intake in mice, and a knockin mouse model carrying the same mutation in one NPS patient developed extreme leanness and hypophagia that resemble the patient (Duerrschmid et al., 2017). In humans, elevated asprosin levels are associated with obesity and metabolic disorders. For example, circulating asprosin levels are significantly higher in obese adults and children than in non-obese subjects; in addition, children with insulin resistance (IR) have higher asprosin levels than a non-IR group (Wang et al., 2019a; Wang et al., 2019b). Importantly, the asprosin level increases in accordance with increasing BMI; on the other hand, the asprosin amount decreases as BMI decreases (Ugur and Aydin, 2019). Thus, these results indicate that asprosin plays an important role in regulating body weight balance via its actions on melanocortin neurons, and that altered asprosin levels in humans may account for dysregulations of body weight balance.

2.8 CONCLUSIONS

The combination of human genetic/metabolic studies and basic animal neuroendocrinology studies have started to reveal the fundamental genetic basis and the neuroendocrine mechanisms that regulate body weight homeostasis. As discussed above, many genetic variants associated with human obesity disrupt the brain melanocortin system through various mechanisms. These include impaired development of melanocortin neurons, reduced or increased production of melanocortin ligands or their activities, altered excitability of melanocortin neurons, and/or deficits in the upstream or downstream signaling of melanocortin neurons. These findings highlight the critical importance of the brain melanocortin system in the regulation of energy balance in humans (Figure 2.1). It is worth mentioning that most of these studies took advantage of combined human genetics and mouse genetics to provide compelling evidence for the cause of a human disease and the underlying mechanisms. Since most of the obesity-associated human variants affect genes that are enriched in the brain (Locke et al., 2015), we suggest that if we can bring together the diverse expertise in human obesity research and basic neuroendocrinology, much more can be learned about obesity development and mechanisms not only in animals but also in humans.

In addition to advancing our understanding of the causes and mechanisms of human obesity, these studies also facilitate the development of novel treatments for the disease. Indeed, several of these genetic obese disorders, e.g. patients with leptin deficiency, are now treatable (Farooqi et al., 1999). In addition, as most MC4R mutation carriers are heterozygous, MC4R agonists could be used to treat obesity in these individuals. A variety of peptides and small chemical MC4R agonists have been

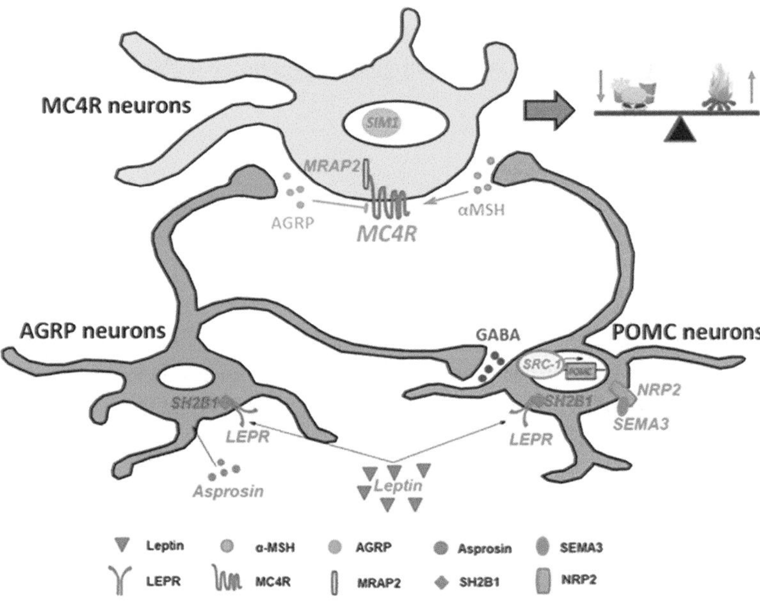

FIGURE 2.1 A simplified summary of the brain melanocortin system including the key components that are affected by known human genetic variants (red text). α-MSH: α-melanocyte stimulating hormone; AGRP: agouti-related peptide; GABA: γ-aminobutyric acid; LEPR: leptin receptor; MC4R: melanocortin 4 receptor; MRAP2: melanocortin 2 receptor accessory protein 2; NRP2: neuropilin-2 receptor; POMC: pro-opiomelanocortin; SEMA3: semaphorin 3; SH2B1: Src homology 2B adaptor protein 1; SIM1: single-minded 1; SRC-1: steroid receptor co-activator-1.

developed and shown to reduce food intake and body weight in rodents (Goncalves et al., 2018), although many of these agonists also cause cardiovascular side effects due to MC4R-related sympathetic activation (Fani et al., 2014; Goncalves et al., 2018; Kuhnen et al., 2019). However, a synthetic eight amino acid cyclic MC4R agonist peptide, setmelanotide (RM-493), has been demonstrated to effectively induce biased signaling of MC4R, and therefore produce weight-lowering benefits without causing adverse effects in heart rate and blood pressure (Chen et al., 2015; Collet et al., 2017). Importantly, setmelanotide treatment of severely obese LEPR-deficient individuals shows substantial and durable reductions in hyperphagia and body weight over 45–61 weeks (Clement et al., 2018). Currently, setmelanotide is at the phase 3 clinical trial stage for the treatment of various human obesity syndromes, including POMC deficiency, LEPR deficiency, Bardet-Biedl syndrome, Alström syndrome, and other obesity with an impaired MC4R pathway (Kuhnen et al., 2019; Sharma et al., 2019). Interestingly, CRISPR-mediated activation (CRISPRa) gene therapy was recently utilized to increase the functions of the remaining copy of the haploinsufficient gene (Matharu et al., 2019). It has been demonstrated that CRISPRa targeting of the SIM1 promoter or its distant hypothalamic enhancer can increase SIM1 expression from the endogenous functional allele, which leads to reductions in body weight in heterozygous SIM1 knockout mice. Similarly, CRISPRa-mediated enhancement of the MC4R allele can rescue obesity in MC4R haploinsufficient mice (Matharu et al., 2019). Thus, these findings provide a framework to further develop the CRISPRa as a potential tool to treat gene dosage-related obesity.

REFERENCES

Ahmed, Z., and Pillay, T.S. (2003). Adapter protein with a pleckstrin homology (PH) and an Src homology 2 (SH2) domain (APS) and SH2-B enhance insulin-receptor autophosphorylation, extracellular-signal-regulated kinase and phosphoinositide 3-kinase-dependent signalling. *The Biochemical Journal 371*, 405–412.

Andermann, M.L., and Lowell, B.B. (2017). Toward a Wiring Diagram Understanding of Appetite Control. *Neuron 95*, 757–778.

Appleyard, S.M., Bailey, T.W., Doyle, M.W., Jin, Y.H., Smart, J.L., Low, M.J., and Andresen, M.C. (2005). Proopiomelanocortin neurons in nucleus tractus solitarius are activated by visceral afferents: regulation by cholecystokinin and opioids. *The Journal of Neuroscience: The Official Journal of the Society for Neuroscience 25*, 3578–3585.

Argyropoulos, G., Rankinen, T., Bai, F., Rice, T., Province, M.A., Leon, A.S., Skinner, J.S., Wilmore, J.H., Rao, D.C., and Bouchard, C. (2003). The agouti-related protein and body fatness in humans. *International Journal of Obesity and Related Metabolic Disorders : Journal of the International Association for the Study of Obesity 27*, 276–280.

Argyropoulos, G., Rankinen, T., Neufeld, D.R., Rice, T., Province, M.A., Leon, A.S., Skinner, J.S., Wilmore, J.H., Rao, D.C., and Bouchard, C. (2002). A polymorphism in the human agouti-related protein is associated with late-onset obesity. *The Journal of Clinical Endocrinology and Metabolism 87*, 4198–4202.

Asai, M., Ramachandrappa, S., Joachim, M., Shen, Y., Zhang, R., Nuthalapati, N., Ramanathan, V., Strochlic, D.E., Ferket, P., Linhart, K., et al. (2013). Loss of function of the melanocortin 2 receptor accessory protein 2 is associated with mammalian obesity. *Science 341*, 275–278.

Atasoy, D., Betley, J.N., Su, H.H., and Sternson, S.M. (2012). Deconstruction of a neural circuit for hunger. *Nature 488*, 172–177.

Bai, F., Rankinen, T., Charbonneau, C., Belsham, D.D., Rao, D.C., Bouchard, C., and Argyropoulos, G. (2004). Functional dimorphism of two hAgRP promoter SNPs in linkage disequilibrium. *Journal of Medical Genetics 41*, 350–353.

Baldini, G., and Phelan, K.D. (2019). The melanocortin pathway and control of appetite-progress and therapeutic implications. *The Journal of Endocrinology 241*, R1–R33.

Balthasar, N., Dalgaard, L.T., Lee, C.E., Yu, J., Funahashi, H., Williams, T., Ferreira, M., Tang, V., McGovern, R.A., Kenny, C.D., et al. (2005). Divergence of melanocortin pathways in the control of food intake and energy expenditure. *Cell 123*, 493–505.

Baron, M., Maillet, J., Huyvaert, M., Dechaume, A., Boutry, R., Loiselle, H., Durand, E., Toussaint, B., Vaillant, E., Philippe, J., et al. (2019). Loss-of-function mutations in MRAP2 are pathogenic in hyperphagic obesity with hyperglycemia and hypertension. *Nature Medicine 25*, 1733–1738.

Bates, S.H., Stearns, W.H., Dundon, T.A., Schubert, M., Tso, A.W., Wang, Y., Banks, A.S., Lavery, H.J., Haq, A.K., Maratos-Flier, E., et al. (2003). STAT3 signalling is required for leptin regulation of energy balance but not reproduction. *Nature 421*, 856–859.

Bewick, G.A., Gardiner, J.V., Dhillo, W.S., Kent, A.S., White, N.E., Webster, Z., Ghatei, M.A., and Bloom, S.R. (2005). Post-embryonic ablation of AgRP neurons in mice leads to a lean, hypophagic phenotype. *The FASEB Journal 19*, 1680–1682.

Bochukova, E.G., Huang, N., Keogh, J., Henning, E., Purmann, C., Blaszczyk, K., Saeed, S., Hamilton-Shield, J., Clayton-Smith, J., O'Rahilly, S., et al. (2010). Large, rare chromosomal deletions associated with severe early-onset obesity. *Nature 463*, 666–670.

Bonilla, C., Panguluri, R.K., Taliaferro-Smith, L., Argyropoulos, G., Chen, G., Adeyemo, A.A., Amoah, A., Owusu, S., Acheampong, J., Agyenim-Boateng, K., et al. (2006). Agouti-related protein promoter variant associated with leanness and decreased risk for diabetes in West Africans. *International Journal of Obesity 30*, 715–721.

Broberger, C., Johansen, J., Johansson, C., Schalling, M., and Hokfelt, T. (1998). The neuropeptide Y/agouti gene-related protein (AGRP) brain circuitry in normal, anorectic, and monosodium glutamate-treated mice. *Proceedings of the National Academy of Sciences of the United States of America 95*, 15043–15048.

Bronstein, D.M., Schafer, M.K., Watson, S.J., and Akil, H. (1992). Evidence that beta-endorphin is synthesized in cells in the nucleus tractus solitarius: detection of POMC mRNA. *Brain Research 587*, 269–275.

Challis, B.G., Coll, A.P., Yeo, G.S., Pinnock, S.B., Dickson, S.L., Thresher, R.R., Dixon, J., Zahn, D., Rochford, J.J., White, A., et al. (2004). Mice lacking pro-opiomelanocortin are sensitive to high-fat feeding but respond normally to the acute anorectic effects of peptide-YY(3-36). *Proceedings of the National Academy of Sciences of the United States of America 101*, 4695–4700.

Chen, H., Charlat, O., Tartaglia, L.A., Woolf, E.A., Weng, X., Ellis, S.J., Lakey, N.D., Culpepper, J., Moore, K.J., Breitbart, R.E., et al. (1996). Evidence that the diabetes gene encodes the leptin receptor: identification of a mutation in the leptin receptor gene in db/db mice. *Cell 84*, 491–495.

Chen, K.Y., Muniyappa, R., Abel, B.S., Mullins, K.P., Staker, P., Brychta, R.J., Zhao, X., Ring, M., Psota, T.L., Cone, R.D., et al. (2015). RM-493, a melanocortin-4 receptor (MC4R) agonist, increases resting energy expenditure in obese individuals. *The Journal of Clinical Endocrinology and Metabolism 100*, 1639–1645.

Chua, S.C., Jr., Chung, W.K., Wu-Peng, X.S., Zhang, Y., Liu, S.M., Tartaglia, L., and Leibel, R.L. (1996). Phenotypes of mouse diabetes and rat fatty due to mutations in the OB (leptin) receptor. *Science 271*, 994–996.

Clement, K., Biebermann, H., Farooqi, I.S., Van der Ploeg, L., Wolters, B., Poitou, C., Puder, L., Fiedorek, F., Gottesdiener, K., Kleinau, G., et al. (2018). MC4R agonism promotes durable weight loss in patients with leptin receptor deficiency. *Nature Medicine 24*, 551–555.

Clement, K., Vaisse, C., Lahlou, N., Cabrol, S., Pelloux, V., Cassuto, D., Gourmelen, M., Dina, C., Chambaz, J., Lacorte, J.M., et al. (1998). A mutation in the human leptin receptor gene causes obesity and pituitary dysfunction. *Nature 392*, 398–401.

Collet, T.H., Dubern, B., Mokrosinski, J., Connors, H., Keogh, J.M., Mendes de Oliveira, E., Henning, E., Poitou-Bernert, C., Oppert, J.M., Tounian, P., et al. (2017). Evaluation of a melanocortin-4 receptor (MC4R) agonist (Setmelanotide) in MC4R deficiency. *Molecular metabolism 6*, 1321–1329.

Cone, R.D. (2006). Studies on the physiological functions of the melanocortin system. *Endocrine Reviews 27*, 736–749.

Cowley, M.A., Pronchuk, N., Fan, W., Dinulescu, D.M., Colmers, W.F., and Cone, R.D. (1999). Integration of NPY, AGRP, and melanocortin signals in the hypothalamic paraventricular nucleus: evidence of a cellular basis for the adipostat. *Neuron 24*, 155–163.

Cowley, M.A., Smart, J.L., Rubinstein, M., Cerdan, M.G., Diano, S., Horvath, T.L., Cone, R.D., and Low, M.J. (2001). Leptin activates anorexigenic POMC neurons through a neural network in the arcuate nucleus. *Nature 411*, 480–484.

Dores, R.M., Liang, L., Davis, P., Thomas, A.L., and Petko, B. (2016). 60 YEARS OF POMC: Melanocortin receptors: evolution of ligand selectivity for melanocortin peptides. *Journal of Molecular Endocrinology 56*, T119–T133.

Duan, C., Yang, H., White, M.F., and Rui, L. (2004). Disruption of the SH2-B gene causes age-dependent insulin resistance and glucose intolerance. *Molecular and Cellular Biology 24*, 7435–7443.

Duerrschmid, C., He, Y., Wang, C., Li, C., Bournat, J.C., Romere, C., Saha, P.K., Lee, M.E., Phillips, K.J., Jain, M., et al. (2017). Asprosin is a centrally acting orexigenic hormone. *Nature Medicine 23*, 1444–1453.

Elias, C.F., Lee, C., Kelly, J., Aschkenasi, C., Ahima, R.S., Couceyro, P.R., Kuhar, M.J., Saper, C.B., and Elmquist, J.K. (1998). Leptin activates hypothalamic CART neurons projecting to the spinal cord. *Neuron 21*, 1375–1385.

Ericson, M.D., and Haskell-Luevano, C. (2018). A Review of Single-Nucleotide Polymorphisms in Orexigenic Neuropeptides Targeting G Protein-Coupled Receptors. *ACS Chemical Neuroscience 9*, 1235–1246.

Fairbrother, U., Kidd, E., Malagamuwa, T., and Walley, A. (2018). Genetics of Severe Obesity. *Current Diabetes Reports 18*, 85.

Faivre, L., Cormier-Daire, V., Lapierre, J.M., Colleaux, L., Jacquemont, S., Genevieve, D., Saunier, P., Munnich, A., Turleau, C., Romana, S., et al. (2002). Deletion of the SIM1 gene (6q16.2) in a patient with a Prader-Willi-like phenotype. *Journal of Medical Genetics 39*, 594–596.

Fan, W., Boston, B.A., Kesterson, R.A., Hruby, V.J., and Cone, R.D. (1997). Role of melanocortinergic neurons in feeding and the agouti obesity syndrome. *Nature 385*, 165–168.

Fan, W., Ellacott, K.L., Halatchev, I.G., Takahashi, K., Yu, P., and Cone, R.D. (2004). Cholecystokinin-mediated suppression of feeding involves the brainstem melanocortin system. *Nature Neuroscience 7*, 335–336.

Fani, L., Bak, S., Delhanty, P., van Rossum, E.F., and van den Akker, E.L. (2014). The melanocortin-4 receptor as target for obesity treatment: a systematic review of emerging pharmacological therapeutic options. *International Journal of Obesity 38*, 163–169.

Farooqi, I.S., Drop, S., Clements, A., Keogh, J.M., Biernacka, J., Lowenbein, S., Challis, B.G., and O'Rahilly, S. (2006). Heterozygosity for a POMC-null mutation and increased obesity risk in humans. *Diabetes 55*, 2549–2553.

Farooqi, I.S., Jebb, S.A., Langmack, G., Lawrence, E., Cheetham, C.H., Prentice, A.M., Hughes, I.A., McCamish, M.A., and O'Rahilly, S. (1999). Effects of recombinant leptin therapy in a child with congenital leptin deficiency. *The New England Journal of Medicine 341*, 879–884.

Farooqi, I.S., Keogh, J.M., Yeo, G.S., Lank, E.J., Cheetham, T., and O'Rahilly, S. (2003). Clinical spectrum of obesity and mutations in the melanocortin 4 receptor gene. *The New England Journal of Medicine 348*, 1085–1095.

Farooqi, I.S., and O'Rahilly, S. (2000). *The Genetics of Obesity in Humans.*

Farooqi, I.S., and O'Rahilly, S. (2008). Mutations in ligands and receptors of the leptin-melanocortin pathway that lead to obesity. *Nature Clinical Practice Endocrinology & Metabolism 4*, 569–577.

Fekete, C., Sarkar, S., Rand, W.M., Harney, J.W., Emerson, C.H., Bianco, A.C., and Lechan, R.M. (2002). Agouti-related protein (AGRP) has a central inhibitory action on the hypothalamic-pituitary-thyroid (HPT) axis; comparisons between the effect of AGRP and neuropeptide Y on energy homeostasis and the HPT axis. *Endocrinology 143*, 3846–3853.

Friedman, J. (2016). The long road to leptin. *The Journal of Clinical Investigation 126*, 4727–4734.

Gantz, I., Konda, Y., Tashiro, T., Shimoto, Y., Miwa, H., Munzert, G., Watson, S.J., DelValle, J., and Yamada, T. (1993). Molecular cloning of a novel melanocortin receptor. *The Journal of Biological Chemistry 268*, 8246–8250.

Gautron, L., Elmquist, J.K., and Williams, K.W. (2015). Neural control of energy balance: translating circuits to therapies. *Cell 161*, 133–145.

Ghamari-Langroudi, M., Digby, G.J., Sebag, J.A., Millhauser, G.L., Palomino, R., Matthews, R., Gillyard, T., Panaro, B.L., Tough, I.R., Cox, H.M., et al. (2015). G-protein-independent coupling of MC4R to Kir7.1 in hypothalamic neurons. *Nature 520*, 94–98.

Goncalves, J.P.L., Palmer, D., and Meldal, M. (2018). MC4R Agonists: Structural Overview on Antiobesity Therapeutics. *Trends in Pharmacological Sciences 39*, 402–423.

Graham, M., Shutter, J.R., Sarmiento, U., Sarosi, I., and Stark, K.L. (1997). Overexpression of Agrt leads to obesity in transgenic mice. *Nature Genetics 17*, 273–274.

Greenman, Y., Kuperman, Y., Drori, Y., Asa, S.L., Navon, I., Forkosh, O., Gil, S., Stern, N., and Chen, A. (2013). Postnatal ablation of POMC neurons induces an obese phenotype characterized by decreased food intake and enhanced anxiety-like behavior. *Molecular Endocrinology 27*, 1091–1102.

Grill, H.J., Ginsberg, A.B., Seeley, R.J., and Kaplan, J.M. (1998). Brainstem application of melanocortin receptor ligands produces long-lasting effects on feeding and body weight. *The Journal of Neuroscience: The Official Journal of the Society for Neuroscience 18*, 10128–10135.

Gropp, E., Shanabrough, M., Borok, E., Xu, A.W., Janoschek, R., Buch, T., Plum, L., Balthasar, N., Hampel, B., Waisman, A., et al. (2005). Agouti-related peptide-expressing neurons are mandatory for feeding. *Nature Neuroscience 8*, 1289–1291.

Halaas, J.L., Gajiwala, K.S., Maffei, M., Cohen, S.L., Chait, B.T., Rabinowitz, D., Lallone, R.L., Burley, S.K., and Friedman, J.M. (1995). Weight-reducing effects of the plasma protein encoded by the obese gene. *Science 269*, 543–546.

Heisler, L.K., Jobst, E.E., Sutton, G.M., Zhou, L., Borok, E., Thornton-Jones, Z., Liu, H.Y., Zigman, J.M., Balthasar, N., Kishi, T., et al. (2006). Serotonin reciprocally regulates melanocortin neurons to modulate food intake. *Neuron 51*, 239–249.

Holder, J.L., Jr., Butte, N.F., and Zinn, A.R. (2000). Profound obesity associated with a balanced translocation that disrupts the SIM1 gene. *Human Molecular Genetics 9*, 101–108.

Hummel, K.P., Dickie, M.M., and Coleman, D.L. (1966). Diabetes, a new mutation in the mouse. *Science 153*, 1127–1128.

Huszar, D., Lynch, C.A., Fairchild-Huntress, V., Dunmore, J.H., Fang, Q., Berkemeier, L.R., Gu, W., Kesterson, R.A., Boston, B.A., Cone, R.D., et al. (1997). Targeted disruption of the melanocortin-4 receptor results in obesity in mice. *Cell 88*, 131–141.

Ilnytska, O., and Argyropoulos, G. (2008). The role of the Agouti-Related Protein in energy balance regulation. *Cellular and Molecular Life Sciences: CMLS 65*, 2721–2731.

Kalnina, I., Kapa, I., Pirags, V., Ignatovica, V., Schioth, H.B., and Klovins, J. (2009). Association between a rare SNP in the second intron of human Agouti related protein gene and increased BMI. *BMC Medical Genetics 10*, 63.

Kishi, T., Aschkenasi, C.J., Lee, C.E., Mountjoy, K.G., Saper, C.B., and Elmquist, J.K. (2003). Expression of melanocortin 4 receptor mRNA in the central nervous system of the rat. *Journal of Comparative Neurology 457*, 213–235.

Kitamura, T., Feng, Y., Kitamura, Y.I., Chua, S.C., Jr., Xu, A.W., Barsh, G.S., Rossetti, L., and Accili, D. (2006). Forkhead protein FoxO1 mediates Agrp-dependent effects of leptin on food intake. *Nature Medicine 12*, 534–540.

Koerperich, Z.M., Ericson, M.D., Freeman, K.T., Speth, R.C., Pogozheva, I.D., Mosberg, H.I., and Haskell-Luevano, C. (2020). Incorporation of Agouti-Related Protein (AgRP) Human Single Nucleotide Polymorphisms (SNPs) in the AgRP-Derived Macrocyclic Scaffold c[Pro-Arg-Phe-Phe-Asn-Ala-Phe-dPro] Decreases Melanocortin-4 Receptor Antagonist Potency and Results in the Discovery of Melanocortin-5 Receptor Antagonists. *Journal of Medicinal Chemistry 63*, 2194–2208.

Krude, H., Biebermann, H., Luck, W., Horn, R., Brabant, G., and Gruters, A. (1998). Severe early-onset obesity, adrenal insufficiency and red hair pigmentation caused by POMC mutations in humans. *Nature Genetics 19*, 155–157.

Kublaoui, B.M., Gemelli, T., Tolson, K.P., Wang, Y., and Zinn, A.R. (2008). Oxytocin deficiency mediates hyperphagic obesity of Sim1 haploinsufficient mice. *Molecular Endocrinology 22*, 1723–1734.

Kuhnen, P., Krude, H., and Biebermann, H. (2019). Melanocortin-4 Receptor Signalling: Importance for Weight Regulation and Obesity Treatment. *Trends in Molecular Medicine 25*, 136–148.

Labayen, I., Ruiz, J.R., Moreno, L.A., Ortega, F.B., Beghin, L., DeHenauw, S., Benito, P.J., Diaz, L.E., Ferrari, M., Moschonis, G., et al. (2011). The effect of ponderal index at birth on the relationships between common LEP and LEPR polymorphisms and adiposity in adolescents. *Obesity (Silver Spring) 19*, 2038–2045.

Larsen, L.H., Echwald, S.M., Sorensen, T.I., Andersen, T., Wulff, B.S., and Pedersen, O. (2005). Prevalence of mutations and functional analyses of melanocortin 4 receptor variants identified among 750 men with juvenile-onset obesity. *The Journal of Clinical Endocrinology and Metabolism 90*, 219–224.

Lee, G.H., Proenca, R., Montez, J.M., Carroll, K.M., Darvishzadeh, J.G., Lee, J.I., and Friedman, J.M. (1996). Abnormal splicing of the leptin receptor in diabetic mice. *Nature 379*, 632–635.

Lee, Y.S., Challis, B.G., Thompson, D.A., Yeo, G.S., Keogh, J.M., Madonna, M.E., Wraight, V., Sims, M., Vatin, V., Meyre, D., et al. (2006). A POMC variant implicates beta-melanocyte-stimulating hormone in the control of human energy balance. *Cell Metabolism 3*, 135–140.

Li, P., Tiwari, H.K., Lin, W.Y., Allison, D.B., Chung, W.K., Leibel, R.L., Yi, N., and Liu, N. (2014). Genetic association analysis of 30 genes related to obesity in a European American population. *International Journal of Obesity 38*, 724–729.

Liang, J., Li, L., Jin, X., Xu, B., Pi, L., Liu, S., Zhu, W., Zhang, C., Luan, B., and Gong, L. (2018). Pharmacological effect of human melanocortin-2 receptor accessory protein 2 variants on hypothalamic melanocortin receptors. *Endocrine 61*, 94–104.

Liu, H., Kishi, T., Roseberry, A.G., Cai, X., Lee, C.E., Montez, J.M., Friedman, J.M., and Elmquist, J.K. (2003). Transgenic mice expressing green fluorescent protein under the control of the melanocortin-4 receptor promoter. *The Journal of Neuroscience 23*, 7143–7154.

Locke, A.E., Kahali, B., Berndt, S.I., Justice, A.E., Pers, T.H., Day, F.R., Powell, C., Vedantam, S., Buchkovich, M.L., Yang, J., et al. (2015). Genetic studies of body mass index yield new insights for obesity biology. *Nature 518*, 197–206.

Lotta, L.A., Mokrosinski, J., Mendes de Oliveira, E., Li, C., Sharp, S.J., Luan, J., Brouwers, B., Ayinampudi, V., Bowker, N., Kerrison, N., et al. (2019). Human Gain-of-Function MC4R Variants Show Signaling Bias and Protect against Obesity. *Cell 177*, 597–607 e599.

Luquet, S., Perez, F.A., Hnasko, T.S., and Palmiter, R.D. (2005). NPY/AgRP neurons are essential for feeding in adult mice but can be ablated in neonates. *Science 310*, 683–685.

Marks, D.L., Boucher, N., Lanouette, C.M., Perusse, L., Brookhart, G., Comuzzie, A.G., Chagnon, Y.C., and Cone, R.D. (2004). Ala67Thr polymorphism in the Agouti-related peptide gene is associated with inherited leanness in humans. *American Journal of Medical Genetics Part A 126A*, 267–271.

Matharu, N., Rattanasopha, S., Tamura, S., Maliskova, L., Wang, Y., Bernard, A., Hardin, A., Eckalbar, W.L., Vaisse, C., and Ahituv, N. (2019). CRISPR-mediated activation of a promoter or enhancer rescues obesity caused by haploinsufficiency. *Science 363*.

Mayfield, D.K., Brown, A.M., Page, G.P., Garvey, W.T., Shriver, M.D., and Argyropoulos, G. (2001). A role for the Agouti-Related Protein promoter in obesity and type 2 diabetes. *Biochemical and Biophysical Research Communications 287*, 568–573.

Mercer, A.J., Hentges, S.T., Meshul, C.K., and Low, M.J. (2013). Unraveling the central proopiomelanocortin neural circuits. *Frontiers in Neuroscience 7*, 19.

Michaud, J.L., Boucher, F., Melnyk, A., Gauthier, F., Goshu, E., Levy, E., Mitchell, G.A., Himms-Hagen, J., and Fan, C.M. (2001). Sim1 haploinsufficiency causes hyperphagia, obesity and reduction of the paraventricular nucleus of the hypothalamus. *Human Molecular Genetics 10*, 1465–1473.

Michaud, J.L., Rosenquist, T., May, N.R., and Fan, C.M. (1998). Development of neuroendocrine lineages requires the bHLH-PAS transcription factor SIM1. *Genes & Development 12*, 3264–3275.

Mizuno, T.M., and Mobbs, C.V. (1999). Hypothalamic agouti-related protein messenger ribonucleic acid is inhibited by leptin and stimulated by fasting. *Endocrinology 140*, 814–817.

Montague, C.T., Farooqi, I.S., Whitehead, J.P., Soos, M.A., Rau, H., Wareham, N.J., Sewter, C.P., Digby, J.E., Mohammed, S.N., Hurst, J.A., et al. (1997). Congenital leptin deficiency is associated with severe early-onset obesity in humans. *Nature 387*, 903–908.

Morton, G.J., Cummings, D.E., Baskin, D.G., Barsh, G.S., and Schwartz, M.W. (2006). Central nervous system control of food intake and body weight. *Nature 443*, 289–295.

Novoselova, T.V., Larder, R., Rimmington, D., Lelliott, C., Wynn, E.H., Gorrigan, R.J., Tate, P.H., Guasti, L., O'Rahilly, S., Clark, A.J., et al. (2016). Loss of Mrap2 is associated with Sim1 deficiency and increased circulating cholesterol. *The Journal of Endocrinology 230*, 13–26.

Ollmann, M.M., Wilson, B.D., Yang, Y.K., Kerns, J.A., Chen, Y., Gantz, I., and Barsh, G.S. (1997). Antagonism of central melanocortin receptors in vitro and in vivo by agouti-related protein. *Science 278*, 135–138.

Pelleymounter, M.A., Cullen, M.J., Baker, M.B., Hecht, R., Winters, D., Boone, T., and Collins, F. (1995). Effects of the obese gene product on body weight regulation in ob/ob mice. *Science 269*, 540–543.

Pritchard, L.E., Turnbull, A.V., and White, A. (2002). Pro-opiomelanocortin processing in the hypothalamus: impact on melanocortin signalling and obesity. *The Journal of Endocrinology 172*, 411–421.

Qian, S., Chen, H., Weingarth, D., Trumbauer, M.E., Novi, D.E., Guan, X., Yu, H., Shen, Z., Feng, Y., Frazier, E., et al. (2002). Neither agouti-related protein nor neuropeptide Y is critically required for the regulation of energy homeostasis in mice. *Molecular Cell Biology 22*, 5027–5035.

Ramachandrappa, S., Raimondo, A., Cali, A.M., Keogh, J.M., Henning, E., Saeed, S., Thompson, A., Garg, S., Bochukova, E.G., Brage, S., et al. (2013). Rare variants in single-minded 1 (SIM1) are associated with severe obesity. *The Journal of Clinical Investigation 123*, 3042–3050.

Ren, D., Li, M., Duan, C., and Rui, L. (2005). Identification of SH2-B as a key regulator of leptin sensitivity, energy balance, and body weight in mice. *Cell Metabolism 2*, 95–104.

Ren, D., Xu, J.H., Bi, Y., Zhang, Z., Zhang, R., Li, Y., Hu, J., Guo, Z., Niu, W., Yang, F., et al. (2019). Association study between LEPR, MC4R polymorphisms and overweight/obesity in Chinese Han adolescents. *Gene 692*, 54–59.

Ren, D., Zhou, Y., Morris, D., Li, M., Li, Z., and Rui, L. (2007). Neuronal SH2B1 is essential for controlling energy and glucose homeostasis. *The Journal of Clinical Investigation 117*, 397–406.

Romere, C., Duerrschmid, C., Bournat, J., Constable, P., Jain, M., Xia, F., Saha, P.K., Del Solar, M., Zhu, B., York, B., et al. (2016). Asprosin, a Fasting-Induced Glucogenic Protein Hormone. *Cell 165*, 566–579.

Sarkar, S., Legradi, G., and Lechan, R.M. (2002). Intracerebroventricular administration of alpha-melanocyte stimulating hormone increases phosphorylation of CREB in TRH- and CRH-producing neurons of the hypothalamic paraventricular nucleus. *Brain Research 945*, 50–59.

Schonnop, L., Kleinau, G., Herrfurth, N., Volckmar, A.L., Cetindag, C., Muller, A., Peters, T., Herpertz, S., Antel, J., Hebebrand, J., et al. (2016). Decreased melanocortin-4 receptor function conferred by an infrequent variant at the human melanocortin receptor accessory protein 2 gene. *Obesity (Silver Spring) 24*, 1976–1982.

Schwartz, M.W., Seeley, R.J., Woods, S.C., Weigle, D.S., Campfield, L.A., Burn, P., and Baskin, D.G. (1997). Leptin increases hypothalamic pro-opiomelanocortin mRNA expression in the rostral arcuate nucleus. *Diabetes 46*, 2119–2123.

Seeley, R.J., Yagaloff, K.A., Fisher, S.L., Burn, P., Thiele, T.E., van Dijk, G., Baskin, D.G., and Schwartz, M.W. (1997). Melanocortin receptors in leptin effects. *Nature 390*, 349.

Sharma, S., Garfield, A.S., Shah, B., Kleyn, P., Ichetovkin, I., Moeller, I.H., Mowrey, W.R., and Van der Ploeg, L.H.T. (2019). Current Mechanistic and Pharmacodynamic Understanding of Melanocortin-4 Receptor Activation. *Molecules 24*.

Shen, W.J., Yao, T., Kong, X., Williams, K.W., and Liu, T. (2017). Melanocortin neurons: Multiple routes to regulation of metabolism. *Biochimica et Biophysica Acta, Molecular Basis of Disease 1863*, 2477–2485.

Smart, J.L., Tolle, V., and Low, M.J. (2006). Glucocorticoids exacerbate obesity and insulin resistance in neuron-specific proopiomelanocortin-deficient mice. *The Journal of Clinical Investigation 116*, 495–505.

Sözen, M.A., de Jonge, L.H.M., Greenway, F., Ravussin, E., Smith, S.R., and Argyropoulos, G. (2007). A rare mutation in AgRP, +79G>A, affects promoter activity. *European Journal of Clinical Nutrition 61*, 809–812.

Swart, I., Jahng, J.W., Overton, J.M., and Houpt, T.A. (2002). Hypothalamic NPY, AGRP, and POMC mRNA responses to leptin and refeeding in mice. *American Journal of Physiology. Regulatory, Integrative and Comparative Physiology 283*, R1020–R1026.

Takahashi, K.A., and Cone, R.D. (2005). Fasting induces a large, leptin-dependent increase in the intrinsic action potential frequency of orexigenic arcuate nucleus neuropeptide Y/Agouti-related protein neurons. *Endocrinology 146*, 1043–1047.

Toda, C., Santoro, A., Kim, J.D., and Diano, S. (2017). POMC Neurons: From Birth to Death. *Annual Review of Physiology 79*, 209–236.

Tolson, K.P., Gemelli, T., Gautron, L., Elmquist, J.K., Zinn, A.R., and Kublaoui, B.M. (2010). Postnatal Sim1 deficiency causes hyperphagic obesity and reduced Mc4r and oxytocin expression. *The Journal of Neuroscience 30*, 3803–3812.

Traurig, M., Mack, J., Hanson, R.L., Ghoussaini, M., Meyre, D., Knowler, W.C., Kobes, S., Froguel, P., Bogardus, C., and Baier, L.J. (2009). Common variation in SIM1 is reproducibly associated with BMI in Pima Indians. *Diabetes 58*, 1682–1689.

Turcot, V., Lu, Y., Highland, H.M., Schurmann, C., Justice, A.E., Fine, R.S., Bradfield, J.P., Esko, T., Giri, A., Graff, M., et al. (2018). Protein-altering variants associated with body mass index implicate pathways that control energy intake and expenditure in obesity. *Nature Genetics 50*, 26–41.

Ugur, K., and Aydin, S. (2019). Saliva and Blood Asprosin Hormone Concentration Associated with Obesity. *International Journal of Endocrinology 2019*, 2521096.

Vaisse, C., Clement, K., Guy-Grand, B., and Froguel, P. (1998). A frameshift mutation in human MC4R is associated with a dominant form of obesity. *Nature Genetics 20*, 113–114.

van der Klaauw, A.A., Croizier, S., Mendes de Oliveira, E., Stadler, L.K.J., Park, S., Kong, Y., Banton, M.C., Tandon, P., Hendricks, A.E., Keogh, J.M., et al. (2019). Human Semaphorin 3 Variants Link Melanocortin Circuit Development and Energy Balance. *Cell 176*, 729–742 e718.

van Rossum, C.T., Pijl, H., Adan, R.A., Hoebee, B., and Seidell, J.C. (2006). Polymorphisms in the NPY and AGRP genes and body fatness in Dutch adults. *International Journal of Obesity 30*, 1522–1528.

Villa, A., Urioste, M., Bofarull, J.M., and Martinez-Frias, M.L. (1995). De novo interstitial deletion q16.2q21 on chromosome 6. *American Journal of Medical Genetics 55*, 379–383.

Wahl, S., Drong, A., Lehne, B., Loh, M., Scott, W.R., Kunze, S., Tsai, P.C., Ried, J.S., Zhang, W., Yang, Y., et al. (2017). Epigenome-wide association study of body mass index, and the adverse outcomes of adiposity. *Nature 541*, 81–86.

Wang, C.Y., Lin, T.A., Liu, K.H., Liao, C.H., Liu, Y.Y., Wu, V.C., Wen, M.S., and Yeh, T.S. (2019a). Serum asprosin levels and bariatric surgery outcomes in obese adults. *International Journal of Obesity 43*, 1019–1025.

Wang, D., He, X., Zhao, Z., Feng, Q., Lin, R., Sun, Y., Ding, T., Xu, F., Luo, M., and Zhan, C. (2015). Whole-brain mapping of the direct inputs and axonal projections of POMC and AgRP neurons. *Frontiers in Neuroanatomy 9*, 40.

Wang, J.C., Turner, L., Lomax, B., and Eydoux, P. (2008). A 5-Mb microdeletion at 6q16.1-q16.3 with SIM gene deletion and obesity. *American Journal of Medical Genetics Part A 146A*, 2975–2978.

Wang, M., Yin, C., Wang, L., Liu, Y., Li, H., Li, M., Yi, X., and Xiao, Y. (2019b). Serum Asprosin Concentrations Are Increased and Associated with Insulin Resistance in Children with Obesity. *Annals of Nutrition & Metabolism 75*, 205–212.

Xu, Y., Elmquist, J.K., and Fukuda, M. (2011). Central nervous control of energy and glucose balance: focus on the central melanocortin system. *Annals of the New York Academy of Sciences 1243*, 1–14.

Yang, Y., van der Klaauw, A.A., Zhu, L., Cacciottolo, T.M., He, Y., Stadler, L.K.J., Wang, C., Xu, P., Saito, K., Hinton, A., Jr., et al. (2019). Steroid receptor coactivator-1 modulates the function of Pomc neurons and energy homeostasis. *Nature Communications 10*, 1718.

Yaswen, L., Diehl, N., Brennan, M.B., and Hochgeschwender, U. (1999). Obesity in the mouse model of pro-opiomelanocortin deficiency responds to peripheral melanocortin. *Nature Medicine 5*, 1066–1070.

Yeo, G.S., Farooqi, I.S., Aminian, S., Halsall, D.J., Stanhope, R.G., and O'Rahilly, S. (1998). A frameshift mutation in MC4R associated with dominantly inherited human obesity. *Nature Genetics 20*, 111–112.

Zhan, C., Zhou, J., Feng, Q., Zhang, J.E., Lin, S., Bao, J., Wu, P., and Luo, M. (2013). Acute and long-term suppression of feeding behavior by POMC neurons in the brainstem and hypothalamus, respectively. *The Journal of Neuroscience 33*, 3624–3632.

Zhang, Y., Proenca, R., Maffei, M., Barone, M., Leopold, L., and Friedman, J.M. (1994). Positional cloning of the mouse obese gene and its human homologue. *Nature 372*, 425–432.

3 Neurotransmitter Co-transmission in Brain Control of Feeding and Body Weight

Jing Cai, Ryan M. Cassidy, Jessie Morrill and Qingchun Tong

The University of Texas Health Science Center, USA

CONTENTS

3.1 INTRODUCTION

In all living organisms, the ability to harness energy is essential for survival. For a multi-organ system, different organs function in a coordinated fashion to perform distinct functions and maintain energy balance. Energy balance is depicted as the balance between food intake and energy expenditure, including internal heat production and external labor and energy storage (Lowell and Bachman, 2003). Obesity results from a disrupted energy balance with more energy intake than expenditure. According to recent estimates, approximately 40% of Americans are categorized as obese, and recent findings also suggest that obesity prevalence is increasing in children and adults alike (Ward et al., 2019). Although both social and pharmacological interventions are being pursued, it remains a challenge to reverse the prevalence of increasing obesity. This dire situation demands a clear understanding of body weight regulation. It is now widely accepted that the brain controls both feeding and energy expenditure, and therefore holds the key to controlling body weight. Neurons within the hypothalamus are known to sense nutritional status indicators from peripheral metabolic organs and have a profound effect on body weight homeostasis by engaging a diverse group of downstream neurons (Cone, 2005; Elmquist et al., 2005; Saper et al., 2002). As neuron function relies on neurotransmission, understanding the role of neurotransmission represents a key step in delineating neural pathways underlying brain mechanisms for energy balance. Neurotransmitters can be classified as either classical neurotransmitters (amino acids, monoamines, and acetylcholine) or neuropeptides.

Amino acids are the most abundant neurotransmitters in the central nervous system (CNS), and the most prevalent ones are glutamate and gamma aminobutyric acid (GABA), the major brain excitatory and inhibitory neurotransmitters, respectively. Both neurotransmitters can produce fast action through their ionotropic receptors and therefore also called fast-acting neurotransmitters. Acetylcholine (Ach) is another neurotransmitter used by discrete groups of neurons. Dopamine (DA), epinephrine (E), norepinephrine (NE), serotonin (5-HT), and histamine are monoamine neurotransmitters used by specialized neurons. The release of amino acid, monoamine, and Ach neurotransmitters is mediated by presynaptic fusion of small core vesicles and requires specific synthesis and transportation machinery. The expression of these transportation molecular machineries is used as a marker for specific neurotransmitter neuron types regarding their capability to release the corresponding neurotransmitter. Interestingly, the expression of a specific vesicular transporter seems to be sufficient, at least with the availability of the corresponding neurotransmitter, for the neuron to release the neurotransmitter (Takamori et al., 2001). Neuropeptides are typically used by discrete groups of neurons, and normally categorized as neuromodulators because of their slow kinetic action (van den Pol, 2012). While the release of classical neurotransmitters has been elucidated in the literature, less is known about the mechanisms underlying neuropeptide release. Much information on peptide release can be gained from extensive studies on endocrine pancreatic hormonal release including insulin and glucagon. Although it is known that peptides are stored in large dense granules, it is not clear whether peptide-containing granules require the same presynaptic machinery used by small vesicle mediated release. Evidence also shows that peptides can undergo volume release, i.e. they can be released from soma and exert actions in an autocrine or paracrine manner (Fuxe et al., 2007; Fuxe et al., 2005). However, the mechanism underlying the volume release of peptides is not yet clear.

It has historically been accepted that each neuron releases only a single neurotransmitter. However, this view has increasingly been challenged by observations suggesting co-transmission between neuropeptides and classical neurotransmitters, or between two classical neurotransmitters (El Mestikawy et al., 2011; Vaaga et al., 2014) (Figure 3.1). This may occur within one action potential (Tritsch et al., 2016), typically when more than two types of neurotransmitter are packaged into the same vesicles or through synchronous fusion of different vesicles filled with different neurotransmitters to the membrane (Tritsch et al., 2016). "Co-release" refers to a single neuron releasing more than one neurotransmitters under one action potential. The function of neurotransmitter co-release is unknown but may enhance synaptic transmission. Co-transmission is more broad than co-release, as neurotransmitters are not necessarily released under one action potential (Vaaga et al., 2014). The functional importance of a dual- (or multi-) transmitter extends beyond actions on postsynaptic receptors, due in part to differential spatial and temporal profiles of each neurotransmitter. Co-transmission increases the flexibility of a neuronal circuit as one neuron can release different neurotransmitters on different targets (Nusbaum et al., 2017; Sigvardt et al., 1986; Tritsch et al., 2016; Zhang et al., 2015). For example, neurons can release different neurotransmitters, which can bind with different receptors under different firing patterns. (Fuzesi et al., 2016).

Research in past decades has identified important brain neurons that regulate feeding and energy expenditure, most of which are located in the hypothalamus. Compared to fast-acting neurotransmitters, the approaches to study the function of peptides including pharmacology, specific targeting in the brain and mouse genetic models are relatively easier to achieve, and thus, most of the earlier studies on body weight regulation focus on the function of neuropeptides (Kalra and Kalra, 2004; van den Pol, 2003, 2012). These neuropeptides include agouti-related protein (AgRP), neuropeptide Y (NPY), proopiomelanocortin (POMC) peptides, orexin, and melanin concentrating hormones (MCH). Important peptides outside the hypothalamus include glucagon-like peptide 1 (GLP1), which is mostly located in the hindbrain (Hayes and Schmidt, 2016). The function of these neuropeptides in mediating feeding behavior and body weight regulation has been well studied recently.

For fast-acting neurotransmitter glutamate and GABA, due to their universal presence in the brain, the characterization of their roles is largely limited to *in vitro* recording and *in vivo* pharmacology; it has been difficult to delineate their function in specific groups of neurons (van den Pol, 2003). With the development of the approach that can achieve specific manipulation of gene expression selectively in distinct groups of neurons, mouse models with neuron-specific alterations in the release of fast-acting neurotransmitters or the function of their receptors can be generated. The first model concerns the specific deletion of NMDAR1 subunit in the CA1 hippocampal neurons, revealing an important role of glutamatergic inputs to these neurons in learning and memory (Tsien et al., 1996). Within the brain areas involved in energy homeostasis, a number of animal models have been generated from specific subsets of hypothalamic or hindbrain neurons with disrupted glutamate or GABA release (Tong et al., 2008; Xu et al., 2013). These models, especially with the recent availability of optogenetics and chemogenetics, have been extensively used to interrogate the role of fast-acting neurotransmitters in feeding and body weight regulation.

This chapter will focus on the role of co-transmission in the context of the brain control of feeding, energy expenditure, and body weight regulation. We will focus on neurons that release mixed neuropeptides and classical neurotransmitters, and also on those releasing more than one classical neurotransmitter.

3.2 CO-TRANSMISSION IN THE ARCUATE NUCLEUS NEURONS

The arcuate nucleus of the hypothalamus (Arc) is an important region involved in regulating body weight, metabolism, the cardiovascular system, and fertility

(Andermann and Lowell, 2017; Egan et al., 2017; Rahmouni, 2016). The Arc contains well studied AgRP and POMC neurons (Andermann and Lowell, 2017; Munzberg and Myers, 2005; Myers et al., 2008), in addition to other less characterized neurons.

3.2.1 AgRP Neurons

Extensive results demonstrate that AgRP neurons in the Arc are critical regulators of feeding and food-seeking behavior (Cone, 2005; Flier, 2006; Ollmann et al., 1997). These neurons directly sense changes in nutritional status through hormonal signaling by leptin, insulin, ghrelin, and others. Activation of these neurons induces the release of three known transmitters (GABA, AgRP, and NPY) to drive feeding (Krashes et al., 2013). Acute activation of AgRP neurons in mice is sufficient to induce feeding and associated food-seeking behaviors (Atasoy et al., 2012), whereas AgRP lesions in adult mice lead to starvation (Bewick et al., 2005; Gropp et al., 2005; Luquet et al., 2005; Xu et al., 2005), although recent work suggests that chronic inhibition of this group of neurons fails to cause body weight changes (Zhu et al., 2020).

AgRP is selectively produced by Arc AgRP neurons and is up-regulated in obese mice (Shutter et al., 1997). Consistent with the role of AgRP neurons in feeding, brain NPY and AgRP action induces feeding (Elmquist et al., 2005). Overexpression of AgRP in a transgenic mouse model or intracerebroventricular (ICV) injection of the peptide leads to hyperphagia, reduced energy expenditure, and obesity (Graham et al., 1997; Rossi et al., 1998; Small et al., 2001). Interestingly, the effect of a single injection of AgRP to promote feeding is long-lasting, which is different from other orexigenic hormones including ghrelin and NPY (Hagan et al., 2001; Schwartz et al., 2000). Mechanistically, AgRP functions as an antagonist or inverse agonist of the central melanocortin system (Haskell-Luevano and Monck, 2001; Nijenhuis et al., 2001; Tolle and Low, 2008). Unlike AgRP, NPY is widely expressed throughout the body (Lundberg et al., 1982; Tatemoto et al., 1982). It is present in many brain regions including the hippocampus, hypothalamus, amygdala, and cortex (Gray and Morley, 1986; Wahlestedt et al., 1989), as well as peripheral tissues including the sympathetic post-ganglionic neurons, adrenal medulla, pancreas, and spleen (Ericsson et al., 1987; Klimaschewski et al., 1996; Lundberg et al., 1982; Whim, 2006, 2011). Within the Arc, NPY is highly colocalized with AgRP in AgRP neurons (Hahn et al., 1998). NPY receptors are G protein coupled receptors and their activation usually causes inhibitory responses (Loh et al., 2015). ICV administration of NPY also significantly increases feeding behavior and reduces energy expenditure; and chronic infusion of NPY can induce obesity due to overeating (Zhang et al., 2019).

Besides AgRP and NPY, the role of GABA has also been speculated to be important (van den Pol, 2003). With Cre-loxP technology, disruption of GABA release from AgRP neurons is achieved by inactivating the vesicular GABA transporter (VGAT), which leads to increased energy expenditure and resistance to diet induced obesity (Tong et al., 2008). The importance of GABA is supported by the reversal of starvation from adult AgRP neuron lesion by restoring GABA action in various AgRP neuron downstream sites, especially the parabrachial nucleus (PBN) (Wu et al., 2009).

There is a strong interest in understanding how the co-transmission of the three known neurotransmitters mediates AgRP neuron function. First, these three neurotransmitters seem to act in parallel, i.e. having an independent role on acting on downstream neurons. This is supported by the action of AgRP and NPY on their respective receptors of downstream neurons, as well as recent optogenetic studies on GABA and its specific postsynaptic neurons (Krashes et al., 2013). AgRP functions as an antagonist (or reverse agonist) on the melanocortin receptors 3 and 4, especially MC4Rs on paraventricular hypothalamic (PVH) neurons, thereby reducing the activity of these neurons to increase feeding and reduce energy expenditure (Fan et al., 1997; Ollmann et al., 1997). NPY potently increases feeding through various NPY receptors in PVH neurons (Aramakis et al., 1996). Specific optogenetic activation of AgRP neurons to the PVH projections potently promotes feeding, which can be blocked by GABA-A receptor antagonists and NPY receptor antagonists, further demonstrating a parallel function of these two neurotransmitters in promoting feeding (Atasoy et al., 2012). It is worth noting that AgRP neurons also release all three neurotransmitters to other brain sites, especially the PBN, where GABA release appears to mediate the majority of the action (Wu et al., 2009).

A combination of activation of AgRP neurons and loss of neurotransmitter release represents a powerful way to interrogate the functional relationship between different neurotransmitters released from AgRP neurons. With chemogenetic activation of AgRP neurons, the loss of NPY, GABA release, or MC4R deficiency (loss of AgRP effect) causes differential effects on acute feeding, with distinct effects on different phases, suggesting a role for these neurotransmitters in different phases of feeding behavior: initiation, maintenance, or termination (Krashes et al., 2013). Interestingly, recent studies suggest that, in a natural state, activation of AgRP neurons is only required for initiating feeding, and that the maintenance of feeding does not require AgRP neuron activation (Chen et al., 2015; Chen et al., 2016). Surprisingly, the activity of AgRP neurons is actually reduced upon feeding or approaching/sensing food (Chen et al., 2015; Chen et al., 2016). Supporting this, acute chemogenetic activation of AgRP neurons with increased Gs-mediating signaling is capable of achieving a long-term increase in feeding over several days (Nakajima et al., 2016). In theory, acute activation of AgRP neurons via clozapine N-oxide (CNO) action on Gs-DREADD may last over several hours and should be able to recruit both fast-acting GABA release and slow-acting AgRP and NPY release. In this regard, it is interesting to note that NPY release is required for a long-lasting effect on feeding during natural feeding behaviors when AgRP neuron activity is low, suggesting a unique role for NPY, which may elicit a long term alteration of the activity of downstream neurons/pathways in mediating such observed long-lasting feeding behavior (Chen et al., 2019). Supporting this, a recent study suggests a predominant role for NPY in mediating AgRP neuron function in feeding and in the hunger-driven suppression of pain sensation (Alhadeff et al., 2018; Engstrom Ruud et al., 2020), confirming a unique role regarding NPY. Further studies on the different roles of NPY, AgRP, and GABA release from AgRP neurons are warranted to delineate the details in terms of potential differences in release kinetics that can explain their distinct roles in mediating AgRP neuron function.

3.2.2 Co-transmission from POMC Neurons

POMC neurons play an important role in body weight homeostasis, as reflected by the massive obesity in both rodents and humans with POMC gene deficiency (Krude et al., 1998; Yaswen et al., 1999). POMC neurons are known to release several peptides that are products of post-translational modification from the same POMC precursor protein, including alpha-MSH, beta-endorphin, and adrenocorticotropic hormone (ACTH). Studies based on reporter mice suggest that few POMC neurons express VGLUT2 or VGAT, markers for glutamatergic or GABAergic neurons respectively (Vong et al., 2011). However, recent studies suggest a subset of POMC neurons release glutamate while another subset release GABA (Dicken et al., 2012; Hentges et al., 2009; Jarvie and Hentges, 2012), and the number of glutamate and GABA-releasing neurons changes during developmental maturation (Dennison et al., 2016). In addition, anatomic data suggest that a subset of POMC neurons express VChAT (Durr et al., 2007; Meister et al., 2006), a marker for cholinergic neurons. However, the physiological functions of these potential classical neurotransmitters released from POMC neurons have not been well demonstrated yet.

Alpha-MSH, released from POMC neurons, functions as an endogenous agonist for MC4Rs, and therefore plays a critical role in body weight regulation (Thody, 1999). In contrast, beta-endorphin, another cleavage product from the same POMC precursor, has been shown to be implicated in orexigenic feeding regulation (Silva et al., 2001). Strikingly, it has been suggested that alpha-MSH and beta-endorphin coexist in the same axonal projections (Mercer et al., 2013), which raises the question as to how these peptides, if released from the same axon, produce opposite effects on feeding. Further studies on their potential differential receptor expression patterns may provide some insights. Nevertheless, mice with knockout of the whole POMC gene are obese with hyperphagia (Yaswen et al., 1999), suggesting that the effect of loss of alpha-MSH is dominant over those of beta-endorphin. In addition, as an opioid, beta-endorphin can modulate feeding behaviors based on energy balance status and is involved in cannabinoid-induced feeding (Koch et al., 2015; Low et al., 2003). Besides POMC peptides, a subset of POMC neurons also release cocaine- and amphetamine-regulated transcript (CART), another peptide shown to play a role in feeding (Elias et al., 1999; Kristensen et al., 1998). However, the effect of CART on feeding and body weight appears to be mild, and little is known about its mechanism, including its receptors.

Contrary to the demonstrated salient role of AgRP neurons in feeding, the role of POMC neurons in acute feeding behavior seems to be mild. Acute activation of POMC neurons through either optogenetics or chemogenetics fails to produce obvious effects on feeding, and chronic manipulations on activity of these neurons elicit only mild effects on feeding and body weight (Aponte et al., 2011; Zhan et al., 2013). In contrast, acute activation of nucleus tractus solitarius (NTS) POMC neurons produces an immediate reduction in food intake (Zhan et al., 2013). Consistent with the massive obesity in POMC KO mice (Yaswen et al., 1999), ablation of POMC neurons also produces massive obesity with increased feeding and reduced energy expenditure (Greenman et al., 2013). Thus, it appears that Arc POMC neurons are required but may not be sufficient in the regulation of body weight.

3.3 CO-TRANSMISSION FROM PARAVENTRICULAR HYPOTHALAMIC NEURONS

The paraventricular hypothalamus (PVH) is a key integrative center with an important function in feeding, energy expenditure, and body weight regulation. The PVH integrates hormonal and synaptic inputs from various other brain sites, and its function is mediated by downstream neuroendocrine and autonomic nerve projections. The importance of the PVH function is reflected by massive obesity from PVH lesions through either physical damage or precise genetic approaches (Aravich and Sclafani, 1983; Holder et al., 2000; Tolson et al., 2010; Xi et al., 2012).

One major characteristic of the PVH is the diversity of neuron types with distinct functions. Earlier studies with a major focus on peptides have identified important peptides used by and released from PVH neurons. These peptides include oxytocin, vasopressin (AVP), corticotropin-release hormone (CRH), and thyroid-releasing hormone (TRH). One unique feature of the PVH is a subset of these neurons which can be categorized as neuroendocrine cells, i.e. they function through releasing hormones into blood. These neurons include a subset of oxytocin and AVP neurons, which directly release oxytocin and AVP to the blood circulation in the posterior pituitary, and CRH and TRH neurons, which release CRH and TRH respectively to the anterior pituitary to regulate hypothalamic-pituitary adrenal and hypothalamic-pituitary thyroid axes. It is important to point out that a subset of these peptidergic neurons may not be neuroendocrine cells, but function through projections to other brain sites. Notably, within PVH neurons, the main body-weight-regulating function of the PVH appears to be mediated by melanocotin 4 receptors (MC4R) and prodynorphin neurons (Li et al., 2019). MC4R-expressing neurons in the PVH are the major downstream neurons of arcuate POMC neurons which regulate feeding and body weight (Cone, 2005; Elmquist et al., 2005).

For feeding and body weight regulation, PVH peptides seem not be required. Mice with knockout of each of these peptides fail to develop obvious obesity or body weight changes, suggesting that these peptides are not required for normal body weight regulation (Jacobson, 1999; Wu et al., 2012; Yamada et al., 1997). However, changes in feeding can be observed from pharmacological studies with these peptides or related agonists. For example, pharmacologic activation of the oxytocin pathway inhibits feeding through projections to the hindbrain area (Blevins et al., 2004), suggesting a sufficient role of this peptide. In addition to peptides, PVH neurons release fast-acting neurotransmitters. The vast majority of PVH neurons express vesicular glutamate transporter 2 (VGLUT2) and use glutamate as neurotransmitter while another subset of PVH neurons express VGAT and use GABA as neurotransmitter (Jiang et al., 2018; Xu et al., 2013). Compared to peptides, the role of classical neurotransmitters has received much less attention but is proven to be more important. Disruption of glutamate release from PVH neurons through deletion of VGLUT2 specifically from the PVH causes obesity and completely reverses beneficial effects in reducing body weight by restoration of PVH MC4R expression in MC4R KO mice (Xu et al., 2013). Studies show that these neurons function through projections to the hindbrain or the lateral septum (Shah et al., 2014; Xu et al., 2019).

Recent studies have expanded the investigation on glutamate release from individual groups of PVH neurons. Although the physiological role of glutamate release from CRH neurons in body weight remains to be demonstrated, this release directly activates downstream lateral hypothalamic neurons and may contribute to stress-related behaviors (Fuzesi et al., 2016; Hrabovszky et al., 2005; Romanov et al., 2017). The fast action of glutamate helps animals respond more quickly to environmental cues and is essential for survival (Fuzesi et al., 2016). Glutamate release from TRH neurons serves as an important upstream signal to activate AgRP neurons and promote feeding (Hrabovszky et al., 2005; Krashes et al., 2014). Recent results show that PVH neurons also send a unique projection to the ventral part of the lateral septum (LSv), a forebrain site known to regulate emotion and aggression (Xu et al., 2019). In addition, optogenetic activation of PVH to midbrain projections also inhibits feeding and promotes defense-related behaviors, which also requires glutamate release (Mangieri et al., 2019). Thus, it appears that glutamate is the major neurotransmitter that PVH neurons use to exert its function.

It is currently unknown how peptide and glutamate co-transmission from PVH neurons is coordinated to mediate PVH function. One possibility is that neuropeptides and glutamate contribute to different aspects of PVH function. For example, CRH knockout dramatically reduces hypothalamus–pituitary–adrenal (HPA) axis activity and causes defects in adrenal development (Muglia et al., 1995). Although further studies are required, given the presumed intact glutamate neurotransmission, these results suggest that glutamate release fails to compensate for the loss of CRH action. This is intriguing as pituitary ACTH cells (the target of CRH released from the PVH) express glutamate receptors (Zemkova and Stojilkovic, 2018). For both neuroendocrine oxytocin and vasopressin neurons, as both peptides are released directly from terminals to blood circulation in the posterior pituitary, their physiological roles in lactation/uterus contraction (oxytocin) and blood osmolarity (vasopressin) are well-established (Mavani et al., 2015; Nishimori et al., 1996). It is interesting to note that axons in the posterior pituitary contain both large granules and small dense core vesicles (Figure 3.1), suggesting that PVH projections to the posterior pituitary, including oxytocin and vasopressin, are capable of releasing glutamate. Additional studies are warranted to examine the potential importance of glutamate release from these terminals in addition to the role of neuropeptides and their receptors.

Interestingly, evidence suggests that peptides may undergo volume release from soma and in turn modulate the activity of PVH neurons in an autocrine or paracrine manner, which is consistent with the expression of peptide receptors in the PVH

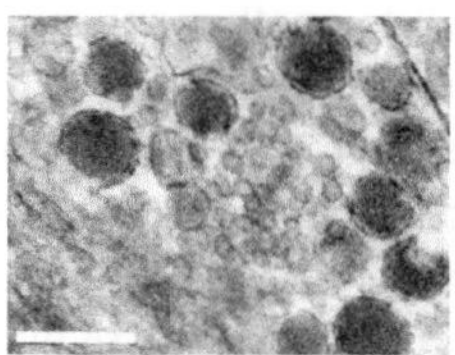

FIGURE 3.1 Co-existence of large granules and small dense core vesicles in axons in the posterior pituitary. Electron microscopic picture illustrating small vesicles and large granules in the same axon terminals. Scale bar = 200nm.

(Jiang et al., 2018). The volume release may play a modulatory role on the release of both peptides and glutamate release from terminals. In addition, PVH neurons have also been shown to innervate each other, especially between the two hemisphere neurons via glutamatergic neurotransmission (Boudaba and Tasker, 2006). This excitatory transmission may help propagate excitation among PVH neurons, enabling amplification of peptide release from terminals (Boudaba and Tasker, 2006).

3.4 CO-TRANSMISSION FROM LATERAL HYPOTHALAMIC NEURONS

The lateral hypothalamus is another important brain region for feeding and body weight regulation, as reflected by hypophagia and leanness caused by earlier lesion studies (Anand and Brobeck, 1951; Teitelbaum and Epstein, 1962). As in other hypothalamic areas, initial studies focus on the identification and function of neuropeptides. The most studied neuropeptides from the lateral hypothalamus (LH) are orexin and MCH. Recent studies also demonstrate the importance of neurotensin in feeding and body weight regulation (Schroeder and Leinninger, 2018). Notably, the majority of LH neurons do not express any known peptides. In contrast, most, if not all, LH neurons release either glutamate or GABA as a neurotransmitter as both VGLUT2 and VGAT are abundantly expressed in non-overlapping LH neurons. It appears that orexin and MCH neurons are glutamatergic whereas neurotensin neurons are more complex, being either glutamatergic (van den Pol, 2012) or GABAergic (Leinninger et al., 2011). Based on the projection patterns of orexin and MCH immunohistochemistry, these neurons project diffusively to numerous brain sites (Bittencourt et al., 1992; Elias et al., 1998; Peyron et al., 1998). However, most studies on these neurons only focus on a few brain sites. Thus, functional understanding of these neurons is largely incomplete.

Orexin neurons are known for the function of inducing arousal (Chemelli et al., 1999; Sakurai, 2007). Orexin regulates feeding behavior, its central application during light period promotes feeding (Edwards et al., 1999; Haynes et al., 2002; Haynes et al., 2000; Sakurai et al., 1998). Immunochemistry studies also show that orexin neurons innervate numerous feeding-related brain regions (Sakurai et al., 2005; Yoshida et al., 2006). This is consistent with subsequent pharmacogenetic studies, in which acute stimulation of orexin neurons increases food intake, water intake, as well as locomotor activity (Inutsuka et al., 2014). However, some studies show that orexin deficiency leads to obesity (Hara et al., 2001; Hara et al., 2005). It remains to be determined whether long-term and short-term effects of orexin could be different. Most orexin neurons are glutamatergic (Rosin et al., 2003; Torrealba et al., 2003). Recent studies prove that glutamate and orexin co-transmission is not redundant. These two neurotransmitters activate different output spikes in the same histamine neurons in regulating arousal (Schone et al., 2014; Schone et al., 2012). It has also been demonstrated that glutamate release from orexin neurons activates PVH CRH neurons and regulates arousal-related activation of the HPA axis (Bonnavion et al., 2015). However, despite intense studies on orexin neuron function, most studies focus on orexin itself and its receptors, and the role of glutamate release from these neurons is largely neglected.

Earlier studies suggest that MCH has a role in increasing feeding as the MCH KO mice exhibit lower body weight and are resistant to diet-induced obesity (Alon and

Friedman, 2006; Shimada et al., 1998). This claim is also supported by pharmacological studies with MCH or its receptor agonists or antagonists (Mashiko et al., 2005; Qu et al., 1996; Rossi et al., 1997; Shearman et al., 2003). In addition, MCH neurons are also important for normal glucose homeostasis (Burdakov et al., 2005; Kong et al., 2010). In contrast to the previous report that MCH neurons were GABAergic (Del Cid-Pellitero and Jones, 2012; Jego et al., 2013), recent evidence suggests that these neurons are glutamatergic (Chee et al., 2015). In electrophysiological recordings, MCH neurons project to the lateral septum and release glutamate, which activates a local self-innervating GABAergic network (Chee et al., 2015). Functionally, both MCH and glutamate release are required for the role of MCH neurons in the regulation of body weight (Schneeberger et al., 2018). Projections from MCH neurons to the ventral tegmental area (VTA) have been demonstrated to regulate reward-related feeding behavior (Domingos et al., 2013; Schneeberger et al., 2018). Interestingly, only glutamate but not MCH is required for reward feeding behavior (Schneeberger et al., 2018).

Neurotensin (NT) was first identified in the hypothalamic tissue (Carraway and Leeman, 1973), but has been found to be widely expressed in the brain and involved in the modulation of a variety of neural pathways and physiological processes. Central administration of NT reduces food intake (Cooke et al., 2009; Hawkins, 1986; Luttinger et al., 1982). LH NT neurons represent a small portion of brain NT-expressing neurons, and have been well studied in the context of feeding and body weight regulation. Acute activation of LH NT neurons increases locomotor activity and energy expenditure, and reduces food intake, consistent with the effects of the direct application of NT (Kurt et al., 2019; Woodworth et al., 2017). Genetic ablation of LH NT neurons leads to increased adiposity, decreased energy expenditure, and downregulation of orexin, which is essential in body weight homeostasis (Brown et al., 2019). A group of LH NT neurons are capable of sensing leptin through a leptin receptor (LepR) and potentially mediate leptin action on body weight involving local orexin neurons and downstream midbrain dopamine neurons (Brown et al., 2017; Leinninger et al., 2009; Leinninger et al., 2011). LepR-expressing NT neurons co-release GABA and modulate orexin neuronal activity through a GABAergic mechanism or a GABA-independent mechanism (Furutani et al., 2013; Goforth et al., 2014; Leinninger et al., 2011). Interestingly, NT neurons project to the VTA and increase the activity of VTA dopamine neurons through neurotensin receptor 1 (NTR1) (Leinninger et al., 2011; Opland et al., 2013; Patterson et al., 2015; Woodworth et al., 2017). Activation of this projection increases reward behaviors through NTR1-induced potentiation of glutamate receptor action (Kempadoo et al., 2013). However, as it appears that these neurons also release GABA (Omelchenko and Sesack, 2009), how GABA release is involved in this activation is unknown. It is speculated that some collaterals from this projection may regulate VTA local GABA neurons, thereby indirectly increasing VTA neuron activity (Nieh et al., 2016).

Recent studies have revealed important functions of GABAergic and glutamatergic LH neurons. Compared to peptide function, GABAergic and glutamatergic LH neurons, as a whole, play a much more definite role in feeding-related behaviors. Activation of LH GABAergic neurons promotes feeding, increasing both consummatory and hedonic feeding with positive valence (Jennings et al., 2015; Nieh et al., 2016). This effect may be partially mediated by GABAergic projections to the VTA and basal forebrain (Cassidy et al., 2019; Nieh et al., 2016). Consistent with the role of LH GABAergic neurons in promoting feeding, specific activation of the projections of these neurons in the periaqueductal gray elicits predatory behaviors, an action required for feeding (Li et al., 2018). In contrast, activation of LH glutamatergic neurons inhibits feeding associated with negative valance, which is partially mediated by glutamatergic projections to the lateral habenula (Stamatakis et al., 2016). Interestingly, both LH glutamatergic and GABAergic neurons send direct projections to the PVH, in which GABAergic projections elicit voracious feeding, while activation of glutamatergic projections inhibits feeding and promotes behavioral signs of stress-related negative emotions (Mangieri et al., 2018). Of note, these two types of projections antagonize each other on feeding and by the associated behaviors, suggesting that LH glutamatergic and GABAergic neurons may be alternately activated during different physiological states (Mangieri et al., 2018).

Despite the emerging concept of co-transmission, the investigation of LH neurons on neuropeptides and classical neurotransmitters remains largely segregated. It appears that the effect induced by the release of classical neurotransmitters from LH neurons is much greater than that of neuropeptides. It will be interesting to learn how LH neuropeptides interact with the function of classical neurotransmitters released from their own or neighboring neurons.

3.5 CO-TRANSMISSION FROM VTA DA NEURONS

DA neurons in the VTA have been extensively studied and well demonstrated to play an essential role in the reward system, and the role of DA and DA receptors in downstream neurons is also well documented (Bromberg-Martin et al., 2010; Watabe-Uchida et al., 2017). However, emerging data suggest that DA can co-release with GABA and glutamate from VTA DA neurons. Given the known role of VTA DA neurons in feeding and body weight regulation (Cassidy and Tong, 2017; Rossi and Stuber, 2018), it is important to know the potential implication of co-transmission from these neurons in energy balance regulation.

A subset of DA neurons in the VTA release glutamate onto striatal spiny projection neurons and cholinergic interneurons (Chuhma et al., 2018; Stuber et al., 2010; Tecuapetla et al., 2010). These neurons converge at the midline of the VTA, and glutamate released by these neurons is key in development, facilitating axonal growth, and survival and synaptic plasticity in drug addiction (Fortin et al., 2012; Papathanou et al., 2018). Conditional knockout of VGLUT2 in mature DA neurons will impact excitatory outputs and reduce action potentials in the nucleus accumbens (Hnasko et al., 2012). Some ultrastructural studies also show that the release of dopamine and glutamate occurs in the same axon but in different sub-regions (Zhang et al., 2015). The aversion induced by activation of these fibers on GABAergic interneurons in the nucleus accumbens is promoted by both glutamate- and GABA-receptor signaling (Qi et al., 2016).

It has been suggested that the glutamatergic phenotype (i.e. VGLUT2 expression) of VTA DA neurons may have a developmental origin. When VGLUT2-Cre mice were crossed with floxed vesicular monoamine transporter 2 (VMAT2) mice, the resulting

VGLUT2-Cre::Vmat2$^{f/f}$ mice died at around two to three weeks of age (Figure 3.2), recapitulating the phenotype of VMAT2 KO mice and mice with specific VMAT2 knockout in tyrosine hydroxylase (TH) neurons (Hnasko et al., 2012). In these mice, VMAT2 is largely deleted in the VTA, suggesting that the vast majority of DA neurons express VGLUT2 during development. Consistently, VTA DA neurons express abundant VGLUT2 in an early developmental time, but much less VGLUT2 expression in adult mice, suggesting that the VGLUT2 expression program is turned off during development (Steinkellner et al., 2018). This turn-off program is very important for DA neuron survival as overexpression of VGLUT2 in these neurons of adult mice leads to neuronal death (Steinkellner et al., 2018). Thus, it is clear that turning off VGLUT2 expression is an essential part of VTA DA neuron development. However, it is still unknown why these neurons are glutamatergic during neonatal development.

In addition to glutamate, VTA DA neurons are also capable of releasing GABA. With the channelrhodopsin 2 (ChR2) assisted circuit mapping (CRACM) method, optogenetic stimulation of VTA DA neuronal projections at the nucleus accumbens (NAc) reliably elicits DA-mediated postsynaptic currents with typical slow kinetics in striatal projection neurons and GABA-mediated postsynaptic inhibitory currents (Tritsch et al., 2014). Surprisingly, this GABA release is not mediated by the known VGAT but VMAT2 instead, which is capable of accumulating GABA in the vesicle independent of VGAT (Tritsch et al., 2014). Intriguingly, the source of intracellular GABA is not derived from conventional GABA synthesizing enzymes – GABA decarboxylase (GAD) 65 or 67 – but rather is derived from reuptake by GABA transporters or aldehyde dehydrogenase 1a1 (ALDH 1a1), which is a metabolic enzyme highly expressed in VTA DA neurons (Kim et al., 2015; Tritsch et al., 2014). GABA co-release from VTA DA neurons is physiologically functional and important, as demonstrated by the mouse model, with loss of GABA from these neurons by deletion of ALDH1a1 showing defects in alcohol addiction (Kim et al., 2015). There is another subset of TH neurons that release GABA, which project to the glutamatergic neurons in the LHb and release GABA in a VGAT-dependent manner.

Despite intensive research on co-transmission from VTA DA neurons, many interesting questions remain. It is still uncertain whether DA and glutamate or GABA can be co-released from the same vesicle (Trudeau and El Mestikawy, 2018), or to what

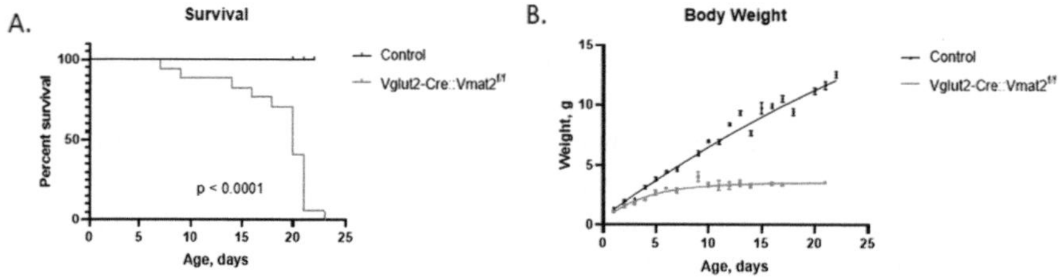

FIGURE 3.2 Neonatal knockout of VMAT2 in VGLUT2 neurons leads to death. Data was collected in pups from mouse breeding between VGLUT2-Cre::VMAT22$^{f/+}$ (heterozygous for VMATmat2 floxed alleles) and VMAT2$^{f/f}$ (homozygous for VMAT2 floxed alleles). Survival curve (A) and body weight (B) of VGLUT2-Cre::VMAT2f/f (i.e. VMAT2 KO) mice and their littermates; ***n*** = 17–20. VGLUT2-Cre mouse line expresses Cre driven by the endogenous VGLUT2 gene (i.e. VGLUT2-Ires-Cre).

extent glutamate or GABA mediates the DA neuron function (Wang et al., 2017; Zell et al., 2020). It will be interesting to determine whether DA and glutamate/GABA mediate the distinct functions of DA neurons during different physiological conditions, especially different feeding states.

3.6 CO-RELEASE FROM HINDBRAIN GLP1 NEURONS

Glucagon-like peptide 1 (GLP1) is one of the cleavage products of the preproglucagon peptide expressed in various peripheral tissues and the brain. Important preproglucagon peripheral sites include pancreatic alpha cells (glucagon) and gut (GLP1 and GLP2). In the brain, GLP1 is expressed in a few groups of neurons at various sites with the hindbrain being the main location of GLP1 (Holt et al., 2019). GLP1 is defined as an incretin hormone, which is broadly involved in improving glucose homeostasis, reducing feeding and regulating body weight and other metabolism-related functions and has been extensively explored for treatment against metabolic diseases (Andersen et al., 2018; Fava, 2014; Madsbad and Holst, 2014; Turton et al., 1996). Hindbrain GLP1 neurons send projections to a variety of brain regions to regulate feeding and body weight. These regions include typically known feeding-regulating hypothalamic neurons such as PVH neurons and POMC neurons in the Arc, as well as other brain sites including the lateral septum (Llewellyn-Smith et al., 2013; Llewellyn-Smith et al., 2011; Rinaman, 2010; Tauchi et al., 2008; Terrill et al., 2016; Vrang et al., 2007). Consistently, GLP1 receptors have been identified in these brain areas and the application of receptor pharmacology reveals the importance of endogenous GLP1 receptors in feeding, body weight, and other physiological processes related to changes in the activity of these neurons (Cork et al., 2015; Merchenthaler et al., 1999; Sandoval et al., 2008). For example, GLP1 or the GLP1 receptor agonist in the PVH inhibits feeding and, importantly, GLP1 receptor-expressing neurons in the PVH represent a key group of feeding-inhibiting neurons (Adams et al., 2018; McMahon and Wellman, 1998). Surprisingly, the specific activation of GLP1 receptors in the lateral septum (mostly the dorsal part), a known region involved in aggression and emotion control, strongly inhibits feeding (Terrill et al., 2016). As LSv neurons also receive direct inputs from the PVH to inhibit feeding (Xu et al., 2019), the lateral septum may integrate feeding-related inputs from multiple brain sites to co-regulate feeding and related emotional states.

In addition to GLP1, the hindbrain GLP1 neurons also express VGLUT2 and release glutamate (Zheng et al., 2015). Similar to other brain neurons releasing both peptides and fast-acting neurotransmitters, the role of glutamate release is much less appreciated in GLP1 neurons. Optogenetic stimulation of hindbrain GLP1 neuron terminals in the Arc shows that POMC neurons receive both GLP1 and glutamate inputs from hindbrain GLP1 neurons (He et al., 2019). However, the contribution by glutamatergic inputs to POMC neurons remains untested. Probably, the most well studied co-release of glutamate and GLP1 is the hindbrain GLP1 neurons to the PVH. Using a combination of mouse genetics, optogenetics, biochemistry, and *in vitro* electrophysiology, a recent study has nicely demonstrated that GLP1 action on PVH neurons amplifies glutamatergic action onto these neurons: GLP1 increases trafficking of AMPA receptor subunits to neuronal membranes and strengthens the action of glutamatergic inputs from presynaptic neurons (Liu et al., 2017). An intriguing observation is that disruption of glutamate release specifically from hindbrain GLP1 neurons causes no apparent phenotype on feeding and body weight, much less than that observed from disruption of GLP1 (Liu et al., 2017). One potential reason could be that lack of glutamate release from GLP1 neurons could invoke compensatory responses from other presynaptic glutamatergic neurons. Nevertheless, one major role of GLP1 is to serve as a modulator to gauge the strength of glutamatergic action on the postsynaptic neurons. More studies are required to examine whether a similar mechanism operates in GLP1 neuron projections in other brain neurons and as to whether there are additional pathways in which glutamate and GLP1 interact in mediating the function of GLP1 neurons.

3.7 SUMMARY

In this chapter, we have introduced recent developments in co-transmission on key body-weight-regulating neurons that are shown to release more than one neurotransmitter. There is an increasing number of neurons that are capable of co-neurotransmission. Examples include dorsal raphe serotoninergic neurons, a subset of which express VGLUT3 and release glutamate (Commons and Valentino, 2002), and striatal cholinergic neurons, a subset of which also express VGLUT3 and release glutamate (Gras et al., 2002). It is also worth noting that the nodose ganglion is known to release multiple neuropeptides, including substance P and calcitonin gene-related peptide, and express VGLUT2 and release glutamate (Lawrence, 1995; Saha et al., 1995; Schaffar et al., 1997). Co-transmission of glutamate and peptides from nodose neurons to neurons in the nucleus of solidary tract and dorsal motor vagus neurons is well characterized in *in vitro* electrophysiological studies (Babic et al., 2012). Thus, this chapter may serve as a prologue in the effort of delineating the physiological significance of co-transmission.

Efforts toward understanding the function of co-transmission are highly significant. As discussed in this chapter, the current research efforts on the role of neurotransmitters in this area are still largely segregated, with most focus on peptides, monoamines, amino acids, or Ach. With the emerging techniques that allow *in vivo* monitoring of neuropeptides, monoamines, and amino acids on postsynaptic neurons with fluorescence measurements (Leopold et al., 2019; Wang et al., 2018), it is anticipated that more rapid progress will be made in the near future on the physiological significance of co-transmission. Extensive studies on neuropeptide function have tried to target peptide action for drug treatments, but most fail. One of the underlying reasons is that it is difficult to appreciate the impact elicited by peptide action on co-transmitted neurotransmitters. Understanding co-transmission is imperative to appreciate the functional relationship between the co-transmitted signals and the full physiological effects.

ACKNOWLEDGMENTS

Research in the Tong lab was supported by grants NIH R01 DK114279, R21NS108091, R01DK109934, R01DK120858, and DOD W81XWH-19-1-0429.

REFERENCES

Adams, J.M., Pei, H., Sandoval, D.A., Seeley, R.J., Chang, R.B., Liberles, S.D., and Olson, D.P. (2018). Liraglutide modulates appetite and body weight through glucagon-Like peptide 1 receptor-expressing glutamatergic neurons. *Diabetes 67*, 1538–1548.

Alhadeff, A.L., Su, Z., Hernandez, E., Klima, M.L., Phillips, S.Z., Holland, R.A., Guo, C., Hantman, A.W., De Jonghe, B.C., and Betley, J.N. (2018). A neural circuit for the suppression of pain by a competing need state. *Cell 173*, 140–152 e115.

Alon, T., and Friedman, J.M. (2006). Late-onset leanness in mice with targeted ablation of melanin concentrating hormone neurons. *J Neurosci 26*, 389–397.

Anand, B.K., and Brobeck, J.R. (1951). Hypothalamic control of food intake in rats and cats. *Yale J Biol Med 24*, 123–140.

Andermann, M.L., and Lowell, B.B. (2017). Toward a wiring diagram understanding of appetite control. *Neuron 95*, 757–778.

Andersen, A., Lund, A., Knop, F.K., and Vilsboll, T. (2018). Glucagon-like peptide 1 in health and disease. *Nat Rev Endocrinol 14*, 390–403.

Aponte, Y., Atasoy, D., and Sternson, S.M. (2011). AGRP neurons are sufficient to orchestrate feeding behavior rapidly and without training. *Nat Neurosci 14*, 351–355.

Aramakis, V.B., Stanley, B.G., and Ashe, J.H. (1996). Neuropeptide Y receptor agonists: multiple effects on spontaneous activity in the paraventricular hypothalamus. *Peptides 17*, 1349–1357.

Aravich, P.F., and Sclafani, A. (1983). Paraventricular hypothalamic lesions and medial hypothalamic knife cuts produce similar hyperphagia syndromes. *Behav Neurosci 97*, 970–983.

Atasoy, D., Betley, J.N., Su, H.H., and Sternson, S.M. (2012). Deconstruction of a neural circuit for hunger. *Nature 488*, 172–177.

Babic, T., Troy, A.E., Fortna, S.R., and Browning, K.N. (2012). Glucose-dependent trafficking of 5-HT3 receptors in rat gastrointestinal vagal afferent neurons. *Neurogastroenterol Motil 24*, e476–e488.

Bewick, G.A., Gardiner, J.V., Dhillo, W.S., Kent, A.S., White, N.E., Webster, Z., Ghatei, M.A., and Bloom, S.R. (2005). Post-embryonic ablation of AgRP neurons in mice leads to a lean, hypophagic phenotype. *FASEB journal: official publication of the Federation of American Societies for Experimental Biology 19*, 1680–1682.

Bittencourt, J.C., Presse, F., Arias, C., Peto, C., Vaughan, J., Nahon, J.L., Vale, W., and Sawchenko, P.E. (1992). The melanin-concentrating hormone system of the rat brain: an immuno- and hybridization histochemical characterization. *J Comp Neurol 319*, 218–245.

Blevins, J.E., Schwartz, M.W., and Baskin, D.G. (2004). Evidence that paraventricular nucleus oxytocin neurons link hypothalamic leptin action to caudal brain stem nuclei controlling meal size. *Am J Physiol Regul Integr Comp Physiol 287*, R87–R96.

Bonnavion, P., Jackson, A.C., Carter, M.E., and de Lecea, L. (2015). Antagonistic interplay between hypocretin and leptin in the lateral hypothalamus regulates stress responses. *Nat Commun 6*, 6266.

Boudaba, C., and Tasker, J.G. (2006). Intranuclear coupling of hypothalamic magnocellular nuclei by glutamate synaptic circuits. *Am J Physiol Regul Integr Comp Physiol 291*, R102–R111.

Bromberg-Martin, E.S., Matsumoto, M., and Hikosaka, O. (2010). Dopamine in motivational control: rewarding, aversive, and alerting. *Neuron 68*, 815–834.

Brown, J.A., Bugescu, R., Mayer, T.A., Gata-Garcia, A., Kurt, G., Woodworth, H.L., and Leinninger, G.M. (2017). Loss of action via neurotensin-leptin receptor neurons disrupts leptin and Ghrelin-Mediated control of energy balance. *Endocrinology 158*, 1271–1288.

Brown, J.A., Wright, A., Bugescu, R., Christensen, L., Olson, D.P., and Leinninger, G.M. (2019). Distinct subsets of lateral hypothalamic neurotensin neurons are activated by leptin or dehydration. *Sci Rep 9*, 1873.

Burdakov, D., Gerasimenko, O., and Verkhratsky, A. (2005). Physiological changes in glucose differentially modulate the excitability of hypothalamic melanin-concentrating hormone and orexin neurons in situ. *J Neurosci 25*, 2429–2433.

Carraway, R., and Leeman, S.E. (1973). The isolation of a new hypotensive peptide, neurotensin, from bovine hypothalami. *J Biol Chem 248*, 6854–6861.

Cassidy, R.M., Lu, Y., Jere, M., Tian, J.B., Xu, Y., Mangieri, L.R., Felix-Okoroji, B., Selever, J., Xu, Y., Arenkiel, B.R., et al. (2019). A lateral hypothalamus to basal forebrain neurocircuit promotes feeding by suppressing responses to anxiogenic environmental cues. *Sci Adv 5*, eaav1640.

Cassidy, R.M., and Tong, Q. (2017). Hunger and satiety gauge reward sensitivity. *Front Endocrinol (Lausanne) 8*, 104.

Chee, M.J., Arrigoni, E., and Maratos-Flier, E. (2015). Melanin-concentrating hormone neurons release glutamate for feedforward inhibition of the lateral septum. *J Neurosci 35*, 3644–3651.

Chemelli, R.M., Willie, J.T., Sinton, C.M., Elmquist, J.K., Scammell, T., Lee, C., Richardson, J.A., Williams, S.C., Xiong, Y., Kisanuki, Y., et al. (1999). Narcolepsy in orexin knockout mice: molecular genetics of sleep regulation. *Cell 98*, 437–451.

Chen, Y., Essner, R.A., Kosar, S., Miller, O.H., Lin, Y.C., Mesgarzadeh, S., and Knight, Z.A. (2019). Sustained NPY signaling enables AgRP neurons to drive feeding. *elife 8*.

Chen, Y., Lin, Y.C., Kuo, T.W., and Knight, Z.A. (2015). Sensory detection of food rapidly modulates arcuate feeding circuits. *Cell 160*, 829–841.

Chen, Y., Lin, Y.C., Zimmerman, C.A., Essner, R.A., and Knight, Z.A. (2016). Hunger neurons drive feeding through a sustained, positive reinforcement signal. *elife 5*.

Chuhma, N., Mingote, S., Yetnikoff, L., Kalmbach, A., Ma, T., Ztaou, S., Sienna, A.C., Tepler, S., Poulin, J.F., Ansorge, M., et al. (2018). Dopamine neuron glutamate cotransmission evokes a delayed excitation in lateral dorsal striatal cholinergic interneurons. *Elife 7*.

Commons, K.G., and Valentino, R.J. (2002). Cellular basis for the effects of substance P in the periaqueductal gray and dorsal raphe nucleus. *J Comp Neurol 447*, 82–97.

Cone, R.D. (2005). Anatomy and regulation of the central melanocortin system. *Nat Neurosci 8*, 571–578.

Cooke, J.H., Patterson, M., Patel, S.R., Smith, K.L., Ghatei, M.A., Bloom, S.R., and Murphy, K.G. (2009). Peripheral and central administration of xenin and neurotensin suppress food intake in rodents. *Obesity (Silver Spring) 17*, 1135–1143.

Cork, S.C., Richards, J.E., Holt, M.K., Gribble, F.M., Reimann, F., and Trapp, S. (2015). Distribution and characterisation of Glucagon-like peptide-1 receptor expressing cells in the mouse brain. *Mol Metab 4*, 718–731.

Del Cid-Pellitero, E., and Jones, B.E. (2012). Immunohistochemical evidence for synaptic release of GABA from melanin-concentrating hormone containing varicosities in the locus coeruleus. *Neuroscience 223*, 269–276.

Dennison, C.S., King, C.M., Dicken, M.S., and Hentges, S.T. (2016). Age-dependent changes in amino acid phenotype and the role of glutamate release from hypothalamic proopiomelanocortin neurons. *J Comp Neurol 524*, 1222–1235.

Dicken, M.S., Tooker, R.E., and Hentges, S.T. (2012). Regulation of GABA and glutamate release from proopiomelanocortin neuron terminals in intact hypothalamic networks. *J Neurosci 32*, 4042–4048.

Domingos, A.I., Sordillo, A., Dietrich, M.O., Liu, Z.W., Tellez, L.A., Vaynshteyn, J., Ferreira, J.G., Ekstrand, M.I., Horvath, T.L., de Araujo, I.E., et al. (2013). Hypothalamic melanin concentrating hormone neurons communicate the nutrient value of sugar. *elife 2*, e01462.

Durr, K., Norsted, E., Gomuc, B., Suarez, E., Hannibal, J., and Meister, B. (2007). Presence of pituitary adenylate cyclase-activating polypeptide (PACAP) defines a subpopulation of hypothalamic POMC neurons. *Brain Res 1186*, 203–211.

Edwards, C.M., Abusnana, S., Sunter, D., Murphy, K.G., Ghatei, M.A., and Bloom, S.R. (1999). The effect of the orexins on food intake: comparison with neuropeptide Y, melanin-concentrating hormone and galanin. *J Endocrinol 160*, R7–12.

Egan, O.K., Inglis, M.A., and Anderson, G.M. (2017). Leptin signaling in AgRP neurons modulates puberty onset and adult fertility in mice. *J Neurosci 37*, 3875–3886.

El Mestikawy, S., Wallen-Mackenzie, A., Fortin, G.M., Descarries, L., and Trudeau, L.E. (2011). From glutamate co-release to vesicular synergy: vesicular glutamate transporters. *Nat Rev Neurosci 12*, 204–216.

Elias, C.F., Aschkenasi, C., Lee, C., Kelly, J., Ahima, R.S., Bjorbaek, C., Flier, J.S., Saper, C.B., and Elmquist, J.K. (1999). Leptin differentially regulates NPY and POMC neurons projecting to the lateral hypothalamic area. *Neuron 23*, 775–786.

Elias, C.F., Saper, C.B., Maratos-Flier, E., Tritos, N.A., Lee, C., Kelly, J., Tatro, J.B., Hoffman, G.E., Ollmann, M.M., Barsh, G.S., et al. (1998). Chemically defined projections linking the mediobasal hypothalamus and the lateral hypothalamic area. *J Comp Neurol 402*, 442–459.

Elmquist, J.K., Coppari, R., Balthasar, N., Ichinose, M., and Lowell, B.B. (2005). Identifying hypothalamic pathways controlling food intake, body weight, and glucose homeostasis. *J Comp Neurol 493*, 63–71.

Engstrom Ruud, L., Pereira, M.M.A., de Solis, A.J., Fenselau, H., and Bruning, J.C. (2020). NPY mediates the rapid feeding and glucose metabolism regulatory functions of AgRP neurons. *Nat Commun 11*, 442.

Ericsson, A., Schalling, M., McIntyre, K.R., Lundberg, J.M., Larhammar, D., Seroogy, K., Hokfelt, T., and Persson, H. (1987). Detection of neuropeptide Y and its mRNA in megakaryocytes: enhanced levels in certain autoimmune mice. *Proc Natl Acad Sci U S A 84*, 5585–5589.

Fan, W., Boston, B.A., Kesterson, R.A., Hruby, V.J., and Cone, R.D. (1997). Role of melanocortinergic neurons in feeding and the agouti obesity syndrome. *Nature 385*, 165–168.

Fava, S. (2014). Glucagon-like peptide 1 and the cardiovascular system. *Curr Diabetes Rev 10*, 302–310.

Flier, J.S. (2006). AgRP in energy balance: will the real AgRP please stand up? *Cell Metab 3*, 83–85.

Fortin, G.M., Bourque, M.J., Mendez, J.A., Leo, D., Nordenankar, K., Birgner, C., Arvidsson, E., Rymar, V.V., Berube-Carriere, N., Claveau, A.M., et al. (2012). Glutamate corelease promotes growth and survival of midbrain dopamine neurons. *J Neurosci 32*, 17477–17491.

Furutani, N., Hondo, M., Kageyama, H., Tsujino, N., Mieda, M., Yanagisawa, M., Shioda, S., and Sakurai, T. (2013). Neurotensin co-expressed in orexin-producing neurons in the lateral hypothalamus plays an important role in regulation of sleep/wakefulness states. *PLoS One 8*, e62391.

Fuxe, K., Dahlstrom, A., Hoistad, M., Marcellino, D., Jansson, A., Rivera, A., Diaz-Cabiale, Z., Jacobsen, K., Tinner-Staines, B., Hagman, B., et al. (2007). From the Golgi-Cajal mapping to the transmitter-based characterization of the neuronal networks leading to two modes of brain communication: wiring and volume transmission. *Brain Res Rev 55*, 17–54.

Fuxe, K., Rivera, A., Jacobsen, K.X., Hoistad, M., Leo, G., Horvath, T.L., Staines, W., De la Calle, A., and Agnati, L.F. (2005). Dynamics of volume transmission in the brain. Focus on catecholamine and opioid peptide communication and the role of uncoupling protein 2. *J Neural Transm (Vienna) 112*, 65–76.

Fuzesi, T., Daviu, N., Wamsteeker Cusulin, J.I., Bonin, R.P., and Bains, J.S. (2016). Hypothalamic CRH neurons orchestrate complex behaviours after stress. *Nat Commun 7*, 11937.

Goforth, P.B., Leinninger, G.M., Patterson, C.M., Satin, L.S., and Myers, M.G., Jr. (2014). Leptin acts via lateral hypothalamic area neurotensin neurons to inhibit orexin neurons by multiple GABA-independent mechanisms. *J Neurosci 34*, 11405–11415.

Graham, M., Shutter, J.R., Sarmiento, U., Sarosi, I., and Stark, K.L. (1997). Overexpression of Agrt leads to obesity in transgenic mice. *Nat Genet 17*, 273–274.

Gras, C., Herzog, E., Bellenchi, G.C., Bernard, V., Ravassard, P., Pohl, M., Gasnier, B., Giros, B., and El Mestikawy, S. (2002). A third vesicular glutamate transporter expressed by cholinergic and serotoninergic neurons. *J Neurosci 22*, 5442–5451.

Gray, T.S., and Morley, J.E. (1986). Neuropeptide Y: anatomical distribution and possible function in mammalian nervous system. *Life Sci 38*, 389–401.

Greenman, Y., Kuperman, Y., Drori, Y., Asa, S.L., Navon, I., Forkosh, O., Gil, S., Stern, N., and Chen, A. (2013). Postnatal ablation of POMC neurons induces an obese phenotype characterized by decreased food intake and enhanced anxiety-like behavior. *Mol Endocrinol 27*, 1091–1102.

Gropp, E., Shanabrough, M., Borok, E., Xu, A.W., Janoschek, R., Buch, T., Plum, L., Balthasar, N., Hampel, B., Waisman, A., et al. (2005). Agouti-related peptide-expressing neurons are mandatory for feeding. *Nat Neurosci 8*, 1289–1291.

Hagan, M.M., Rushing, P.A., Benoit, S.C., Woods, S.C., and Seeley, R.J. (2001). Opioid receptor involvement in the effect of AgRP- (83-132) on food intake and food selection. *Am J Physiol Regul Integr Comp Physiol 280*, R814–R821.

Hahn, T.M., Breininger, J.F., Baskin, D.G., and Schwartz, M.W. (1998). Coexpression of Agrp and NPY in fasting-activated hypothalamic neurons. *Nat Neurosci 1*, 271–272.

Hara, J., Beuckmann, C.T., Nambu, T., Willie, J.T., Chemelli, R.M., Sinton, C.M., Sugiyama, F., Yagami, K., Goto, K., Yanagisawa, M., et al. (2001). Genetic ablation of orexin neurons in mice results in narcolepsy, hypophagia, and obesity. *Neuron 30*, 345–354.

Hara, J., Yanagisawa, M., and Sakurai, T. (2005). Difference in obesity phenotype between orexin-knockout mice and orexin neuron-deficient mice with same genetic background and environmental conditions. *Neurosci Lett 380*, 239–242.

Haskell-Luevano, C., and Monck, E.K. (2001). Agouti-related protein functions as an inverse agonist at a constitutively active brain melanocortin-4 receptor. *Regul Pept 99*, 1–7.

Hawkins, M.F. (1986). Central nervous system neurotensin and feeding. *Physiol Behav 36*, 1–8.

Hayes, M.R., and Schmidt, H.D. (2016). GLP-1 influences food and drug reward. *Curr Opin Behav Sci 9*, 66–70.

Haynes, A.C., Chapman, H., Taylor, C., Moore, G.B., Cawthorne, M.A., Tadayyon, M., Clapham, J.C., and Arch, J.R. (2002). Anorectic, thermogenic and anti-obesity activity of a selective orexin-1 receptor antagonist in ob/ob mice. *Regul Pept 104*, 153–159.

Haynes, A.C., Jackson, B., Chapman, H., Tadayyon, M., Johns, A., Porter, R.A., and Arch, J.R. (2000). A selective orexin-1 receptor antagonist reduces food consumption in male and female rats. *Regul Pept 96*, 45–51.

He, Z., Gao, Y., Lieu, L., Afrin, S., Cao, J., Michael, N.J., Dong, Y., Sun, J., Guo, H., and Williams, K.W. (2019). Direct and indirect effects of liraglutide on hypothalamic POMC and NPY/AgRP neurons - Implications for energy balance and glucose control. *Mol Metab 28*, 120–134.

Hentges, S.T., Otero-Corchon, V., Pennock, R.L., King, C.M., and Low, M.J. (2009). Proopiomelanocortin expression in both GABA and glutamate neurons. *J Neurosci 29*, 13684–13690.

Hnasko, T.S., Hjelmstad, G.O., Fields, H.L., and Edwards, R.H. (2012). Ventral tegmental area glutamate neurons: electrophysiological properties and projections. *J Neurosci 32*, 15076–15085.

Holder, J.L., Jr., Butte, N.F., and Zinn, A.R. (2000). Profound obesity associated with a balanced translocation that disrupts the SIM1 gene. *Hum Mol Genet 9*, 101–108.

Holt, M.K., Richards, J.E., Cook, D.R., Brierley, D.I., Williams, D.L., Reimann, F., Gribble, F.M., and Trapp, S. (2019). Preproglucagon neurons in the nucleus of the solitary tract are the main source of brain GLP-1, mediate stress-Induced hypophagia, and limit unusually large intakes of food. *Diabetes 68*, 21–33.

Hrabovszky, E., Halasz, J., Meelis, W., Kruk, M.R., Liposits, Z., and Haller, J. (2005). Neurochemical characterization of hypothalamic neurons involved in attack behavior: glutamatergic dominance and co-expression of thyrotropin-releasing hormone in a subset of glutamatergic neurons. *Neuroscience 133*, 657–666.

Inutsuka, A., Inui, A., Tabuchi, S., Tsunematsu, T., Lazarus, M., and Yamanaka, A. (2014). Concurrent and robust regulation of feeding behaviors and metabolism by orexin neurons. *Neuropharmacology 85*, 451–460.

Jacobson, L. (1999). Glucocorticoid replacement, but not corticotropin-releasing hormone deficiency, prevents adrenalectomy-induced anorexia in mice. *Endocrinology 140*, 310–317.

Jarvie, B.C., and Hentges, S.T. (2012). Expression of GABAergic and glutamatergic phenotypic markers in hypothalamic proopiomelanocortin neurons. *J Comp Neurol 520*, 3863–3876.

Jego, S., Glasgow, S.D., Herrera, C.G., Ekstrand, M., Reed, S.J., Boyce, R., Friedman, J., Burdakov, D., and Adamantidis, A.R. (2013). Optogenetic identification of a rapid eye movement sleep modulatory circuit in the hypothalamus. *Nat Neurosci 16*, 1637–1643.

Jennings, J.H., Ung, R.L., Resendez, S.L., Stamatakis, A.M., Taylor, J.G., Huang, J., Veleta, K., Kantak, P.A., Aita, M., Shilling-Scrivo, K., et al. (2015). Visualizing hypothalamic network dynamics for appetitive and consummatory behaviors. *Cell 160*, 516–527.

Jiang, Z., Rajamanickam, S., and Justice, N.J. (2018). Local Corticotropin-Releasing Factor Signaling in the Hypothalamic Paraventricular Nucleus. *J Neurosci 38*, 1874–1890.

Kalra, S.P., and Kalra, P.S. (2004). NPY and cohorts in regulating appetite, obesity and metabolic syndrome: beneficial effects of gene therapy. *Neuropeptides 38*, 201–211.

Kempadoo, K.A., Tourino, C., Cho, S.L., Magnani, F., Leinninger, G.M., Stuber, G.D., Zhang, F., Myers, M.G., Deisseroth, K., de Lecea, L., et al. (2013). Hypothalamic neurotensin projections promote reward by enhancing glutamate transmission in the VTA. *J Neurosci 33*, 7618–7626.

Kim, J.I., Ganesan, S., Luo, S.X., Wu, Y.W., Park, E., Huang, E.J., Chen, L., and Ding, J.B. (2015). Aldehyde dehydrogenase 1a1 mediates a GABA synthesis pathway in midbrain dopaminergic neurons. *Science 350*, 102–106.

Klimaschewski, L., Kummer, W., and Heym, C. (1996). Localization, regulation and functions of neurotransmitters and neuromodulators in cervical sympathetic ganglia. *Microsc Res Tech 35*, 44–68.

Koch, M., Varela, L., Kim, J.G., Kim, J.D., Hernandez-Nuno, F., Simonds, S.E., Castorena, C.M., Vianna, C.R., Elmquist, J.K., Morozov, Y.M., et al. (2015). Hypothalamic POMC neurons promote cannabinoid-induced feeding. *Nature 519*, 45–50.

Kong, D., Vong, L., Parton, L.E., Ye, C., Tong, Q., Hu, X., Choi, B., Bruning, J.C., and Lowell, B.B. (2010). Glucose stimulation of hypothalamic MCH neurons involves K(ATP) channels, is modulated by UCP2, and regulates peripheral glucose homeostasis. *Cell Metab 12*, 545–552.

Krashes, M.J., Shah, B.P., Koda, S., and Lowell, B.B. (2013). Rapid versus delayed stimulation of feeding by the endogenously released AgRP neuron mediators GABA, NPY, and AgRP. *Cell Metab 18*, 588–595.

Krashes, M.J., Shah, B.P., Madara, J.C., Olson, D.P., Strochlic, D.E., Garfield, A.S., Vong, L., Pei, H., Watabe-Uchida, M., Uchida, N., et al. (2014). An excitatory paraventricular nucleus to AgRP neuron circuit that drives hunger. *Nature 507*, 238–242.

Kristensen, P., Judge, M.E., Thim, L., Ribel, U., Christjansen, K.N., Wulff, B.S., Clausen, J.T., Jensen, P.B., Madsen, O.D., Vrang, N., et al. (1998). Hypothalamic CART is a new anorectic peptide regulated by leptin. *Nature 393*, 72–76.

Krude, H., Biebermann, H., Luck, W., Horn, R., Brabant, G., and Gruters, A. (1998). Severe early-onset obesity, adrenal insufficiency and red hair pigmentation caused by POMC mutations in humans. *Nat Genet 19*, 155–157.

Kurt, G., Woodworth, H.L., Fowler, S., Bugescu, R., and Leinninger, G.M. (2019). Activation of lateral hypothalamic area neurotensin-expressing neurons promotes drinking. *Neuropharmacology 154*, 13–21.

Lawrence, A.J. (1995). Neurotransmitter mechanisms of rat vagal afferent neurons. *Clin Exp Pharmacol Physiol 22*, 869–873.

Leinninger, G.M., Jo, Y.H., Leshan, R.L., Louis, G.W., Yang, H., Barrera, J.G., Wilson, H., Opland, D.M., Faouzi, M.A., Gong, Y., et al. (2009). Leptin acts via leptin receptor-expressing lateral hypothalamic neurons to modulate the mesolimbic dopamine system and suppress feeding. *Cell Metab 10*, 89–98.

Leinninger, G.M., Opland, D.M., Jo, Y.H., Faouzi, M., Christensen, L., Cappellucci, L.A., Rhodes, C.J., Gnegy, M.E., Becker, J.B., Pothos, E.N., et al. (2011). Leptin action via neurotensin neurons controls orexin, the mesolimbic dopamine system and energy balance. *Cell Metab 14*, 313–323.

Leopold, A.V., Shcherbakova, D.M., and Verkhusha, V.V. (2019). Fluorescent biosensors for neurotransmission and neuromodulation: engineering and applications. *Front Cell Neurosci 13*, 474.

Li, M.M., Madara, J.C., Steger, J.S., Krashes, M.J., Balthasar, N., Campbell, J.N., Resch, J.M., Conley, N.J., Garfield, A.S., and Lowell, B.B. (2019). The paraventricular hypothalamus regulates satiety and prevents obesity via two genetically distinct circuits. *Neuron 102*, 653–667 e656.

Li, Y., Zeng, J., Zhang, J., Yue, C., Zhong, W., Liu, Z., Feng, Q., and Luo, M. (2018). Hypothalamic circuits for predation and evasion. *Neuron 97*, 911–924 e915.

Liu, J., Conde, K., Zhang, P., Lilascharoen, V., Xu, Z., Lim, B.K., Seeley, R.J., Zhu, J.J., Scott, M.M., and Pang, Z.P. (2017). Enhanced AMPA receptor trafficking mediates the anorexigenic effect of endogenous glucagon-like peptide-1 in the paraventricular hypothalamus. *Neuron 96*, 897–909 e895.

Llewellyn-Smith, I.J., Gnanamanickam, G.J., Reimann, F., Gribble, F.M., and Trapp, S. (2013). Preproglucagon (PPG) neurons innervate neurochemically identified autonomic neurons in the mouse brainstem. *Neuroscience 229*, 130–143.

Llewellyn-Smith, I.J., Reimann, F., Gribble, F.M., and Trapp, S. (2011). Preproglucagon neurons project widely to autonomic control areas in the mouse brain. *Neuroscience 180*, 111–121.

Loh, K., Herzog, H., and Shi, Y.C. (2015). Regulation of energy homeostasis by the NPY system. *Trends Endocrinol Metab 26*, 125–135.

Low, M.J., Hayward, M.D., Appleyard, S.M., and Rubinstein, M. (2003). State-dependent modulation of feeding behavior by proopiomelanocortin-derived beta-endorphin. *Ann N Y Acad Sci 994*, 192–201.

Lowell, B.B., and Bachman, E.S. (2003). Beta-Adrenergic receptors, diet-induced thermogenesis, and obesity. *J Biol Chem 278*, 29385–29388.

Lundberg, J.M., Terenius, L., Hokfelt, T., Martling, C.R., Tatemoto, K., Mutt, V., Polak, J., Bloom, S., and Goldstein, M. (1982). Neuropeptide Y (NPY)-like immunoreactivity in peripheral noradrenergic neurons and effects of NPY on sympathetic function. *Acta Physiol Scand 116*, 477–480.

Luquet, S., Perez, F.A., Hnasko, T.S., and Palmiter, R.D. (2005). NPY/AgRP neurons are essential for feeding in adult mice but can be ablated in neonates. *Science 310*, 683–685.

Luttinger, D., King, R.A., Sheppard, D., Strupp, J., Nemeroff, C.B., and Prange, A.J., Jr. (1982). The effect of neurotensin on food consumption in the rat. *Eur J Pharmacol 81*, 499–503.

Madsbad, S., and Holst, J.J. (2014). GLP-1 as a mediator in the remission of type 2 diabetes after gastric bypass and sleeve gastrectomy surgery. *Diabetes 63*, 3172–3174.

Mangieri, L.R., Jiang, Z., Lu, Y., Xu, Y., Cassidy, R.M., Justice, N., Xu, Y., Arenkiel, B.R., and Tong, Q. (2019). Defensive behaviors driven by a hypothalamic-ventral midbrain circuit. *eNeuro 6*.

Mangieri, L.R., Lu, Y., Xu, Y., Cassidy, R.M., Xu, Y., Arenkiel, B.R., and Tong, Q. (2018). A neural basis for antagonistic control of feeding and compulsive behaviors. *Nat Commun 9*, 52.

Mashiko, S., Ishihara, A., Gomori, A., Moriya, R., Ito, M., Iwaasa, H., Matsuda, M., Feng, Y., Shen, Z., Marsh, D.J., et al. (2005). Antiobesity effect of a melanin-concentrating hormone 1 receptor antagonist in diet-induced obese mice. *Endocrinology 146*, 3080–3086.

Mavani, G.P., DeVita, M.V., and Michelis, M.F. (2015). A review of the nonpressor and nonantidiuretic actions of the hormone vasopressin. *Front Med (Lausanne) 2*, 19.

McMahon, L.R., and Wellman, P.J. (1998). PVN infusion of GLP-1-(7-36) amide suppresses feeding but does not induce aversion or alter locomotion in rats. *Am J Phys 274*, R23–R29.

Meister, B., Gomuc, B., Suarez, E., Ishii, Y., Durr, K., and Gillberg, L. (2006). Hypothalamic proopiomelanocortin (POMC) neurons have a cholinergic phenotype. *Eur J Neurosci 24*, 2731–2740.

Mercer, A.J., Hentges, S.T., Meshul, C.K., and Low, M.J. (2013). Unraveling the central proopiomelanocortin neural circuits. *Front Neurosci 7*, 19.

Merchenthaler, I., Lane, M., and Shughrue, P. (1999). Distribution of pre-pro-glucagon and glucagon-like peptide-1 receptor messenger RNAs in the rat central nervous system. *J Comp Neurol 403*, 261–280.

Muglia, L., Jacobson, L., Dikkes, P., and Majzoub, J.A. (1995). Corticotropin-releasing hormone deficiency reveals major fetal but not adult glucocorticoid need. *Nature 373*, 427–432.

Munzberg, H., and Myers, M.G., Jr. (2005). Molecular and anatomical determinants of central leptin resistance. *Nat Neurosci 8*, 566–570.

Myers, M.G., Cowley, M.A., and Munzberg, H. (2008). Mechanisms of leptin action and leptin resistance. *Annu Rev Physiol 70*, 537–556.

Nakajima, K., Cui, Z., Li, C., Meister, J., Cui, Y., Fu, O., Smith, A.S., Jain, S., Lowell, B.B., Krashes, M.J., et al. (2016). Gs-coupled GPCR signalling in AgRP neurons triggers sustained increase in food intake. *Nat Commun 7*, 10268.

Nieh, E.H., Vander Weele, C.M., Matthews, G.A., Presbrey, K.N., Wichmann, R., Leppla, C.A., Izadmehr, E.M., and Tye, K.M. (2016). Inhibitory Input from the Lateral Hypothalamus to the Ventral Tegmental Area Disinhibits Dopamine Neurons and Promotes Behavioral Activation. *Neuron 90*, 1286–1298.

Nijenhuis, W.A., Oosterom, J., and Adan, R.A. (2001). AgRP(83-132) acts as an inverse agonist on the human-melanocortin-4 receptor. *Mol Endocrinol 15*, 164–171.

Nishimori, K., Young, L.J., Guo, Q., Wang, Z., Insel, T.R., and Matzuk, M.M. (1996). Oxytocin is required for nursing but is not essential for parturition or reproductive behavior. *Proc Natl Acad Sci U S A 93*, 11699–11704.

Nusbaum, M.P., Blitz, D.M., and Marder, E. (2017). Functional consequences of neuropeptide and small-molecule co-transmission. *Nat Rev Neurosci 18*, 389–403.

Ollmann, M.M., Wilson, B.D., Yang, Y.K., Kerns, J.A., Chen, Y., Gantz, I., and Barsh, G.S. (1997). Antagonism of central melanocortin receptors in vitro and in vivo by agouti-related protein. *Science 278*, 135–138.

Omelchenko, N., and Sesack, S.R. (2009). Ultrastructural analysis of local collaterals of rat ventral tegmental area neurons: GABA phenotype and synapses onto dopamine and GABA cells. *Synapse 63*, 895–906.

Opland, D., Sutton, A., Woodworth, H., Brown, J., Bugescu, R., Garcia, A., Christensen, L., Rhodes, C., Myers, M., Jr., and Leinninger, G. (2013). Loss of neurotensin receptor-1 disrupts the control of the mesolimbic dopamine system by leptin and promotes hedonic feeding and obesity. *Mol Metab 2*, 423–434.

Papathanou, M., Creed, M., Dorst, M.C., Bimpisidis, Z., Dumas, S., Pettersson, H., Bellone, C., Silberberg, G., Luscher, C., and Wallen-Mackenzie, A. (2018). Targeting VGLUT2 in mature dopamine neurons decreases mesoaccumbal glutamatergic transmission and identifies a role for glutamate co-release in synaptic plasticity by increasing baseline AMPA/NMDA ratio. *Front Neural Circuits 12*, 64.

Patterson, C.M., Wong, J.M., Leinninger, G.M., Allison, M.B., Mabrouk, O.S., Kasper, C.L., Gonzalez, I.E., Mackenzie, A., Jones, J.C., Kennedy, R.T., et al. (2015). Ventral tegmental area neurotensin signaling links the lateral hypothalamus to locomotor activity and striatal dopamine efflux in male mice. *Endocrinology 156*, 1692–1700.

Peyron, C., Tighe, D.K., van den Pol, A.N., de Lecea, L., Heller, H.C., Sutcliffe, J.G., and Kilduff, T.S. (1998). Neurons containing hypocretin (orexin) project to multiple neuronal systems. *J Neurosci 18*, 9996–10015.

Qi, J., Zhang, S., Wang, H.L., Barker, D.J., Miranda-Barrientos, J., and Morales, M. (2016). VTA glutamatergic inputs to nucleus accumbens drive aversion by acting on GABAergic interneurons. *Nat Neurosci 19*, 725–733.

Qu, D., Ludwig, D.S., Gammeltoft, S., Piper, M., Pelleymounter, M.A., Cullen, M.J., Mathes, W.F., Przypek, R., Kanarek, R., and Maratos-Flier, E. (1996). A role for melanin-concentrating hormone in the central regulation of feeding behaviour. *Nature 380*, 243–247.

Rahmouni, K. (2016). Cardiovascular regulation by the arcuate nucleus of the hypothalamus: neurocircuitry and signaling systems. *Hypertension 67*, 1064–1071.

Rinaman, L. (2010). Ascending projections from the caudal visceral nucleus of the solitary tract to brain regions involved in food intake and energy expenditure. *Brain Res 1350*, 18–34.

Romanov, R.A., Zeisel, A., Bakker, J., Girach, F., Hellysaz, A., Tomer, R., Alpar, A., Mulder, J., Clotman, F., Keimpema, E., et al. (2017). Molecular interrogation of hypothalamic organization reveals distinct dopamine neuronal subtypes. *Nat Neurosci 20*, 176–188.

Rosin, D.L., Weston, M.C., Sevigny, C.P., Stornetta, R.L., and Guyenet, P.G. (2003). Hypothalamic orexin (hypocretin) neurons express vesicular glutamate transporters VGLUT1 or VGLUT2. *J Comp Neurol 465*, 593–603.

Rossi, M., Choi, S.J., O'Shea, D., Miyoshi, T., Ghatei, M.A., and Bloom, S.R. (1997). Melanin-concentrating hormone acutely stimulates feeding, but chronic administration has no effect on body weight. *Endocrinology 138*, 351–355.

Rossi, M., Kim, M.S., Morgan, D.G., Small, C.J., Edwards, C.M., Sunter, D., Abusnana, S., Goldstone, A.P., Russell, S.H., Stanley, S.A., et al. (1998). A C-terminal fragment of Agouti-related protein increases feeding and antagonizes the effect of alpha-melanocyte stimulating hormone in vivo. *Endocrinology 139*, 4428–4431.

Rossi, M.A., and Stuber, G.D. (2018). Overlapping brain circuits for homeostatic and hedonic feeding. *Cell Metab 27*, 42–56.

Saha, S., Batten, T.F., and McWilliam, P.N. (1995). Glutamate-immunoreactivity in identified vagal afferent terminals of the cat: a study combining horseradish peroxidase tracing and postembedding electron microscopic immunogold staining. *Exp Physiol 80*, 193–202.

Sakurai, T. (2007). The neural circuit of orexin (hypocretin): maintaining sleep and wakefulness. *Nat Rev Neurosci 8*, 171–181.

Sakurai, T., Amemiya, A., Ishii, M., Matsuzaki, I., Chemelli, R.M., Tanaka, H., Williams, S.C., Richarson, J.A., Kozlowski, G.P., Wilson, S., et al. (1998). Orexins and orexin receptors: a family of hypothalamic neuropeptides and G protein-coupled receptors that regulate feeding behavior. *Cell 92*, 1 page following 696.

Sakurai, T., Nagata, R., Yamanaka, A., Kawamura, H., Tsujino, N., Muraki, Y., Kageyama, H., Kunita, S., Takahashi, S., Goto, K., et al. (2005). Input of orexin/hypocretin neurons revealed by a genetically encoded tracer in mice. *Neuron 46*, 297–308.

Sandoval, D.A., Bagnol, D., Woods, S.C., D'Alessio, D.A., and Seeley, R.J. (2008). Arcuate glucagon-like peptide 1 receptors regulate glucose homeostasis but not food intake. *Diabetes 57*, 2046–2054.

Saper, C.B., Chou, T.C., and Elmquist, J.K. (2002). The need to feed: homeostatic and hedonic control of eating. *Neuron 36*, 199–211.

Schaffar, N., Rao, H., Kessler, J.P., and Jean, A. (1997). Immunohistochemical detection of glutamate in rat vagal sensory neurons. *Brain Res 778*, 302–308.

Schneeberger, M., Tan, K., Nectow, A.R., Parolari, L., Caglar, C., Azevedo, E., Li, Z., Domingos, A., and Friedman, J.M. (2018). Functional analysis reveals differential effects of glutamate and MCH neuropeptide in MCH neurons. *Mol Metab 13*, 83–89.

Schone, C., Apergis-Schoute, J., Sakurai, T., Adamantidis, A., and Burdakov, D. (2014). Coreleased orexin and glutamate evoke nonredundant spike outputs and computations in histamine neurons. *Cell Rep 7*, 697–704.

Schone, C., Cao, Z.F., Apergis-Schoute, J., Adamantidis, A., Sakurai, T., and Burdakov, D. (2012). Optogenetic probing of fast glutamatergic transmission from hypocretin/orexin to histamine neurons in situ. *J Neurosci 32*, 12437–12443.

Schroeder, L.E., and Leinninger, G.M. (2018). Role of central neurotensin in regulating feeding: Implications for the development and treatment of body weight disorders. *Biochim Biophys Acta Mol basis Dis 1864*, 900–916.

Schwartz, M.W., Woods, S.C., Porte, D., Jr., Seeley, R.J., and Baskin, D.G. (2000). Central nervous system control of food intake. *Nature 404*, 661–671.

Shah, B.P., Vong, L., Olson, D.P., Koda, S., Krashes, M.J., Ye, C., Yang, Z., Fuller, P.M., Elmquist, J.K., and Lowell, B.B. (2014). MC4R-expressing glutamatergic neurons in the paraventricular hypothalamus regulate feeding and are synaptically connected to the parabrachial nucleus. *Proc Natl Acad Sci U S A 111*, 13193–13198.

Shearman, L.P., Camacho, R.E., Sloan Stribling, D., Zhou, D., Bednarek, M.A., Hreniuk, D.L., Feighner, S.D., Tan, C.P., Howard, A.D., Van der Ploeg, L.H., et al. (2003). Chronic MCH-1 receptor modulation alters appetite, body weight and adiposity in rats. *Eur J Pharmacol 475*, 37–47.

Shimada, M., Tritos, N.A., Lowell, B.B., Flier, J.S., and Maratos-Flier, E. (1998). Mice lacking melanin-concentrating hormone are hypophagic and lean. *Nature 396*, 670–674.

Shutter, J.R., Graham, M., Kinsey, A.C., Scully, S., Luthy, R., and Stark, K.L. (1997). Hypothalamic expression of ART, a novel gene related to agouti, is up-regulated in obese and diabetic mutant mice. *Genes Develop 11*, 593–602.

Sigvardt, K.A., Rothman, B.S., Brown, R.O., and Mayeri, E. (1986). The bag cells of Aplysia as a multitransmitter system: identification of alpha bag cell peptide as a second neurotransmitter. *J Neurosci 6*, 803–813.

Silva, R.M., Hadjimarkou, M.M., Rossi, G.C., Pasternak, G.W., and Bodnar, R.J. (2001). Beta-endorphin-induced feeding: pharmacological characterization using selective opioid antagonists and antisense probes in rats. *J Pharmacol Exp Ther 297*, 590–596.

Small, C.J., Kim, M.S., Stanley, S.A., Mitchell, J.R., Murphy, K., Morgan, D.G., Ghatei, M.A., and Bloom, S.R. (2001). Effects of chronic central nervous system administration of agouti-related protein in pair-fed animals. *Diabetes 50*, 248–254.

Stamatakis, A.M., Van Swieten, M., Basiri, M.L., Blair, G.A., Kantak, P., and Stuber, G.D. (2016). Lateral Hypothalamic Area Glutamatergic Neurons and Their Projections to the Lateral Habenula Regulate Feeding and Reward. *J Neurosci 36*, 302–311.

Steinkellner, T., Zell, V., Farino, Z.J., Sonders, M.S., Villeneuve, M., Freyberg, R.J., Przedborski, S., Lu, W., Freyberg, Z., and Hnasko, T.S. (2018). Role for VGLUT2 in selective vulnerability of midbrain dopamine neurons. *J Clin Invest 128*, 774–788.

Stuber, G.D., Hnasko, T.S., Britt, J.P., Edwards, R.H., and Bonci, A. (2010). Dopaminergic terminals in the nucleus accumbens but not the dorsal striatum corelease glutamate. *J Neurosci 30*, 8229–8233.

Takamori, S., Rhee, J.S., Rosenmund, C., and Jahn, R. (2001). Identification of differentiation-associated brain-specific phosphate transporter as a second vesicular glutamate transporter (VGLUT2). *J Neurosci 21*, RC182.

Tatemoto, K., Carlquist, M., and Mutt, V. (1982). Neuropeptide Y--a novel brain peptide with structural similarities to peptide YY and pancreatic polypeptide. *Nature 296*, 659–660.

Tauchi, M., Zhang, R., D'Alessio, D.A., Stern, J.E., and Herman, J.P. (2008). Distribution of glucagon-like peptide-1 immunoreactivity in the hypothalamic paraventricular and supraoptic nuclei. *J Chem Neuroanat 36*, 144–149.

Tecuapetla, F., Patel, J.C., Xenias, H., English, D., Tadros, I., Shah, F., Berlin, J., Deisseroth, K., Rice, M.E., Tepper, J.M., et al. (2010). Glutamatergic signaling by mesolimbic dopamine neurons in the nucleus accumbens. *J Neurosci 30*, 7105–7110.

Teitelbaum, P., and Epstein, A.N. (1962). The lateral hypothalamic syndrome: recovery of feeding and drinking after lateral hypothalamic lesions. *Psychol Rev 69*, 74–90.

Terrill, S.J., Jackson, C.M., Greene, H.E., Lilly, N., Maske, C.B., Vallejo, S., and Williams, D.L. (2016). Role of lateral septum glucagon-like peptide 1 receptors in food intake. *Am J Physiol Regul Integr Comp Physiol 311*, R124–R132.

Thody, A.J. (1999). alpha-MSH and the regulation of melanocyte function. *Ann N Y Acad Sci 885*, 217–229.

Tolle, V., and Low, M.J. (2008). In vivo evidence for inverse agonism of Agouti-related peptide in the central nervous system of proopiomelanocortin-deficient mice. *Diabetes 57*, 86–94.

Tolson, K.P., Gemelli, T., Gautron, L., Elmquist, J.K., Zinn, A.R., and Kublaoui, B.M. (2010). Postnatal Sim1 deficiency causes hyperphagic obesity and reduced Mc4r and oxytocin expression. *J Neurosci 30*, 3803–3812.

Tong, Q., Ye, C.P., Jones, J.E., Elmquist, J.K., and Lowell, B.B. (2008). Synaptic release of GABA by AgRP neurons is required for normal regulation of energy balance. *Nat Neurosci 11*, 998–1000.

Torrealba, F., Yanagisawa, M., and Saper, C.B. (2003). Colocalization of orexin a and glutamate immunoreactivity in axon terminals in the tuberomammillary nucleus in rats. *Neuroscience 119*, 1033–1044.

Tritsch, N.X., Granger, A.J., and Sabatini, B.L. (2016). Mechanisms and functions of GABA co-release. *Nat Rev Neurosci 17*, 139–145.

Tritsch, N.X., Oh, W.J., Gu, C., and Sabatini, B.L. (2014). Midbrain dopamine neurons sustain inhibitory transmission using plasma membrane uptake of GABA, not synthesis. *Elife 3*, e01936.

Trudeau, L.E., and El Mestikawy, S. (2018). Glutamate cotransmission in cholinergic, GABAergic and monoamine systems: contrasts and commonalities. *Front Neural Circuits 12*, 113.

Tsien, J.Z., Huerta, P.T., and Tonegawa, S. (1996). The essential role of hippocampal CA1 NMDA receptor-dependent synaptic plasticity in spatial memory. *Cell 87*, 1327–1338.

Turton, M.D., O'Shea, D., Gunn, I., Beak, S.A., Edwards, C.M., Meeran, K., Choi, S.J., Taylor, G.M., Heath, M.M., Lambert, P.D., et al. (1996). A role for glucagon-like peptide-1 in the central regulation of feeding. *Nature 379*, 69–72.

Vaaga, C.E., Borisovska, M., and Westbrook, G.L. (2014). Dual-transmitter neurons: functional implications of co-release and co-transmission. *Curr Opin Neurobiol 29*, 25–32.

van den Pol, A.N. (2003). Weighing the role of hypothalamic feeding neurotransmitters. *Neuron 40*, 1059–1061.

van den Pol, A.N. (2012). Neuropeptide transmission in brain circuits. *Neuron 76*, 98–115.

Vong, L., Ye, C., Yang, Z., Choi, B., Chua, S., Jr., and Lowell, B.B. (2011). Leptin action on GABAergic neurons prevents obesity and reduces inhibitory tone to POMC neurons. *Neuron 71*, 142–154.

Vrang, N., Hansen, M., Larsen, P.J., and Tang-Christensen, M. (2007). Characterization of brainstem preproglucagon projections to the paraventricular and dorsomedial hypothalamic nuclei. *Brain Res 1149*, 118–126.

Wahlestedt, C., Ekman, R., and Widerlov, E. (1989). Neuropeptide Y (NPY) and the central nervous system: distribution effects and possible relationship to neurological and psychiatric disorders. *Prog Neuro-Psychopharmacol Biol Psychiatry 13*, 31–54.

Wang, D.V., Viereckel, T., Zell, V., Konradsson-Geuken, A., Broker, C.J., Talishinsky, A., Yoo, J.H., Galinato, M.H., Arvidsson, E., Kesner, A.J., et al. (2017). Disrupting glutamate co-transmission does not affect acquisition of conditioned behavior reinforced by dopamine neuron activation. *Cell Rep 18*, 2584–2591.

Wang, H., Jing, M., and Li, Y. (2018). Lighting up the brain: genetically encoded fluorescent sensors for imaging neurotransmitters and neuromodulators. *Curr Opin Neurobiol 50*, 171–178.

Ward, Z.J., Bleich, S.N., Cradock, A.L., Barrett, J.L., Giles, C.M., Flax, C., Long, M.W., and Gortmaker, S.L. (2019). Projected U.S. State-Level prevalence of adult obesity and severe obesity. *N Engl J Med 381*, 2440–2450.

Watabe-Uchida, M., Eshel, N., and Uchida, N. (2017). Neural circuitry of reward prediction error. *Annu Rev Neurosci 40*, 373–394.

Whim, M.D. (2006). Near simultaneous release of classical and peptide cotransmitters from chromaffin cells. *J Neurosci 26*, 6637–6642.

Whim, M.D. (2011). Pancreatic beta cells synthesize neuropeptide Y and can rapidly release peptide co-transmitters. *PLoS One 6*, e19478.

Woodworth, H.L., Beekly, B.G., Batchelor, H.M., Bugescu, R., Perez-Bonilla, P., Schroeder, L.E., and Leinninger, G.M. (2017). Lateral hypothalamic neurotensin neurons orchestrate dual weight loss behaviors via distinct mechanisms. *Cell Rep 21*, 3116–3128.

Wu, Q., Boyle, M.P., and Palmiter, R.D. (2009). Loss of GABAergic signaling by AgRP neurons to the parabrachial nucleus leads to starvation. *Cell 137*, 1225–1234.

Wu, Z., Xu, Y., Zhu, Y., Sutton, A.K., Zhao, R., Lowell, B.B., Olson, D.P., and Tong, Q. (2012). An obligate role of oxytocin neurons in diet induced energy expenditure. *PLoS One 7*, e45167.

Xi, D., Gandhi, N., Lai, M., and Kublaoui, B.M. (2012). Ablation of Sim1 neurons causes obesity through hyperphagia and reduced energy expenditure. *PLoS One 7*, e36453.

Xu, A.W., Kaelin, C.B., Morton, G.J., Ogimoto, K., Stanhope, K., Graham, J., Baskin, D.G., Havel, P., Schwartz, M.W., and Barsh, G.S. (2005). Effects of hypothalamic neurodegeneration on energy balance. *PLoS Biol 3*, e415.

Xu, Y., Lu, Y., Cassidy, R.M., Mangieri, L.R., Zhu, C., Huang, X., Jiang, Z., Justice, N.J., Xu, Y., Arenkiel, B.R., et al. (2019). Identification of a neurocircuit underlying regulation of feeding by stress-related emotional responses. *Nat Commun 10*, 3446.

Xu, Y., Wu, Z., Sun, H., Zhu, Y., Kim, E.R., Lowell, B.B., Arenkiel, B.R., Xu, Y., and Tong, Q. (2013). Glutamate mediates the function of melanocortin receptor 4 on Sim1 neurons in body weight regulation. *Cell Metab 18*, 860–870.

Yamada, M., Saga, Y., Shibusawa, N., Hirato, J., Murakami, M., Iwasaki, T., Hashimoto, K., Satoh, T., Wakabayashi, K., Taketo, M.M., et al. (1997). Tertiary hypothyroidism and hyperglycemia in mice with targeted disruption of the thyrotropin-releasing hormone gene. *Proceedings of the National Academy of Sciences of the United States of America 94*, 10862–10867.

Yaswen, L., Diehl, N., Brennan, M.B., and Hochgeschwender, U. (1999). Obesity in the mouse model of pro-opiomelanocortin deficiency responds to peripheral melanocortin. *Nat Med 5*, 1066–1070.

Yoshida, K., McCormack, S., Espana, R.A., Crocker, A., and Scammell, T.E. (2006). Afferents to the orexin neurons of the rat brain. *J Comp Neurol 494*, 845–861.

Zell, V., Steinkellner, T., Hollon, N.G., Warlow, S.M., Souter, E., Faget, L., Hunker, A.C., Jin, X., Zweifel, L.S., and Hnasko, T.S. (2020). VTA glutamate neuron activity drives positive reinforcement absent dopamine co-release. *Neuron*

Zemkova, H., and Stojilkovic, S.S. (2018). Neurotransmitter receptors as signaling platforms in anterior pituitary cells. *Mol Cell Endocrinol 463*, 49–64.

Zhan, C., Zhou, J., Feng, Q., Zhang, J.E., Lin, S., Bao, J., Wu, P., and Luo, M. (2013). Acute and long-term suppression of feeding behavior by POMC neurons in the brainstem and hypothalamus, respectively. *J Neurosci 33*, 3624–3632.

Zhang, L., Hernandez-Sanchez, D., and Herzog, H. (2019). Regulation of feeding-related behaviors by arcuate neuropeptide Y neurons. *Endocrinology 160*, 1411–1420.

Zhang, S., Qi, J., Li, X., Wang, H.L., Britt, J.P., Hoffman, A.F., Bonci, A., Lupica, C.R., and Morales, M. (2015). Dopaminergic and glutamatergic microdomains in a subset of rodent mesoaccumbens axons. *Nat Neurosci 18*, 386–392.

Zheng, H., Cai, L., and Rinaman, L. (2015). Distribution of glucagon-like peptide 1-immunopositive neurons in human caudal medulla. *Brain Struct Funct 220*, 1213–1219.

Zhu, C., Jiang, Z., Xu, Y., Cai, Z.L., Jiang, Q., Xu, Y., Xue, M., Arenkiel, B.R., Wu, Q., Shu, G., et al. (2020). Profound and redundant functions of arcuate neurons in obesity development. *Nat Metab*

4 Brain Glucagon-Like Peptide 1 Receptor Influence on Feeding Behavior

Diana L. Williams, Lisa R. Anderson, Isabel I. Coiduras and Calyn B. Maske
Florida State University, USA

CONTENTS

4.1 INTRODUCTION

Glucagon-like peptide 1 (GLP-1) is best known as an incretin hormone released by L-cells in the small intestine, but a large body of literature beginning in the 1990s demonstrates that brain-derived GLP-1 and activation of its receptor (GLP-1R) potently suppresses feeding and influences other behaviors that impact energy balance. This chapter focuses on the role of brain GLP-1Rs in these functions, with an emphasis on the methods that help disentangle the behavioral mechanisms for changes in food intake.

The GLP-1R is a G-protein coupled receptor (GPCR) that was originally identified in pancreatic β-cells, and it is expressed in a variety of tissues. Brain expression of the GLP-1R was first confirmed in rodents (Campos et al. 1994) and later shown in other species including humans (Farr et al. 2016). The GLP-1R is expressed widely in nuclei traditionally associated with autonomic function, energy balance and feeding, endocrine control, stress responses, and reward and motivation (Merchenthaler et al. 1999; Cork et al. 2015) and thus it is no surprise that GLP-1R agonists have a broad range of physiologic and behavioral effects.

4.2 AGONISTS FOR THE BRAIN GLP-1R

GLP-1, the primary endogenous ligand for the GLP-1R in mammals, is a cleavage product of the preproglucagon (PPG) precursor peptide. PPG is expressed in pancreatic α-cells, where it is post-translationally processed to glucagon and a major proglucagon fragment, but in the intestine and brain, PPG is instead processed to glicentin or oxyntomodulin (OXM), GLP-1, and GLP-2 (Müller et al. 2019). Both gut and brain-derived GLP-1 have roles in energy balance, but the main endogenous source of ligand for brain GLP-1Rs is PPG neurons, located in the caudal brainstem nucleus of the solitary tract (NTS) and the medullary reticular formation (MRF). PPG neurons project widely throughout the brain to most areas where GLP-1Rs are expressed.

GLP-1 released from the intestine can cross the blood–brain barrier (Kastin et al. 2002), but it is unlikely to be a significant source to the brain under normal circumstances. The half-life of the biologically active form, GLP-$1^{7-36NH2}$, is extremely short (< 1 min) due to rapid degradation by dipeptidyl peptidase IV (DPP-IV) (Holst and Deacon 2005). Blockade of brain GLP-1Rs by intracerebroventricular (icv) injection of the antagonist, exendin (9-39) (Ex9-39), attenuates the ability of icv-injected GLP-1 to suppress feeding but not intraperitoneal (IP) GLP-1 in the rat, suggesting that even if some amount of GLP-1 from the periphery makes it into the brain, it does not stimulate GLP-1Rs sufficiently to contribute to the ingestive behavioral effect (Williams et al. 2009). This may be true in humans, as well, because intravenous (IV) infusion of GLP-1 significantly suppressed intake of an *ad libitum* test meal in control individuals, but had no effect in people who had previously undergone truncal vagotomy (Plamboeck et al. 2013).

Though GLP-1, itself, is the most prominent endogenous ligand, oxyntomodulin (OXM) also binds to and activates the GLP-1R. Exogenous administration of OXM suppresses food intake, so this agonist could play a role in the feeding effects of GLP-1Rs. However, OXM binds to the GLP-1R with much weaker affinity and lower efficacy than GLP-1 (reviewed in Pocai 2012). Biologically active OXM is rapidly degraded, so intestinally released OXM is less likely to be a major source of ligand to brain GLP-1Rs than that released by PPG neurons.

Given the evidence for the relevance of PPG neurons as the ligand source, it is important to understand what drives the activity of these cells. PPG neurons receive excitatory vagal afferent input (Hisadome et al. 2010) and are also activated by the gastrointestinal (GI) hormone cholecystokinin (CCK) (Hisadome et al. 2011; Rinaman 1999a). Consumption of large mixed macronutrient meals or gastric distension by balloon induces c-Fos in PPG neurons (Kreisler and Rinaman 2016; Holt et al. 2019; Vrang et al. 2003). The adiposity hormone, leptin, depolarizes PPG neurons in the mouse (Hisadome et al. 2010), as well. While these neurons respond to signals relevant to feeding under healthy normal circumstances, they are also activated by noxious stimuli, including LiCl and bacterial lipopolysaccharide (LPS) (Rinaman 1999a), as well as restraint stress (Terrill et al. 2018).

Degradation-resistant GLP-1R agonists have been extremely valuable for research, and several are in clinical use for treatment of type II diabetes and obesity (Aroda 2018). Exendin-4 (Ex4) and liraglutide have been the most commonly used long-lasting agonists in research. Their hours-long half-lives likely explain some of their longer-lasting feeding-suppressive effects (Knudsen and Lau 2019; Parkes et al. 2013). These agonists cross the blood–brain barrier and exert some of their effects on feeding behavior by binding to brain GLP-1Rs, because the longer-lasting intake-suppressive effects of systemic administration can be blocked by 3rd-icv Ex9-39 pretreatment (Kanoski et al. 2011) or neuron-specific GLP-1R knockout (Sisley et al. 2014). Fluorescently labeled versions of these ligands have allowed direct investigation of whether they bind to brain GLP-1Rs after systemic treatment. In the mouse, systemically injected labeled liraglutide and semaglutide, a longer-lasting GLP-1R agonist, have been observed in the circumventricular organs and hypothalamic nuclei, most prominently the arcuate nucleus (ARC) (Gabery et al. 2020; Secher et al. 2014).

4.3 BRAIN GLP-1R EFFECTS ON FOOD INTAKE

Initial reports of central GLP-1 effects on food intake (Turton et al. 1996; Tang-Christensen et al. 1996) launched tremendous interest in the role of brain GLP-1Rs in feeding and energy balance. These influential papers took a straightforward behavioral pharmacology approach; the researchers performed dose responses for GLP-1 injected into the lateral ventricle (Tang-Christensen et al. 1996) or third cerebral ventricle (Turton et al. 1996) of rats, and measured food intake by weighing chow before and at various timepoints after the injection. These experiments demonstrated that pharmacologic administration of GLP-1 to the brain could suppress food intake at far lower doses than would be required for effects when delivered peripherally. However, many questions cannot be answered with these approaches, including whether endogenous GLP-1R activity plays a role in the control of food intake, and what specific brain regions and populations of GLP-1Rs serve this function. Furthermore, measurement of the amount consumed over some period of time provides little information about the behavioral mechanisms through which food intake is suppressed. Do subjects eat less after stimulation of brain GLP-1Rs because they are less hungry, the food tastes less appealing, they feel more satiated by food, they are less motivated to obtain food, they feel nauseous, or some combination of these or other factors? These questions have been addressed with more detailed behavioral analysis.

4.3.1 Does Endogenous Stimulation of Brain GLP-1Rs Play a Role in Feeding Control?

Pharmacologic stimulation of a receptor reveals what can happen when that receptor is activated supra-physiologically, but if we want to understand that receptor's role under normal physiologic conditions, loss-of-function approaches are required. Turton et al. (1996) showed that in the rat, acute 3rd-icv injection of Ex9-39 increased light-phase food intake, suggesting that endogenous activity at brain GLP-1Rs restrains eating at that time. Chronic lateral-icv infusion of Ex9-39 or knockdown of PPG in the NTS by virally delivered short hairpin RNA (shRNA) increased food intake and body weight over a period of several weeks in rats that were maintained on either standard chow or a high-fat diet (HFD) (Barrera et al. 2011). The literature now includes many studies showing that specific brain populations of GLP-1Rs play a physiologic role in the control of feeding.

Several studies using mouse models have reported results that are not entirely consistent with the results in rats. Foremost is the global GLP-1R knockout mouse, which expresses no GLP-1Rs anywhere. These mice have no feeding phenotype, although they do not respond to exogenous GLP-1R agonists (Baggio et al. 2004). More selective receptor knockout models show a similar lack of perturbation of feeding behavior; however, loss of GLP-1Rs in glutamate neurons blocks the hypophagic effect of liraglutide treatment (Adams et al. 2018). Species differences may account for the divergent results, but developmental compensation is another possible explanation, because antagonist injections and shRNA delivery were done in adult subjects. Holt et al. (2019) removed the influence of the endogenous agonist in the brains of adult mice that had developed typically by performing selective lesion or silencing of PPG neurons. Taking advantage of a mouse expressing Cre recombinase in PPG neurons, they selectively expressed diphtheria toxin subunit A by viral injection into the NTS, ablating the NTS PPG neuron population. Using the same mouse model, they also induced expression of an inhibitory designer receptor exclusively activated by designer drugs (DREADD) in the NTS PPG neurons. This allowed acute silencing of PPG neurons by injection of the DREADD ligand, clozapine-N-oxide (CNO). These manipulations had no impact on spontaneous food intake and body weight; however, more substantial homeostatic challenges revealed that silencing or loss of PPG neurons did have an impact. The hyperphagia normally observed during the initial refeeding period after an overnight fast was exacerbated by ablation or silencing of PPG neurons, and PPG neuron ablation impaired the normal satiety response to an unusually large nutrient load. Experiments targeting specific brain sites in mice have shown effects of GLP-1R antagonism on feeding (Williams et al. 2018), so subpopulations of brain GLP-1Rs may play a physiologic role in normal feeding in the mouse.

4.3.2 How Do Brain GLP-1Rs Affect Feeding?

Current data suggest that feeding behavior is suppressed by exogenous or endogenous GLP-1R activation in the caudal NTS (Alhadeff et al. 2017: Hayes et al. 2009; Richard et al. 2015;), lateral parabrachial nucleus (lPBN) (Alhadeff et al. 2014; Richard et al.

2014), dorsal raphe (DR) (Anderberg et al. 2017), lateral dorsal tegmental area (LDTg) (Reiner et al. 2018), ventral tegmental area (VTA) (Alhadeff et al. 2012; Dickson et al. 2012), paraventricular nucleus of the hypothalamus (PVN) (Liu et al. 2017; McMahon and Wellman 1998), lateral hypothalamus (LH) (López-Ferreras et al. 2018), supramammillary nucleus (SuM) (López-Ferreras et al. 2019), paraventricular nucleus of the thalamus (PVT) (Ong et al. 2017), lateral septum (LS) (Terrill et al. 2016; Terrill et al. 2019), bed nucleus of the stria terminalis (BNST) (Williams et al. 2018), ventral hippocampus (vHP) (Hsu et al. 2015), and the nucleus accumbens (NAc) (Alhadeff et al. 2012; Dickson et al. 2012; Dossat et al. 2011). Here, we review examples of brain site-specific studies that prompted new ways of thinking about this system, and highlight important methodological and interpretive issues.

4.3.3 Satiation and Satiety

Based on evidence discussed above that PPG neurons are activated by GI meal-related stimuli, it has been proposed that neural GLP-1 acting at brain GLP-1Rs plays a mediatory role in satiation and/or satiety. These terms are often used interchangeably, but they refer to distinct processes: satiation is the within-meal process leading to meal termination, while satiety occurs during the post-meal period, inhibiting the initiation of the next meal. Suppression of total food intake over a given number of hours could be explained by increased satiation, increased satiety, both, or neither, and examination of the pattern of feeding can provide clues. Effects on meal size suggest an effect on satiation, whereas an effect on meal frequency could implicate satiety. More directly, one can ask whether GLP-1R activity is necessary for the satiating effects of gastric distension or GI nutrient load.

GLP-1Rs are expressed at high density in the NTS, and 4th-icv application of GLP-1 agonists effectively suppress feeding (Hayes et al. 2008). Alhadeff et al. (2017) used virally delivered shRNA to reduce GLP-1R expression in the NTS of rats, and conducted behavioral assessments including meal pattern analysis. They showed that relative to controls, NTS GLP-1R knock-down rats had elevated intake that was entirely accounted for by increased meal size, not meal number, suggesting that NTS GLP-1Rs normally function to promote satiation. Taking a different approach, Hayes et al. (2009) used 4th-icv delivery of Ex9-39, which, due to the rostro-caudal flow of cerebrospinal fluid (CSF), delivers the drug to caudal brainstem structures only, before either intra-duodenal nutrient infusion or gastric balloon distention, and this blockade of hindbrain GLP-1Rs attenuated intake suppression by distention while having no impact on intake suppression by the nutrient load. Thus, NTS GLP-1Rs mediate the effects of some but not all GI negative feedback signals. Several mechanisms for these caudal hindbrain GLP-1R effects on feeding have been identified, implicating PKA, MAPK, and PI3K signaling pathways (Hayes et al. 2011; Rupprecht et al. 2013). NTS GABA neurons appear to play a key role (Fortin et al. 2020), and GLP-1R signaling in NTS astrocytes makes a contribution (Reiner et al. 2016).

Some of the other locations where GLP-1Rs have been associated with satiation and satiety are particularly interesting because they had not previously been considered to play this role. The VTA and NAc are best known for their roles in reward and motivation as part of the mesolimbic dopamine pathway. Both receive projections from PPG neurons (Rinaman 2010) and both have a moderate level of GLP-1R expression (Merchenthaler et al. 1999). Intra-VTA administration of the GLP-1R agonist Ex4 suppresses meal size in rats consuming palatable high-fat food, with only a small effect to reduce the number of meals taken between 12 and 24 h after injection (Mietlicki-Baase et al. 2013). Our laboratory found that blockade of GLP-1Rs in the NAc core subregion increased meal size when rats consumed palatable solutions, without increasing meal frequency, and that intra-NAc Ex9-39 attenuated the satiating effect of intragastric nutrient infusion (Dossat et al. 2013). Mietlicki-Baase et al. (2013, 2014) reported evidence that these effects in the VTA and NAc core are mediated by GLP-1Rs acting presynaptically via the α-amino-3-hydroxy-5-methyl-4-isoxazolepropionic acid (AMPA)/kainate receptors to increase glutamatergic transmission. The LS, laterodorsal tegmental nucleus (LDTg), and PVT, all brain areas more associated with reward than feeding, are all locations at which GLP-1R antagonist treatment, blocking endogenous stimulation, increases meal size selectively (Ong et al. 2017; Reiner et al. 2018; Terrill et al., 2016; Terrill et al., 2019), and in the vHP, GLP-1R stimulation selectively decreases meal size (Hsu et al. 2015). Moreover, Ex9-39 injected into the LS or LDTg can block nutrient preload-induced satiety (Reiner et al. 2018; Terrill et al., 2016; Terrill et al., 2019).

4.3.4 Food Reward and Motivation

With GLP-1R expression identified in the nuclei of the mesolimbic reward pathway, an obvious question was whether GLP-1R stimulation affects food reward. The term "food reward" is often used broadly to include palatability and motivation to obtain food, and can include food as a reinforcer or unconditioned stimulus for learned associations and cues. There are a host of behavioral approaches to tease apart these various aspects of reward, and for investigation of brain GLP-1R contributions, most work has focused on the motivation for palatable food, assessed by the operant responding on a progressive ratio (PR) schedule. The PR schedule allows researchers to ask how much effort the subject is willing to put forth to obtain the food reinforcer because the number of responses required to obtain the food increases for each successive reinforcement. Another frequently used approach is conditioned place preference (CPP), where palatable food becomes associated with a specific environment. The rodent undergoes training in which one side of a two-sided chamber is paired with that food, while the other side is not. Time spent in each side of the chamber is assessed in pre- and post-training tests during which the subject has access to both, importantly, with no food present. More time spent in the food-paired side in the post-training test is interpreted as evidence of the rewarding value of the food.

GLP-1R activation at a number of different brain sites has a significant effect on food reward assessed by these approaches. The first evidence of this was from a study by Dickson et al. (2012), which showed first that 3rd-icv GLP-1R stimulation by Ex4 suppressed PR responding for sucrose reinforcers, and then demonstrated that either intra-VTA or NAc injection of Ex4, at lower doses, could suppress PR responding as well. The PVT is yet another brain area where GLP-1R stimulation via Ex4 injection suppresses PR responding for sucrose, and Ong et al. (2017) found that intra-PVT Ex4 also blocked the expression of high-fat diet-induced CPP. It is still unknown whether endogenous GLP-1R stimulation in the VTA, NAc, or PVT suppresses motivation for food, or if these are exclusively pharmacologic effects. Our laboratory took a different approach to look at endogenous GLP-1R activation in the NAc, examining the microstructure of licking for sucrose solutions in rats, and we found that intra-NAc Ex9-39 induced patterns of licking behavior consistent with the idea that GLP-1Rs in this nucleus suppress food palatability (Dossat et al. 2013). We have also investigated LS GLP-1Rs and found that in rats and mice, intra-LS Ex9-39 increases PR responding for sucrose (Terrill et al. 2016; Terrill et al. 2019), supporting a physiologic role for the LS receptors in motivation. The vHP is an interesting example of another brain area at which GLP-1R activation suppressed food-motivated behavior as measured by PR responding for a high-fat, high-sucrose pellet reward, but in this location, GLP-1R agonist injection had no impact on the expression of a palatable food-induced CPP (Hsu et al. 2015). This distinction in the vHP highlights the diversity of function of GLP-1Rs at different sites, and emphasizes the importance of using multiple complementary methods. The vHP is also an unusual site for GLP-1R action in that this area receives no PPG neuron projections, so the means by which an endogenous agonist accesses the vHP is unclear, though a volume transmission mechanism has been proposed (Hsu et al. 2015).

Research on the role of GLP-1Rs in the LH offers a lesson regarding potential sex differences: an effect in males does not necessarily generalize to females. The vast majority of work on brain GLP-1R effects examined male subjects only, but estrogens increase sensitivity to lateral-icv GLP-1 or Ex4 effects on feeding and motivation in females (Maske et al. 2017; Richard et al. 2016). Site-specific LH GLP-1R activation, on the other hand, suppressed PR responding for sucrose in both male and female rats, but only at higher doses in females (López-Ferreras et al. 2018). The difference was more pronounced with blockade or virally delivered shRNA knockdown of LH GLP-1Rs, which potently increased PR responding in males yet had no effect in females (López-Ferreras et al. 2018).

Finally, GLP-1Rs can suppress food reward in brain areas not previously considered to have a role in these functions. NTS activation of GLP-1Rs can suppress PR responding for sucrose pellets as well as expression of a high-fat palatable food-induced CPP (Alhadeff and Grill 2014; Richard et al. 2015). This seems to be a physiologic function of these receptors, because shRNA-mediated knockdown of GLP-1Rs in the NTS increased PR responding for sucrose (Alhadeff et al. 2017). These effects may be mediated through NTS projections to the VTA and subsequent modulation of mesolimbic reward pathway activity (Richard et al. 2015). Similar results have been obtained for the lPBN, another area often considered relevant for homeostatic control of eating but not for food reward (Alhadeff et al. 2014). These effects may be mediated by a GLP-1R-induced increase in calcitonin gene related peptide (CGRP) expression in the PBN (Richard et al. 2014). These data for NTS and lPBN challenge the view that reward and motivation are functions exclusive to the mesolimbic reward pathway and other forebrain areas.

4.3.5 Feeding Effects Mediated by Hypothalamic Structures

This review would be incomplete without discussion of evidence for a role of hypothalamic GLP-1Rs in feeding control, given the dense PPG neuron projections throughout the hypothalamus, GLP-1R expression in these areas, and their longstanding association with energy homeostasis. However, there has been considerably less detailed behavioral analysis for effects of GLP-1R activity in most hypothalamic nuclei than the others discussed above, with the notable exception of the LH. The PVN was one of the first hypothalamic nuclei to be targeted, and indeed, direct injection of GLP-1 into the PVN suppresses food intake in rats (McMahon and Wellman 1998), while PVN injection of Ex9-39 elevates food intake (Katsurada et al. 2014). Evidence for ARC GLP-1R-induced suppression of feeding is mixed. Sandoval and colleagues (2008) showed that intra-ARC injection of GLP-1 impacted glucose homeostasis but not food intake in rats. In another series of experiments, bilateral infusion of Ex9-39 into the ARC failed to affect feeding on its own, but did block the intake-inhibitory effect of peripheral liraglutide injection, whereas PVN-targeted antagonist treatment failed to block liraglutide's effects (Secher et al. 2014). Together, these data suggest that endogenous stimulation of PVN GLP-1Rs plays a role in feeding control, while the ARC GLP-1Rs may be recruited only by exogenous, pharmacologic levels of stimulation.

Results of studies on hypothalamic GLP-1Rs in the mouse have not been entirely consistent. Burmeister and colleagues (2017a) used a transgenic mouse approach to knock out GLP-1R in Nkx2.1-expressing neurons, which are found in a number of hypothalamic nuclei. This resulted in hyperphagia, but that phenotype was not recapitulated by more selective knock-out of GLP-1R in Sim1 neurons (mainly in the PVN) or proopiomelanocortin neurons (POMC, found in the ARC). Species differences between the rat and mouse are possible, but there is potential for developmental compensation in these mouse models. Indeed, loss of GLP-1Rs in the PVN of adult mice yields a different result; Liu et al. (2017) showed that virally mediated knockdown of PVN GLP-1Rs in the adult mouse increased daily food intake.

4.3.6 Nausea, Aversion, and Stress-Induced Hypophagia

For any treatment that suppresses food intake, we must ask whether that intake suppression is due to nausea, malaise, or stress of some kind. GLP-1R agonists cause nausea in humans (Bettge et al. 2017); in rodents, the brain GLP-1 system mediates the aversive effects of noxious stimuli. PPG neurons are activated by IP LiCl and LPS (Lachey et al. 2005; Rinaman 1999a), both interoceptive stressors that suppress food intake. Lateral-icv Ex9-39 pretreatment blocks the intake-suppressive effect of LiCl (Rinaman 1999b), and 4th-icv antagonist pretreatment blocks intake suppression induced by LPS (Grill et al. 2004). The question of whether or not GLP-1R activation in a given brain area suppresses feeding by causing nausea has most often been assessed by conditioned taste aversion (CTA) or pica. CTA is a form of Pavlovian conditioning in which a taste or flavor (often sucrose or saccharin, sometimes fruit-flavored Kool-Aid) is paired with an injection of the nauseating agent, e.g. LiCl. The subject forms an association, and when offered the option to consume fluid of that flavor in the future, the subject declines, typically choosing unflavored water instead. If pairing of a flavor with GLP-1R agonist treatment results in a CTA, that is strong evidence that the drug engages the same brain circuitry as nauseating stimuli like LiCl or LPS. Measuring pica, ingestion of a non-food substance, most often kaolin, is a simpler approach. Rodents will normally consume no kaolin, but a variety of nauseating agents, including LiCl, will induce significant intake. In rats, peripheral liraglutide or Ex4 treatment induces CTA and promotes pica, and these effects can be blocked by 3rd-icv Ex9-39 treatment but not by vagotomy, demonstrating that they are mediated by brain GLP-1Rs (Kanoski et al. 2011). The ability of LiCl to produce pica and CTA, in addition to its suppressive effect on food intake, is blocked by 3rd-icv Ex9-39 treatment in rats, suggesting that endogenous activation of brain GLP-1Rs mediates all of these effects (Seeley et al. 2000). Most of this work has been done in the rat, and there are some species differences, but central GLP-1Rs seem to have a role in nausea in the mouse as well (Lachey et al. 2005).

Does this mean that brain GLP-1R activation suppresses feeding simply by causing nausea? Results of studies targeting specific brain areas suggest that often the feeding and nausea effects can be separated. The list of areas at which GLP-1R activation suppresses feeding yet does not induce pica in rats includes the VTA and NAc (Alhadeff et al. 2012), LDTg (Reiner et al. 2018). lPBN (Alhadeff et al. 2014), PVT (Ong et al. 2017), and the LS (Terrill et al. 2016). PVN GLP-1R activation suppresses feeding without causing a CTA (McMahon and Wellman 1998), as does vHP GLP-1R activation (Hsu et al., 2015). Data for the NTS is inconsistent. Kanoski et al. (2012) reported that medial NTS injection of Ex4 does induce pica and supports the formation of a CTA. However, others reported that Ex4 injected into the NTS can suppress food intake without inducing pica (Alhadeff and Grill 2014; Richard et al. 2015), suggesting that nausea can be uncoupled from feeding control even at this location where GLP-1Rs may be involved in both. A dissociation in the opposite direction is observed at the central nucleus of the amygdala (CeA); intra-CeA GLP-1 injection failed to suppress feeding but did support a CTA, and blockade of GLP-1Rs in the CeA blocked LiCl-induced CTA (Kinzig et al. 2002).

Other forms of stress activate PPG neurons as well, one of the most well-documented being acute restraint stress (Maniscalco et al. 2015; Terrill et al. 2019). This potently suppresses food intake in rodents, and lateral-icv injection of Ex9-39 blocked this effect in rats (Maniscalco et al. 2015). In the mouse, inhibitory DREADD-mediated silencing of PPG neurons attenuated restraint stress-induced anorexia (Holt et al. 2019). Information about the specific brain regions in which GLP-1Rs mediate this effect of stress is limited, but a few locations have been identified. Acute restraint stress-induced hypophagia can be blocked by intra-BNST Ex9-39 pretreatment in the mouse (Williams et al. 2018). In rats, Zheng et al. (2019) used virally delivered shRNA to knock down GLP-1R expression in the anterolateral BNST, and found that this reduced hypophagia induced by more mild stressors, novelty, and elevated open platform exposure. In both rats and mice, intra-LS Ex9-39 injection blunts the hypophagic response to restraint stress (Terrill et al. 2018; Terrill et al. 2019). The contribution of PVN GLP-1Rs has been investigated in mice that lack GLP-1Rs in Sim1 neurons, and although feeding effects were not examined in detail, these mice did not show typical chronic stress-induced body weight loss, suggesting that PVN GLP-1Rs are involved in that response (Ghosal et al. 2017).

4.3.7 Effects of Fasting

Fasting impairs both peripheral and central GLP-1R agonist-induced hypophagia (Sandoval et al. 2012; Williams et al. 2006). This has been hypothesized to be leptin-related, because leptin levels drop substantially with fasting, and physiologic-dose leptin replacement during fasting restores the effectiveness of IP Ex4 (Williams et al. 2006). However, leptin treatment does not augment the effect of 3rd-icv GLP-1 in fasted animals (Sandoval et al. 2012), and evidence suggests that it may instead be brain glucose-sensing that modulates the response to central GLP-1 (Burmeister et al. 2017b; Sandoval et al. 2012). Fasting also has a profound effect on PPG neuron responsivity. Overnight deprivation blocks CCK-, restraint-, and elevated platform stress-induced c-Fos in PPG neurons (Maniscalco and Rinaman 2013; Maniscalco et al. 2015), suggesting that fasting renders GLP-1 less likely to be released to act on its receptors.

4.4 OTHER BEHAVIORAL EFFECTS OF BRAIN GLP-1R STIMULATION

Research on the behavioral effects of GLP-1 has primarily focused on food intake and reward, but GLP-1 has other effects on behavior. It is worth considering how changes in feeding behavior may be coordinated with these, so we will discuss this evidence briefly here.

4.4.1 Water Intake

In the vast majority of research discussed above, water intake was not reported, so information about brain GLP-1R involvement in fluid balance and thirst is limited. Reduced water intake would be expected to accompany the food intake suppression observed after GLP-1 agonist treatment, and this has been reported (Tang-Christensen et al. 1996), but there is evidence that GLP-1 has feeding-independent effects on drinking. A series of studies showed that in rats lateral or 4th-icv injection of Ex4 or liraglutide reduced unstimulated water intake in the absence of food (McKay et al. 2011), as well as water intake induced by either water deprivation or by icv injection of Angiotensin-II (McKay and Daniels 2013). Importantly, they also demonstrated that lateral-icv Ex9-39 injection increased water intake in response to hypertonic saline or water deprivation (McKay et al. 2014). This is striking because water intake is already elevated under those conditions, so blockade of GLP-1Rs increased it further above a high baseline. In the same paper, they showed that PPG mRNA in the NTS was elevated by water consumption, supporting the idea that endogenous production and release of GLP-1 plays a role in the decision to stop drinking, similar to its hypothesized role in meal termination. It remains unclear which brain GLP-1R sites mediate these effects on water intake. Recently in mice, GLP-1R-expressing neurons of the median preoptic nucleus (MnPO) were implicated in thirst satiation (Augustine et al. 2018). These GLP-1R neurons were activated by ingestion of fluids, as measured by calcium imaging, and inhibition of these neurons via DREADD substantially increased drinking. This manipulation silences the neuron, rather than targeting the GLP-1R, so these data do not necessarily implicate GLP-1Rs in the effect on drinking.

4.4.2 Drug and Alcohol Consumption and Reward

Given the anatomy of this system, it is perhaps unsurprising that effects of brain GLP-1 on drug and alcohol seeking and consumption have been investigated and that there is evidence that brain GLP-1R stimulation suppresses these behaviors. In mice, relatively high doses of GLP-1R agonists delivered systemically suppressed CPP induced by amphetamine, cocaine (Graham et al. 2013; Egecioglu et al. 2013b), nicotine (Egecioglu et al. 2013a), or alcohol (Vallöf et al. 2016), and also suppressed the self-administration of cocaine (Sørensen et al. 2015) or alcohol (Vallöf et al. 2016), but notably had no effects on opioid drug self-administration or CPP (Bornebusch et al. 2019). Several studies showed that GLP-1R agonist treatment reduced striatal dopamine release in response to these drugs (e.g. Egecioglu, et al. 2013a; Sørensen et al. 2015;). IP injection of Ex9-39 increases alcohol intake, suggesting that endogenous GLP-1R stimulation limits alcohol consumption (Shirazi et al. 2013). A limited number of studies have looked at specific brain sites for GLP-1R effects on drug and alcohol reward, and the VTA (Schmidt et al. 2016; Shirazi et al. 2013; Schmidt et al. 2016), NTS (Vallöf et al. 2019), LS (Harasta et al. 2015), and interpeduncular nucleus (IPN) (Tuesta et al. 2017) have each been implicated. A role for endogenous GLP-1 in limiting motivation for cocaine is suggested by findings that IV infusion of cocaine induced c-Fos in NTS PPG neurons, and that shRNA-mediated knockdown of GLP-1Rs in the VTA augmented cocaine self-administration (Schmidt et al. 2016). This and other loss-of-function approaches support a role for endogenous GLP-1R activity in the IPN in nicotine avoidance as well (Tuesta et al. 2017).

4.4.3 Sexual Behavior

Mating is a natural reward that engages some of the same circuitry as palatable food and drugs of abuse, so it is perhaps not surprising that in naïve male mice presented with a female in estrus, Ex4 injection into the posterior part of the VTA, NAc shell subregion, and LDTg reduced pre-sex social interaction such as sniffing and following the female, and posterior VTA and LDTg Ex4 also suppressed male mounting behavior (Vestlund and Jerlhag 2020a). The same group also showed that GLP-1Rs in the NTS may have a role, because intra-NTS Ex9-39 blocked the ability of IP Ex4 to suppress these same mating behaviors in male mice (Vestlund and Jerlhag 2020b). Effects in females were not examined in these studies, and these effects in males could be entirely pharmacologic in nature. We speculate that endogenous GLP-1R activity plays a role here as in ingestive behavior and drug reward, but this needs to be tested.

4.4.4 Non-Feeding Stress Responses and Anxiety-Like Behavior

GLP-1R contributions to stress-induced hypophagia were discussed above, but these receptors are involved in other stress responses as well. Ample evidence supports a role for brain GLP-1Rs in HPA responses to stress (Ghosal et al. 2017; Kinzig et al. 2003; Larsen et al. 1997; Tauchi et al. 2008; Zheng et al. 2019), but we focus here on behavior. The elevated plus maze (EPM) is a common tool for investigating stress and anxiety-like behavior in rodents, consisting of a platform several feet above the floor, in a plus shape, with two arms open and the other two enclosed. Placing rodents on the elevated platform stimulates HPA activity, and rodents typically spend more time in the closed arms. Central blockade of GLP-1Rs more than doubled the percentage of time rats spent in the open arms (Kinzig et al. 2003), showing that endogenous activation of these receptors plays a role in the normal inclination toward the closed arms. Knockdown of GLP-1Rs in PVN caused a similar shift in EPM behavior in mice. Knockdown of alBNST GLP-1Rs in rats had no effect on EPM behavior, but did affect responses in the open field and light-enhanced acoustic startle tests (Zheng et al. 2019). The open field test is similar to the EPM in that it relies on rodents' exploratory behavior and avoidance of open areas. Typically, rats spend more time near the walls of the test arena, and alBNST GLP-1R knockdown increased time spent in the center. The acoustic startle test measures the startle response to a loud tone, which is normally enhanced by testing in bright light. Knockdown of alBNST GLP-1Rs eliminated that effect. These complementary tests support a role for BNST GLP-1Rs and show that their function is different from those in the PVN. A role for dorsal raphe (DR) GLP-1Rs has been suggested by findings that intra-DR Ex4 can increase anxiety-like behavior in some of these tests; however, it is unclear whether endogenous activity at DR GLP-1Rs has an effect (Anderberg et al. 2016). Recent data showing sex differences in the effects of GLP-1Rs in the SuM, including an anxiolytic effect of SuM GLP-1R knockdown in females only, highlight the importance of testing both male and female subjects (López-Ferreras et al. 2020).

4.5 CONCLUSIONS

The evidence of a role for brain GLP-1Rs in feeding and food-motivated behavior is overwhelming, and compelling data show GLP-1R involvement in behavioral stress responses and other motivated behaviors including drinking, drug and alcohol seeking, and mating (illustrated in Figure 4.1). Each of these has been studied in isolation, in experiments designed intentionally to target one behavior or another. However, we should consider behavior through a wider lens and recognize that, outside the lab, animals have the option to engage in many different behaviors and must prioritize some over others, especially when some are mutually exclusive. What would activation of the PPG neuron and brain GLP-1R network do to behavior in a natural setting? We suggest that the role of this system is to enable certain interoceptive (GI signals, homeostatic challenges) and environmental cues (signals of possible danger) to broadly suppress exploratory and motivated behavior in the interest of survival. The flexibility to shut this down under fasted conditions would be adaptive; if starvation is a threat, motivation to explore and seek food must remain high. Whether there is selective activation of specific PPG neurons by different types of stimuli, how the multiple GLP-1R-expressing neuron populations that are impacted by endogenous agonist release may interact with each other, and how peripheral GLP-1R signaling is integrated into this system in the brain will all be important future directions (Figure 4.1).

ACKNOWLEDGMENTS

Work in the Williams laboratory is supported by NIH grant R01DK095757 (to D.L.W.); C.B.M. was supported by NIH T32 MH093311 (to P.K. Keel and L.A. Eckel). The authors would like to thank Charles Badland, Program in Neuroscience, for preparation of Figure 4.1.

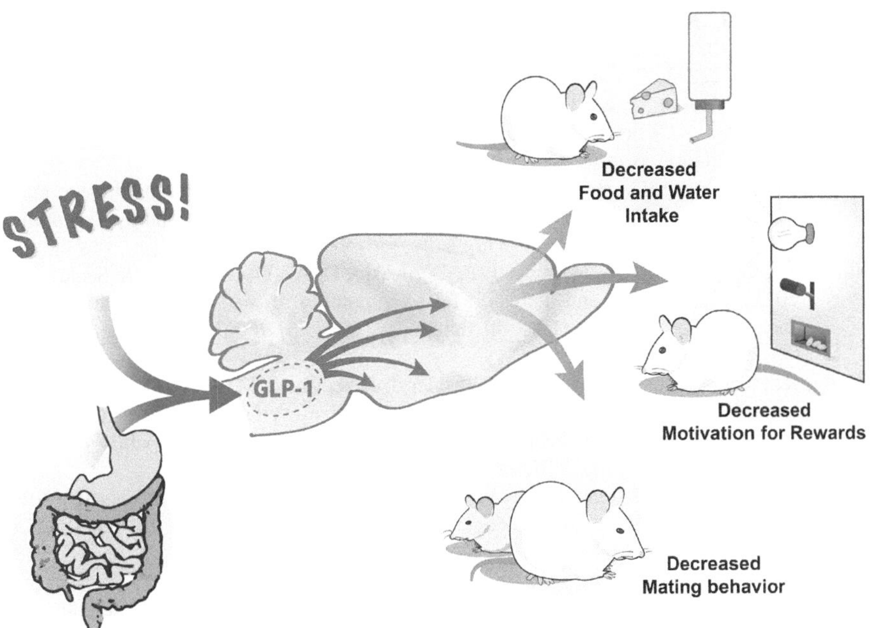

FIGURE 4.1 Illustration of the brain PPG-GLP-1R system's role in behavior. PPG neurons are activated by GI signals or stressors, and GLP-1 stimulation of its receptors throughout the brain then suppresses motivated behavior including but not limited to feeding.

REFERENCES

Adams, J. M., Pei, H., Sandoval, D. A., Seeley, R. J., Chang, R. B., Liberles, S. D., & Olson, D. P. (2018). Liraglutide modulates appetite and body weight through glucagon-like peptide 1 receptor-expressing glutamatergic neurons. *Diabetes*, *67*(8), 1538–1548.

Alhadeff, A. L., Baird, J.-P., Swick, J. C., Hayes, M. R., & Grill, H. J. (2014). Glucagon-like Peptide-1 receptor signaling in the lateral parabrachial nucleus contributes to the control of food intake and motivation to feed. *Neuropsychopharmacology*, *39*(9), 2233–2243.

Alhadeff, A. L., & Grill, H. J. (2014). Hindbrain nucleus tractus solitarius glucagon-like peptide-1 receptor signaling reduces appetitive and motivational aspects of feeding. *American Journal of Physiology. Regulatory, Integrative and Comparative Physiology*, *307*(4), R465–R470.

Alhadeff, A. L., Mergler, B. D., Zimmer, D. J., Turner, C. A., Reiner, D. J., Schmidt, H. D., Grill, H.J., & Hayes, M. R. (2017). Endogenous glucagon-like peptide-1 receptor signaling in the nucleus tractus solitarius is required for food intake control. *Neuropsychopharmacology* *42*(7), 1471–1479.

Alhadeff, A. L., Rupprecht, L. E., & Hayes, M. R. (2012). GLP-1 neurons in the nucleus of the solitary tract project directly to the ventral tegmental area and nucleus accumbens to control for food intake. *Endocrinology*, *153*(2), 647–658. doi:10.1210/en.2011-1443

Anderberg, R. H., Richard, J. E., Eerola, K., López-Ferreras, L., Banke, E., Hansson, C., Nissbrandt, H., Berqquist, F., Gribble, F. M., Reimann, F., et al. (2017). Glucagon-like peptide 1 and its analogs act in the dorsal raphe and modulate central serotonin to reduce appetite and body weight. *Diabetes*, *66*(4), 1062–1073.

Anderberg, R. H., Richard, J. E., Hansson, C., Nissbrandt, H., Bergquist, F., & Skibicka, K. P. (2016). GLP-1 is both anxiogenic and antidepressant; divergent effects of acute and chronic GLP-1 on emotionality. *Psychoneuroendocrinology*, *65*, 54–66.

Aroda, V. R. (2018). A review of GLP-1 receptor agonists: evolution and advancement, through the lens of randomised controlled trials. *Diabetes, Obesity & Metabolism, 20 Suppl 1*, 22–33.

Augustine, V., Gokce, S. K., Lee, S., Wang, B., Davidson, T. J., Reimann, F., Gribble, F., Deisseroth, K., Lois, C., & Oka, Y. (2018). Hierarchical neural architecture underlying thirst regulation. *Nature*, *555*(7695), 204–209.

Baggio, L. L., Huang, Q., Brown, T. J., & Drucker, D. J. (2004). Oxyntomodulin and glucagon-like peptide-1 differentially regulate murine food intake and energy expenditure. *Gastroenterology*, *127*(2), 546–558.

Barrera, J. G., Jones, K. R., Herman, J. P., D'Alessio, D. A., Woods, S. C., & Seeley, R. J. (2011). Hyperphagia and increased fat accumulation in two models of chronic CNS glucagon-like peptide-1 loss of function. *The Journal of Neuroscience*, *31*(10), 3904–3913.

Bettge, K., Kahle, M., Abd El Aziz, M. S., Meier, J. J., & Nauck, M. A. (2017). Occurrence of nausea, vomiting and diarrhoea reported as adverse events in clinical trials studying glucagon-like peptide-1 receptor agonists: A systematic analysis of published clinical trials. *Diabetes, Obesity & Metabolism*, *19*(3), 336–347.

Bornebusch, A. B., Fink-Jensen, A., Wörtwein, G., Seeley, R. J., & Thomsen, M. (2019). Glucagon-like peptide-1 receptor agonist treatment does not reduce abuse-related effects of opioid drugs. *ENeuro*, *6*(2). doi:10.1523/ENEURO.0443-18.2019

Burmeister, M. A., Ayala, J. E., Smouse, H., Landivar-Rocha, A., Brown, J. D., Drucker, D. J., Stoffers, D. A., Sandoval, D. A., Seeley, R. J., & Ayala, J. E. (2017a). The hypothalamic glucagon-like peptide 1 receptor is sufficient but not necessary for the regulation of energy balance and glucose homeostasis in mice. *Diabetes*, 66(2), 372–384.

Burmeister, M. A., Brown, J. D., Ayala, J. E., Stoffers, D. A., Sandoval, D. A., Seeley, R. J., & Ayala, J. E. (2017b). The glucagon-like peptide-1 receptor in the ventromedial hypothalamus reduces short-term food intake in male mice by regulating nutrient sensor activity. *American Journal of Physiology. Endocrinology and Metabolism*, *313*(6), E651–E662.

Campos, R. V., Lee, Y. C., & Drucker, D. J. (1994). Divergent tissue-specific and developmental expression of receptors for glucagon and glucagon-like peptide-1 in the mouse. *Endocrinology*, *134*(5), 2156–2164.

Cork, S. C., Richards, J. E., Holt, M. K., Gribble, F. M., Reimann, F., & Trapp, S. (2015). Distribution and characterisation of Glucagon-like peptide-1 receptor expressing cells in the mouse brain. *Molecular Metabolism*, *4*(10), 718–731.

Dickson, S. L., Shirazi, R. H., Hansson, C., Bergquist, F., Nissbrandt, H., & Skibicka, K. P. (2012). The glucagon-like peptide 1 (GLP-1) analogue, exendin-4, decreases the rewarding value of food: A new role for mesolimbic GLP-1 receptors. *The Journal of Neuroscience*, *32*(14), 4812–4820.

Dossat, A. M., Diaz, R., Gallo, L., Panagos, A., Kay, K., & Williams, D. L. (2013). Nucleus accumbens GLP-1 receptors influence meal size and palatability. *American Journal of Physiology. Endocrinology and Metabolism*, *304*(12), E1314–E1320.

Dossat, A. M., Lilly, N., Kay, K., & Williams, D. L. (2011). Glucagon-like peptide 1 receptors in nucleus accumbens affect food intake. *The Journal of Neuroscience*, *31*(41), 14453–14457.

Egecioglu, E., Engel, J. A., & Jerlhag, E. (2013a). The glucagon-like peptide 1 analogue Exendin-4 attenuates the nicotine-induced locomotor stimulation, accumbal dopamine release, conditioned place preference as well as the expression of locomotor sensitization in mice. *PloS One*, *8*(10), e77284.

Egecioglu, E., Engel, J. A., & Jerlhag, E. (2013b). The glucagon-like peptide 1 analogue, exendin-4, attenuates the rewarding properties of psychostimulant drugs in mice. *PloS One*, *8*(7), e69010.

Farr, O. M., Sofopoulos, M., Tsoukas, M. A., Dincer, F., Thakkar, B., Sahin-Efe, A., Filippaios, A., Bowers, J., Srnka, A., Gavrieli, A., et al. (2016). GLP-1 receptors exist in the parietal cortex, hypothalamus and medulla of human brains and the GLP-1 analogue liraglutide alters brain activity related to highly desirable food cues in individuals with diabetes: A crossover, randomised, placebo-controlled trial. *Diabetologia*, *59*(5), 954–965.

Fortin, S. M., Lipsky, R. K., Lhamo, R., Chen, J., Kim, E., Borner, T., Schmidt, H. D., & Hayes, M. R. (2020). GABA neurons in the nucleus tractus solitarius express GLP-1 receptors and mediate anorectic effects of liraglutide in rats. *Science Translational Medicine*, *12*(533).

Gabery, S., Salinas, C. G., Paulsen, S. J., Ahnfelt-Rønne, J., Alanentalo, T., Baquero, A. F., Buckley, S. T., Farkas, E., Fekete, C., et al. (2020). Semaglutide lowers body weight in rodents via distributed neural pathways. *JCI Insight*, *5*(6).

Ghosal, S., Packard, A. E. B., Mahbod, P., McKlveen, J. M., Seeley, R. J., Myers, B., Ulrich-Lai, Y., Smith, E. P., D'Alessio, D. A., & Herman, J. P. (2017). Disruption of glucagon-like peptide 1 signaling in sim1 neurons reduces physiological and behavioral reactivity to acute and chronic stress. *The Journal of Neuroscience: The Official Journal of the Society for Neuroscience*, *37*(1), 184–193.

Graham, D. L., Erreger, K., Galli, A., & Stanwood, G. D. (2013). GLP-1 analog attenuates cocaine reward. *Molecular Psychiatry*, *18*(9), 961–962.

Grill, H. J., Carmody, J. S., Amanda Sadacca, L., Williams, D. L., & Kaplan, J. M. (2004). Attenuation of lipopolysaccharide anorexia by antagonism of caudal brain stem but not forebrain GLP-1-R. *American Journal of Physiology. Regulatory, Integrative and Comparative Physiology*, *287*(5), R1190–R1193.

Harasta, A. E., Power, J. M., von Jonquieres, G., Karl, T., Drucker, D. J., Housley, G. D., Schneider, M., & Klugmann, M. (2015). Septal glucagon-like peptide 1 receptor expression determines suppression of cocaine-induced behavior. *Neuropsychopharmacology*, *40*(8), 1969–1978.

Hayes, M. R., Bradley, L., & Grill, H. J. (2009). Endogenous hindbrain glucagon-like peptide-1 receptor activation contributes to the control of food intake by mediating gastric satiation signaling. *Endocrinology*, *150*(6), 2654–2659.

Hayes, M. R., Leichner, T. M., Zhao, S., Lee, G. S., Chowansky, A., Zimmer, D., De Jonghe, B. C., Kanoski, S. E., Grill, H. J., & Bence, K. K. (2011). Intracellular signals mediating the food intake-suppressive effects of hindbrain glucagon-like peptide-1 receptor activation. *Cell Metabolism*, *13*(3), 320–330.

Hayes, M. R., Skibicka, K. P., & Grill, H. J. (2008). Caudal brainstem processing is sufficient for behavioral, sympathetic, and parasympathetic responses driven by peripheral and hindbrain glucagon-like-peptide-1 receptor stimulation. *Endocrinology*, *149*(8), 4059–4068.

Hisadome, K., Reimann, F., Gribble, F. M., & Trapp, S. (2011). CCK stimulation of GLP-1 neurons involves α1-adrenoceptor-mediated increase in glutamatergic synaptic inputs. *Diabetes*, *60*(11), 2701–2709.

Hisadome, K., Reimann, F., Gribble, F., & Trapp, S. (2010). Leptin directly depolarizes preproglucagon neurons in the nucleus tractus solitarius: electrical properties of glucagon-like peptide 1 neurons. *Diabetes*, *59*(August), 1890–1898.

Holst, J. J., & Deacon, C. F. (2005). Glucagon-like peptide-1 mediates the therapeutic actions of DPP-IV inhibitors. *Diabetologia*, *48*(4), 612–615.

Holt, M. K., Richards, J. E., Cook, D. R., Brierley, D. I., Williams, D. L., Reimann, F., Gribble, F. M., & Trapp, S. (2019). Preproglucagon neurons in the nucleus of the solitary tract are the main source of brain GLP-1, mediate stress-induced hypophagia, and limit unusually large intakes of food. *Diabetes*, *68*(1), 21–33.

Hsu, T. M., Hahn, J. D., Konanur, V. R., Lam, A., & Kanoski, S. E. (2015). Hippocampal GLP-1 receptors influence food intake, meal size, and effort-based responding for food through volume transmission. *Neuropsychopharmacology*, *40*(2), 327–337.

Kanoski, S. E., Fortin, S. M., Arnold, M., Grill, H. J., & Hayes, M. R. (2011). Peripheral and central GLP-1 receptor populations mediate the anorectic effects of peripherally administered GLP-1 receptor agonists, liraglutide and exendin-4. *Endocrinology*, *152*(8), 3103–3112.

Kanoski, S. E., Rupprecht, L. E., Fortin, S. M., De Jonghe, B. C., & Hayes, M. R. (2012). The role of nausea in food intake and body weight suppression by peripheral GLP-1 receptor agonists exendin-4 and liraglutide. *Neuropharmacology*, *62*(5–6), 1916–1927.

Kastin, A. J., Akerstrom, V., & Pan, W. (2002). Interactions of glucagon-like peptide-1 (GLP-1) with the blood-brain barrier. *Journal of Molecular Neuroscience: MN*, *18*(1–2), 7–14.

Katsurada, K., Maejima, Y., Nakata, M., Kodaira, M., Suyama, S., Iwasaki, Y., Kario, K., & Yada, T. (2014). Endogenous GLP-1 acts on paraventricular nucleus to suppress feeding: Projection from nucleus tractus solitarius and activation of corticotropin-releasing hormone, nesfatin-1 and oxytocin neurons. *Biochemical and Biophysical Research Communications*, *451*(2), 276–281.

Kinzig, K. P., D'Alessio, D. A., Herman, J. P., Sakai, R. R., Vahl, T. P., Figueiredo, H. F., Murphy, E. K., Seeley, R. J., & Figueredo, H. F. (2003). CNS glucagon-like peptide-1 receptors mediate endocrine and anxiety responses to interoceptive and psychogenic stressors. *The Journal of Neuroscience*, *23*(15), 6163–6170.

Kinzig, K. P., D'Alessio, D. A., & Seeley, R. J. (2002). The diverse roles of specific GLP-1 receptors in the control of food intake and the response to visceral illness. *The Journal of Neuroscience*, *22*(23), 10470–10476.

Knudsen, L. B., & Lau, J. (2019). The discovery and development of liraglutide and semaglutide. *Frontiers in Endocrinology*, *10*, 155.

Kreisler, A. D., & Rinaman, L. (2016). Hindbrain glucagon-like peptide-1 neurons track intake volume and contribute to injection stress-induced hypophagia in meal-entrained rats. *American Journal of Physiology - Regulatory, Integrative and Comparative Physiology*, *310*(10), R906–R916.

Lachey, J. L., D'Alessio, D. A., Rinaman, L., Elmquist, J. K., Drucker, D. J., & Seeley, R. J. (2005). The role of central glucagon-like peptide-1 in mediating the effects of visceral illness: Differential effects in rats and mice. *Endocrinology*, *146*(1), 458–462.

Larsen, P. J., Tang-Christensen, M., & Jessop, D. S. (1997). Central administration of glucagon-like peptide-1 activates hypothalamic neuroendocrine neurons in the rat. *Endocrinology*, *138*(10), 4445–4455.

Liu, J., Conde, K., Zhang, P., Lilascharoen, V., Xu, Z., Lim, B. K., Seeley, R. J., Zhu, J. J., Scott, M. M., & Pang, Z. P. (2017). Enhanced AMPA Receptor Trafficking Mediates the Anorexigenic Effect of Endogenous Glucagon-like Peptide-1 in the Paraventricular Hypothalamus. *Neuron*, *96*(4), 897–909.e5.

López-Ferreras, L., Eerola, K., Shevchouk, O. T., Richard, J. E., Nilsson, F. H., Jansson, L. E., Hayes, M. R., & Skibicka, K. P. (2020). The supramammillary nucleus controls anxiety-like behavior; key role of GLP-1R. *Psychoneuroendocrinology*, *119*, 104720.

López-Ferreras, L., Richard, J. E., Noble, E. E., Eerola, K., Anderberg, R. H., Olandersson, K., Taing, L., Kanoski, S. E., Hayes, M. R., & Skibicka, K. P. (2018). Lateral hypothalamic GLP-1 receptors are critical for the control of food reinforcement, *ingestive behavior and body weight. Molecular Psychiatry*, *23*(5), 1157–1168.

López-Ferreras, L., Eerola, K., Mishra, D., Shevchouk, O. T., Richard, J. E., Nilsson, F. H., Hayes, M. R., & Skibicka, K. P. (2019). GLP-1 modulates the supramammillary nucleus-lateral hypothalamic neurocircuit to control ingestive and motivated behavior in a sex divergent manner. *Molecular Metabolism*, *20*, 178–193.

Maniscalco, J. W., & Rinaman, L. (2013). Overnight food deprivation markedly attenuates hindbrain noradrenergic, glucagon-like peptide-1, and hypothalamic neural responses to exogenous cholecystokinin in male rats. *Physiology & Behavior*, *121*, 35–42.

Maniscalco, J. W., Zheng, H., Gordon, P. J., & Rinaman, L. (2015). Negative energy balance blocks neural and behavioral responses to acute stress by "silencing" central glucagon-like peptide 1 signaling in rats. *The Journal of Neuroscience*, *35*(30), 10701–10714.

Maske, C. B., Jackson, C. M., Terrill, S. J., Eckel, L. A., & Williams, D. L. (2017). Estradiol modulates the anorexic response to central glucagon-like peptide 1. *Hormones and Behavior*, *93*, 109–117.

McKay, N. J., & Daniels, D. (2013). Glucagon-like peptide-1 receptor agonist administration suppresses both water and saline intake in rats. *Journal of Neuroendocrinology*, *25*(10), 929–938.

McKay, N. J., Galante, D. L., & Daniels, D. (2014). Endogenous glucagon-like peptide-1 reduces drinking behavior and is differentially engaged by water and food intakes in rats. *The Journal of Neuroscience*, *34*(49), 16417–16423.

McKay, N. J., Kanoski, S. E., Hayes, M. R., & Daniels, D. (2011). Glucagon-like peptide-1 receptor agonists suppress water intake independent of effects on food intake. *American Journal of Physiology. Regulatory, Integrative and Comparative Physiology*, *301*(6), R1755–R1764.

McMahon, L. R., & Wellman, P. J. (1998). PVN infusion of GLP-1-(7-36) amide suppresses feeding but does not induce aversion or alter locomotion in rats. *The American Journal of Physiology*, *274*(1), R23–R29.

Merchenthaler, I., Lane, M., & Shughrue, P. (1999). Distribution of pre-pro-glucagon and glucagon-like peptide-1 receptor messenger RNAs in the rat central nervous system. *The Journal of Comparative Neurology*, *403*(2), 261–280.

Mietlicki-Baase, E. G., Ortinski, P. I., Reiner, D. J., Sinon, C. G., McCutcheon, J. E., Pierce, R. C., Roitman, M. F., & Hayes, M. R. (2014). Glucagon-like peptide-1 receptor activation in the nucleus accumbens core suppresses feeding by increasing glutamatergic AMPA/kainate signaling. *The Journal of Neuroscience*, *34*(20), 6985–6992.

Mietlicki-Baase, E. G., Ortinski, P. I., Rupprecht, L. E., Olivos, D. R., Alhadeff, A. L., Pierce, R. C., & Hayes, M. R. (2013). The food intake-suppressive effects of glucagon-like peptide-1 receptor signaling in the ventral tegmental area are mediated by AMPA/kainate receptors. *American Journal of Physiology. Endocrinology and Metabolism*, *305*(11), E1367–E1374.

Müller, T. D., Finan, B., Bloom, S. R., D'Alessio, D., Drucker, D. J., Flatt, P. R., Fritsche, A., Gribble, F., Grill, H. J., et al. (2019). Glucagon-like peptide 1 (GLP-1). *Molecular Metabolism*, *30*, 72–130.

Ong, Z. Y., Liu, J.-J., Pang, Z. P., & Grill, H. J. (2017). Paraventricular thalamic control of food intake and reward: role of glucagon-like peptide-1 receptor signaling. *Neuropsychopharmacology*, *42*(12), 2387–2397.

Parkes, D. G., Mace, K. F., & Trautmann, M. E. (2013). Discovery and development of exenatide: the first antidiabetic agent to leverage the multiple benefits of the incretin hormone, GLP-1. *Expert Opinion on Drug Discovery*, *8*(2), 219–244.

Plamboeck, A., Veedfald, S., Deacon, C. F., Hartmann, B., Wettergren, A., Svendsen, L. B., Meisner, S., Hovendal, C., Vilsbøll, T., Knop, F. K., et al. (2013). The effect of exogenous GLP-1 on food intake is lost in male truncally vagotomized subjects with pyloroplasty. *American Journal of Physiology. Gastrointestinal and Liver Physiology*, *304*(12), G1117–G1127.

Pocai, A. (2012). Unraveling oxyntomodulin, GLP1's enigmatic brother. *The Journal of Endocrinology*, *215*(3), 335–346.

Reiner, D. J., Leon, R. M., McGrath, L. E., Koch-Laskowski, K., Hahn, J. D., Kanoski, S. E., Mietlicki-Baase, E. G., & Hayes, M. R. (2018). Glucagon-like peptide-1 receptor signaling in the lateral dorsal tegmental nucleus regulates energy balance. *Neuropsychopharmacology: Official Publication of the American College of Neuropsychopharmacology*, *43*(3), 627–637. doi:10.1038/npp.2017.225

Reiner, D. J., Mietlicki-Baase, E. G., McGrath, L. E., Zimmer, D. J., Bence, K. K., Sousa, G. L., Konanur, V. R., Krawczyk, J., Burk, D. H., Kanoski, S. E., et al. (2016). Astrocytes regulate GLP-1 receptor-mediated effects on energy balance. *The Journal of Neuroscience*, *36*(12), 3531–3540.

Richard, J. E., Anderberg, R. H., Göteson, A., Gribble, F. M., Reimann, F., & Skibicka, K. P. (2015). Activation of the GLP-1 receptors in the nucleus of the solitary tract reduces food reward behavior and targets the mesolimbic system. *PloS One*, *10*(3), e0119034.

Richard, J. E., Anderberg, R. H., López-Ferreras, L., Olandersson, K., & Skibicka, K. P. (2016). Sex and estrogens alter the action of glucagon-like peptide-1 on reward. *Biology of Sex Differences*, *7*, 6.

Richard, J. E., Farkas, I., Anesten, F., Anderberg, R. H., Dickson, S. L., Gribble, F. M., Reimann, F., Jansson, J.-O., Liposits, Z., & Skibicka, K. P. (2014). GLP-1 receptor stimulation of the lateral parabrachial nucleus reduces food intake: Neuroanatomical, electrophysiological, *and behavioral evidence. Endocrinology*, *155*(11), 4356–4367.

Rinaman, L. (1999a). Interoceptive stress activates glucagon-like peptide-1 neurons that project to the hypothalamus. *The American Journal of Physiology*, *277*(2), R582–R590.

Rinaman, L. (1999b). A functional role for central glucagon-like peptide-1 receptors in lithium chloride-induced anorexia. *The American Journal of Physiology*, *277*(5), R1537–R1540.

Rinaman, Linda. (2010). Ascending projections from the caudal visceral nucleus of the solitary tract to brain regions involved in food intake and energy expenditure. *Brain Research*, *1350*, 18–34.

Rupprecht, L. E., Mietlicki-Baase, E. G., Zimmer, D. J., McGrath, L. E., Olivos, D. R., & Hayes, M. R. (2013). Hindbrain GLP-1 receptor-mediated suppression of food intake requires a PI3K-dependent decrease in phosphorylation of membrane-bound Akt. *American Journal of Physiology. Endocrinology and Metabolism*, *305*(6), E751–E759.

Sandoval, D., Barrera, J. G., Stefater, M. A., Sisley, S., Woods, S. C., D'Alessio, D. D., & Seeley, R. J. (2012). The anorectic effect of GLP-1 in rats is nutrient dependent. *PloS One*, *7*(12), e51870.

Schmidt, H. D., Mietlicki-Baase, E. G., Ige, K. Y., Maurer, J. J., Reiner, D. J., Zimmer, D. J., Van Nest, D. S., Guercio, L. A., Wimmer, M. E., Olivos, D. R., et al. (2016). Glucagon-like peptide-1 receptor activation in the ventral tegmental area decreases the reinforcing efficacy of cocaine. *Neuropsychopharmacology*, *41*(7), 1917–1928.

Secher, A., Jelsing, J., Baquero, A. F., Hecksher-Sørensen, J., Cowley, M. A., Dalbøge, L. S., Hansen, G., Grove, K. L., Pyke, C., Raun, K., et al. (2014). The arcuate nucleus mediates GLP-1 receptor agonist liraglutide-dependent weight loss. *The Journal of Clinical Investigation*, *124*(10), 4473–4488.

Seeley, R. J., Blake, K., Rushing, P. A., Benoit, S., Eng, J., Woods, S. C., & D'Alessio, D. (2000). The role of CNS glucagon-like peptide-1 (7-36) amide receptors in mediating the visceral illness effects of lithium chloride. *The Journal of Neuroscience*, *20*(4), 1616–1621.

Shirazi, R. H., Dickson, S. L., & Skibicka, K. P. (2013). Gut peptide GLP-1 and its analogue, Exendin-4, decrease alcohol intake and reward. *PloS One*, *8*(4), e61965.

Sisley, S., Gutierrez-Aguilar, R., Scott, M., D'Alessio, D. A., Sandoval, D. A., & Seeley, R. J. (2014). Neuronal GLP1R mediates liraglutide's anorectic but not glucose-lowering effect. *The Journal of Clinical Investigation*, *124*(6), 2456–2463.

Sørensen, G., Reddy, I. A., Weikop, P., Graham, D. L., Stanwood, G. D., Wortwein, G., Galli, A., & Fink-Jensen, A. (2015). The glucagon-like peptide 1 (GLP-1) receptor agonist exendin-4 reduces cocaine self-administration in mice. *Physiology & Behavior*, *149*, 262–268.

Tang-Christensen, M., Larsen, P. J., Göke, R., Fink-Jensen, A., Jessop, D. S., Møller, M., & Sheikh, S. P. (1996). Central administration of GLP-1-(7-36) amide inhibits food and water intake in rats. *The American Journal of Physiology*, *271*(4 Pt 2), R848–R856.

Tauchi, M., Zhang, R., D'Alessio, D. A., Seeley, R. J., & Herman, J. P. (2008). Role of central glucagon-like peptide-1 in hypothalamo-pituitary-adrenocortical facilitation following chronic stress. *Experimental Neurology*, *210*(2), 458–466.

Terrill, S. J., Holt, M. K., Maske, C. B., Abrams, N., Reimann, F., Trapp, S., & Williams, D. L. (2019). Endogenous GLP-1 in lateral septum promotes satiety and suppresses motivation for food in mice. *Physiology & Behavior*, *206*, 191–199.

Terrill, S. J., Jackson, C. M., Greene, H. E., Lilly, N., Maske, C. B., Vallejo, S., & Williams, D. L. (2016). Role of lateral septum glucagon-like peptide 1 receptors in food intake. *American Journal of Physiology. Regulatory, Integrative and Comparative Physiology*, *311*(1), R124–R132.

Terrill, Sarah J., Maske, C. B., & Williams, D. L. (2018). Endogenous GLP-1 in lateral septum contributes to stress-induced hypophagia. *Physiology & Behavior*, *192*, 17–22.

Tuesta, L. M., Chen, Z., Duncan, A., Fowler, C. D., Ishikawa, M., Lee, B. R., Liu, X.-A., Lu, Q., Cameron, M., Hayes, M. R., et al. (2017). GLP-1 acts on habenular avoidance circuits to control nicotine intake. *Nature Neuroscience*, *20*(5), 708–716.

Turton, M. D., O'Shea, D., Gunn, I., Beak, S. A., Edwards, C. M., Meeran, K., Choi, S. J., Taylor, G. M., Heath, M. M., Lambert, P. D., et al. (1996). A role for glucagon-like peptide-1 in the central regulation of feeding. *Nature*, *379*(6560), 69–72.

Vallöf, D., Maccioni, P., Colombo, G., Mandrapa, M., Jörnulf, J. W., Egecioglu, E., Engel, J. A., & Jerlhag, E. (2016). The glucagon-like peptide 1 receptor agonist liraglutide attenuates the reinforcing properties of alcohol in rodents. *Addiction Biology*, *21*(2), 422–437.

Vallöf, D., Vestlund, J., & Jerlhag, E. (2019). Glucagon-like peptide-1 receptors within the nucleus of the solitary tract regulate alcohol-mediated behaviors in rodents. *Neuropharmacology*, *149*, 124–132.

Vestlund, J., & Jerlhag, E. (2020a). The glucagon-like peptide-1 receptor agonist, exendin-4, reduces sexual interaction behaviors in a brain site-specific manner in sexually naïve male mice. *Hormones and Behavior*, *124*, 104778.

Vestlund, J., & Jerlhag, E. (2020b). Glucagon-like peptide-1 receptors and sexual behaviors in male mice. *Psychoneuroendocrinology*, *117*, 104687.

Vrang, N., Phifer, C. B., Corkern, M. M., & Berthoud, H.-R. (2003). Gastric distension induces c-Fos in medullary GLP-1/2-containing neurons. *American Journal of Physiology. Regulatory, Integrative and Comparative Physiology*, *285*(2), R470–R478.

Williams, D. L., Baskin, D. G., & Schwartz, M. W. (2006). Leptin regulation of the anorexic response to glucagon-like peptide-1 receptor stimulation. *Diabetes*, *55*(12), 3387–3393.

Williams, D. L., Baskin, D. G., & Schwartz, M. W. (2009). Evidence that intestinal glucagon-like peptide-1 plays a physiological role in satiety. *Endocrinology*, *150*(4), 1680–1687.

Williams, D. L., Lilly, N. A., Edwards, I. J., Yao, P., Richards, J. E., & Trapp, S. (2018). GLP-1 action in the mouse bed nucleus of the stria terminalis. *Neuropharmacology*, *131*, 83–95.

Zheng, H., Reiner, D. J., Hayes, M. R., & Rinaman, L. (2019). Chronic suppression of glucagon-like peptide-1 receptor (GLP1R) mRNA translation in the rat bed nucleus of the stria terminalis reduces anxiety-like behavior and stress-induced hypophagia, but prolongs stress-induced elevation of plasma corticosterone. *The Journal of Neuroscience*, *39*(14), 2649–2663.

5 Dorsomedial Hypothalamic Regulation of Energy Balance and Glucose Homeostasis

Lessons from Adeno-Associated Virus-Mediated Gene Manipulation

Sheng Bi, Ni Zhang, Kapil Suchal and Jianqiao Zhang

Johns Hopkins University School of Medicine, USA

CONTENTS

5.1 INTRODUCTION

The hypothalamus plays a central role in the regulation of energy balance and glucose homeostasis. The hypothalamus contains various nuclei, such as the arcuate nucleus (ARC), the paraventricular nucleus (PVN), the dorsomedial hypothalamus (DMH), the ventromedial hypothalamus (VMH), and the lateral hypothalamic area (LH). Each of them exerts distinct actions in maintaining energy balance and glucose homeostasis. Beginning with the work of Hetherington and Ranson (1940) and Anand and Brobeck (1951), it has been appreciated that medial hypothalamic lesions result in hyperphagia and obesity, whereas lateral lesions produce hypophagia that, in the absence of nutritional supplementation, results in starvation and death. In combination with results from experiments examining the feeding effects of hypothalamic stimulation, these data served as the basis for Stellar's hypothesis of distinct hunger and satiety centers within the hypothalamus (Stellar, 1954). Since then, particularly with the recent development of various state-of-the-art techniques, we are now able to identify and localize hypothalamic peptide systems that can both stimulate and inhibit food intake or energy expenditure following genetic manipulation of neural signals. For instance, the functions and neural circuits of the ARC have been well studied using these genetic approaches. The ARC contains two distinct populations of neurons: orexigenic neuropeptide agouti-related protein (AgRP)/neuropeptide Y (NPY) neurons and anorexigenic proopiomelanocortin (POMC) neurons (Andermann and Lowell, 2017; Cone, 2006; Elmquist et al., 1999; Friedman, 2014; Morton et al., 2006; Waterson and Horvath, 2015). These two neural systems integrate hormonal (such as leptin and insulin), nutrient, and neural signals to modulate food intake and energy expenditure to maintain energy homeostasis (Andermann and Lowell, 2017; Cone, 2006; Elmquist et al., 1999; Friedman, 2014; Morton et al., 2006; Waterson and Horvath, 2015). The PVN acts as a main output of the hypothalamus and contains various anorexigenic neurons that release neuropeptides/hormones such as oxytocin, corticotropin-releasing hormone (CRH or CRF), and thyrotropin-releasing hormone (TRH) to affect food intake and energy expenditure (Andermann and Lowell, 2017; Cone, 2006; Friedman, 2014; Gautron and Elmquist, 2011; Morton et al., 2006; Waterson and Horvath, 2015). Hypothalamic dysregulation/dysfunctions (such as leptin signaling deficiency resulting from the lack of leptin or leptin receptors) cause obesity, type 2 diabetes, and other metabolic diseases in both rodents and humans.

The DMH is a distinct entity in the hypothalamus. Early hypothalamic studies in rats showed that lesions of the DMH result in hypophagia and reduced body weight (Bernardis et al., 1963), indicating the importance of the DMH in maintaining energy homeostasis. But the neuronal basis of these effects and how DMH neural signals act in the regulation of energy balance have only recently received more attention. The DMH contains a number of energy balance regulation-related neuropeptides, such as NPY, cholecystokinin (CCK), CRF, TRH, and receptors, such as CCK1, melanocortin 4 (MC4), and leptin receptors (LepRb) (Bi et al., 2012). Growing evidence has demonstrated a critical role for DMH peptide signaling in the regulation of energy balance (Bi et al., 2012; Dimicco and Zaretsky, 2007; Morrison et al., 2014; Rezai-Zadeh and Munzberg, 2013), particularly in thermoregulation via affecting brown adipose tissue (BAT) thermogenesis (Chao et al., 2011; Dimicco and Zaretsky, 2007; Dodd et al., 2014; Morrison and Nakamura, 2011; Pinol et al., 2018; Zhang et al., 2011). Our understanding of the glycemic action of the DMH and the mechanism of this action have also significantly increased (Cady et al., 2017; Li et al., 2016; Picard et al., 2016; Zhu et al., 2012). Hence, this chapter aims to outline our recent understanding of how DMH neural signals modulate food intake, energy expenditure, and glucose homeostasis using genetic manipulation approaches, specifically via adeno-associated virus (AAV)-mediated manipulation of DMH neural signals.

5.2 DMH NEURON PROJECTIONS DETERMINED BY AAV-MEDIATED HUMANIZED RENILLA GREEN FLUORESCENT PROTEIN

Over the last two decades, the AAV gene delivery system has widely been used as a means of genetic manipulation in the brain with the features of safety, neuronal- and injection-site-specific infection, and maintaining gene expression for long periods (Okada et al., 2002; Passini et al., 2004). To generate an AAV vector for manipulation of targeted gene expression, the humanized Renilla green fluorescent protein (hrGFP) is commonly inserted and co-produced in the vector as an expression marker. Uniquely, since hrGFP can be efficiently transported from the infected neurons into the axonal projections, researchers have used this feature to conduct neuroanatomical studies to examine the projections of specific neurons in the brain. Gautron et al. (2010) generated a specific AAV vector by encoding an hrGFP that is transcriptionally silenced by a neo cassette flanked by LoxH/LoxP sites, so that the hrGFP is expressed only in neurons with Cre recombinase activity. They delivered this AAV vector unilaterally into the DMH of mice that expresses Cre in neurons expressing the leptin receptors. Consistent with the pattern of DMH projections determined by injections of biotinylated dextran amine, hrGFP-positive axonal projections were found in the PVN, ARC, preoptic area, bed nucleus of the stria terminalis, paraventricular thalamus, periaqueductal gray, and precoeruleus (Gautron et al., 2010). Thus, these results not only identify the projections of DMH LepRb-expressing neurons, but also illustrate a unique conditional tracing approach for neuronal-specific anatomical analysis.

NPY is a potent hypothalamic orexigenic peptide. Within the hypothalamus, NPY-expressing neurons have been identified in the DMH (particularly in the compact subregion) in both rats and primates (Bi, 2013). Although induction of NPY expression in the DMH has been found in certain mouse models of obesity (Guan et al., 1998a; Guan et al., 1998b; Kesterson et al., 1997; Tritos et al., 1998), this expression is undetectable in the DMH of normal weight mice (Bi, 2013). In addition, CCK-1 receptors (CCK1Rs) are found in the DMH of both rats and primates (Hill et al., 1990), but not in mouse DMH (Bi et al., 2004). This difference has been proposed to lead to different phenotypes in body weight control between rats and mice lacking CCK1Rs. While rats lacking CCK1Rs with increased expression of NPY in the DMH develop hyperphagia and obesity, CCK1R knockout mice with undetectable NPY mRNA in the DMH have normal total daily food intake and do not develop obesity (Bi et al., 2004). Thus, because of the similarity of gene expression patterns in the DMH between rats and primates, researchers have conducted studies in rat models to determine the role of DMH NPY in the regulation of energy balance and glucose homeostasis.

Using AAV-mediated hrGFP as an antegrade tracer, neuroanatomical studies have revealed an important projection of DMH NPY neurons to the hindbrain, the central relay that integrates peripheral satiety signals to modulate food intake. In the study, the recombinant vector of AAV-mediated NPY-specific shRNA (AAVshNPY) was generated and unilaterally delivered into the DMH of rats for specific knockdown of NPY (Figure 5.1A–C). As shown in Figure 5.1B, the AAV vector strongly infected neurons within the DMH. Examination of hrGFP and NPY immunostaining fibers revealed that, consistent with the projection of the DMH to the hindbrain (Thompson et al., 1996), hrGFP-positive fibers were well detected in the ipsilateral nucleus solitary tract (NTS) and dorsal motor nucleus of the vagus (DMV) (particularly in the medial and intermediate NTS and lateral DMV) of rats receiving DMH AAV injection (Figure 5.1D). Notably, while NPY fibers (red) were densely detected in the contralateral NTS and DMH, NPY staining fibers were largely abolished in the ipsilateral site (around the hrGFP-staining fiber area) compared to the contralateral site (Figure 5.1E and F), indicating that DMH NPY knockdown silences DMH NPY descending signals to this area (Yang et al., 2009). In support of this projection, additional studies revealed dual hrGFP and NPY staining fibers in the NTS and DMV of rats receiving DMH injection of the control vector containing hrGFP (AAVGFP), indicating that DMH NPY neurons infected by AAVGFP vector transport both NPY signals and the hrGFP marker down to the NTS and DMV (de La Serre et al., 2016). Furthermore, within the NTS, co-staining fibers were found in proximity to catecholaminergic (CA) neurons, suggesting that this DMH NPY projection innervates CA neurons in the NTS (de La Serre et al., 2016). Together, the studies using the AAV vector identify a signaling pathway of DMH NPY neurons projecting to the hindbrain NTS and DMV.

5.3 DETERMINATION OF DMH NEURONAL FUNCTIONS VIA AAV-MEDIATED GENE SILENCING

Since the discovery of RNA interference (RNAi) for gene-specific silencing (Fire et al., 1998), the use of AAV-mediated RNAi has become an important tool for understanding the action of a specific gene at a specific brain site. Using this approach, researchers have determined the functions of DMH neural signals in the regulation of energy balance and glucose homeostasis.

5.3.1 Feeding Effect of DMH NPY

Lesions of the DMH result in hypophagia and decreased body weight in rats (Bernardis et al., 1963), indicating that the main output of the DMH is orexigenic. Consistent with this view, elevation or induction of NPY gene expression in the DMH has been found in rat models with increased energy demands, including lactation (Smith, 1993), chronic food restriction (Bi et al., 2003), and physical exercise (Kawaguchi et al., 2005), and several rodent models of obesity, including the lethal

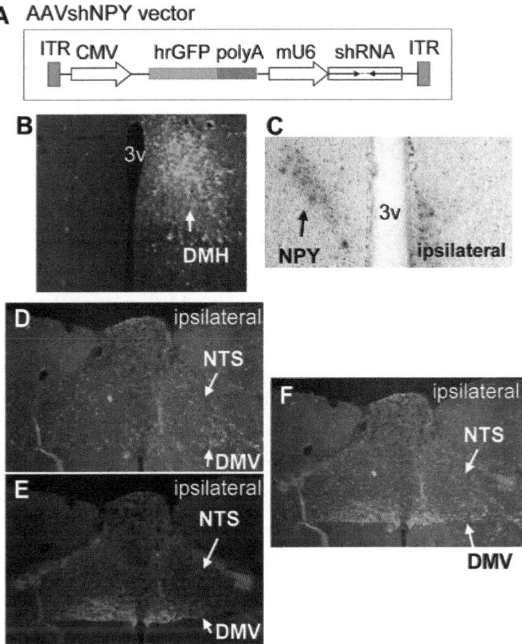

FIGURE 5.1 DMH NPY neurons project to the hindbrain nucleus solitary tract (NTS) and dorsal motor nucleus of the vagus (DMV) in rats. (**A**) Construct of the recombinant vector of AAVshNPY containing hrGFP as an expression marker. (**B**) hrGFP-positive neurons were detected within the DMH of rats receiving unilateral injection of AAVshNPY into the DMH. (**C**) suppression of NPY expression in the ipsilateral DMH was determined by ^{35}S-labeled ***in situ*** hybridization histochemistry compared to the contralateral site. (**D**) hrGFP positive fibers were detected in the ipsilateral NTS and DMV. (**E**) Decreased immunostaining of NPY fibers (red) in the ipsilateral NTS and DMC compared to the contralateral NTS and DMH. (**F**) Merged image of hrGFP positive and NPY fiber staining. Arrows indicate the NTS and DMV areas.

agouti (A^y) (Kesterson et al., 1997), melanocortin-4 receptor (MC4R) knockout (Kesterson et al., 1997), diet-induced obese (Guan et al., 1998a), tubby (Guan et al., 1998b), brown adipose tissue-deficient obese mice (Tritos et al., 1998), and Otsuka Long-Evans Tokushima Fatty (OLETF) rats (Bi et al., 2001; Schroeder et al., 2009). Intriguingly, in contrast to ARC NPY that serves as one of the downstream mediators of leptin's actions, DMH NPY acts independently of leptin. DMH NPY neurons do not co-express LepRbs that are mainly expressed in the ventral and caudal DMH of rats (Bi et al., 2003; Elmquist et al., 1998). NPY gene expression in the DMH is not affected by circulating levels of leptin in fasted rats (Bi et al., 2003) or leptin deficiency in ob/ob mice (Kesterson et al., 1997), while NPY gene expression in the ARC is significantly increased in animals with leptin signaling deficiency (Beck, 2006; Sanacora et al., 1990; Wilding et al., 1993). In fact, DMH NPY signals are affected by CCK, as DMH NPY neurons contain CCK1Rs and NPY expression in the DMH is inhibited by parenchymal microinjection of CCK into the DMH (Bi et al., 2004). Thus, these results indicate that DMH NPY exerts distinct actions different from those of ARC NPY and suggest that DMH NPY acts as an important orexigenic signal in DMH regulation of food intake and energy balance.

To discern the neural mechanism underlying the feeding action of DMH NPY, Yang et al. (2009) had used the approach of AAV-mediated RNAi for knockdown of NPY via delivering AAVshNPY vector into the DMH to assess the effects of DMH NPY knockdown on hyperphagia and obesity in OLETF rats. In support of the hypothesis that NPY overexpression in the DMH contributes to the hyperphagia and obesity of OLETF rats (Bi et al., 2001), data showed that, while OLETF rats became hyperphagic, obese, and had impaired glucose tolerance, DMH NPY knockdown ameliorated these alterations (Yang et al., 2009). In addition, this knockdown produced a nocturnal and meal size-specific feeding effect (Yang et al., 2009). DMH NPY affects within-meal satiation as DMH NPY knockdown resulted in increased feeding inhibitory and NTS c-Fos responses to peripheral administration of satiety signal CCK (Yang et al., 2009). Follow-up studies revealed that DMH NPY descending signals to the NTS affect CCK-induced satiety, at least in part, via modulation of NTS CA neuronal signaling (de La Serre et al., 2016). Thus, the results from studies in rats with DMH NPY knockdown establish a neural pathway of DMH NPY-NTS and DMV in modulating food intake and body weight, indicating that dysregulation of this signaling causes hyperphagia and disordered energy balance leading to obesity.

5.3.2 Thermogenic Effect of DMH NPY

BAT is a non-shivering thermogenic organ that plays an important role in maintaining body temperature. BAT activation combusts energy chemicals (glucose and lipids) and produces heat for protection against cold (Cannon and Nedergaard, 2004). Stimulation of neurons in the DMH evokes non-shivering thermogenesis and elevates core body temperature (Zaretskaia et al., 2002), underscoring the importance of the DMH in the regulation of energy expenditure. Recent studies have provided evidence advancing our understanding of how DMH neural signals regulate BAT thermogenesis, particularly specific DMH neurons have been identified (Chao et al., 2011; Dimicco and Zaretsky, 2007; Dodd et al., 2014; Morrison and Nakamura, 2011; Pinol et al., 2018; Zhang et al., 2011). Manipulation of DMH NPY signals using AAV-mediated RNAi revealed that knockdown of NPY in the DMH of rats results in elevated interscapular BAT (IBAT) temperature and strikingly promotes brown adipocyte development in inguinal white adipose tissue (IWAT) and increases IWAT temperature (Figure 5.2) (Chao et al., 2011). This knockdown leads to increased energy expenditure and enhances cold tolerance in rats in response to a cold environment (Chao et al., 2011). Thus, these data demonstrate a critical role for DMH NPY in the regulation of energy expenditure via modulating browning of WAT and BAT thermogenesis. These results also provide new evidence to interpret early findings that central administration of NPY decreases BAT GDP binding activity (indicating decreased thermogenic activity) (Billington et al., 1991) and suppresses sympathetic activity in the IBAT of rats (Egawa et al., 1991), i.e. elevation of DMH NPY neural signaling leads to an inhibitory action on BAT thermogenesis. There is a remaining question about the neural circuits of DMH NPY thermoregulation in the regulation of energy expenditure and body weight.

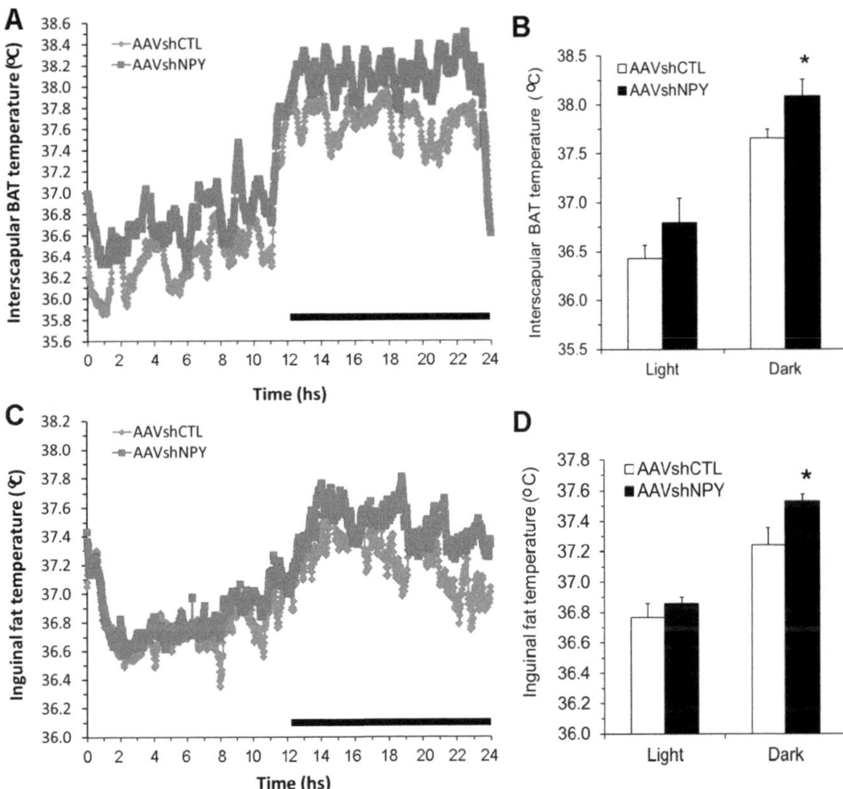

FIGURE 5.2 Effects of DMH NPY knockdown on adipose tissue temperature in rats over a 24 hour period at room temperature. (**A–B**) IBAT temperature. (**C–D**) IWAT temperature. AAVshNPY, rats receiving bilateral DMH injections of AAVshNPY; AAVshCTL, rats receiving bilateral DMH injections of the control vector containing scrambled shRNA. Black bar indicates the dark cycle. Values are mean ± SEM during the light and dark. *P < 0.05 compared to AAVshCTL rats.

Existing evidence has pinpointed potential neuromodulators in modulating DMH NPY thermoregulation. As mentioned above, DMH CCK, but not leptin, has an inhibitory action on DMH NPY neurons through directly interacting with CCK1Rs (Bi et al., 2004; Chen et al., 2008), suggesting that this inhibitory effect on DMH NPY signals may play an important role in modulating IBAT and browning IWAT thermogenesis.

Glucagon-like peptide-1 (GLP-1) is an incretin hormone secreted by intestinal enteroendocrine L-cells postprandially. Centrally, GLP-1 is produced mainly in preproglucagon neurons in the NTS and these preproglucagon neurons project heavily to the PVN and DMH (Rinaman, 1999; Vrang et al., 2007). Of interest, the activation of GLP-1Rs in the DMH of rats via acute microinjection of GLP-1 into the DMH resulted in increases in IBAT and core body temperature as well as a decrease in NPY mRNA expression in the DMH (Lee et al., 2018). In support of this action,

AAV-mediated RNAi for knockdown of GLP-1Rs in the DMH of rats resulted in decreased BAT temperature and energy expenditure and increased expression of NPY in the DMH (Lee et al., 2018), demonstrating that DMH GLP-1 exerts an important role in BAT thermogenesis via activating GLP-1Rs in the DMH and also suggesting that a reduction of DMH NPY signals may underlie this thermogenic effect. *In situ* hybridization histochemistry revealed that the majority of neurons expressing Glp-1r in the DMH of rats are GABAergic and not NPY neurons (Lee et al., 2018), implying that DMH GLP-1 may activate local GABAergic neurons to inhibit DMH NPY signals. It is worth mentioning that in contrast to the findings in rats, acute microinjection of the GLP-1R agonist liraglutide into the DMH of mice did not produce any feeding and thermogenic effects (Beiroa et al., 2014). Since NPY expression is undetectable in the DMH of normal weight mice (Bi, 2013), the negative results from mice may provide additional evidence suggesting the importance or necessity of DMH NPY in the action of DMH GLP-1 in BAT thermoregulation.

In addition, recent studies have shown that DMH MC4R is important for melanocortin regulation of energy expenditure and BAT activation but not food intake in mice (Chen et al., 2017). An induction of NPY expression in the DMH has been found in *Mc4r* knockout mice (Kesterson et al., 1997), implying that this induction may contribute to dysregulation of DMH MC4R signaling in the regulation of thermogenesis and energy expenditure, which merits further investigation.

5.3.3 Glycemic Effect of DMH NPY

While overexpression of NPY in the DMH plays an etiological role in the development of obesity and diabetes of OLETF rats and exacerbates high-fat diet-induced obesity and impaired glucose homeostasis of rats (Yang et al., 2009; Zheng et al., 2013), knockdown of NPY in the DMH ameliorates these alterations (Kim and Bi, 2016; Yang et al., 2009). But whether DMH NPY has a direct effect on glucose homeostasis or the glycemic effect of DMH NPY is secondary to body weight changes remains unanswered. To address this issue, an oral glucose tolerance test was initially carried out. As shown in Figure 5.3A and B, while blood glucose levels in response to an oral glucose challenge did not significantly differ between the two groups of control and NPY knockdown rats with body weight matched, insulin levels were significantly decreased in NPY knockdown rats in both fasting and glucose-challenging conditions (Kim and Bi, 2016), indicating that NPY knockdown rats require less insulin secretion to maintain euglycemia, suggesting that this knockdown increases insulin sensitivity. In contrast, overexpression of NPY in the DMH produces an opposite effect, i.e. rats with DMH NPY overexpression require more insulin secretion to maintain euglycemia (Figure 5.3C and D, Zheng et al., 2013).

The hyperinsulinemic-euglycemic clamp has been widely used as a reference standard for direct determination of insulin sensitivity since it was developed by Defronzo et al. (1979). Using this approach, studies in rats with AAV-mediated knockdown of NPY in the DMH revealed that the glycemic effect of DMH NPY is mainly attributed to increased insulin action on the suppression of hepatic glucose production (HGP), but not through glucose uptake in peripheral tissues including

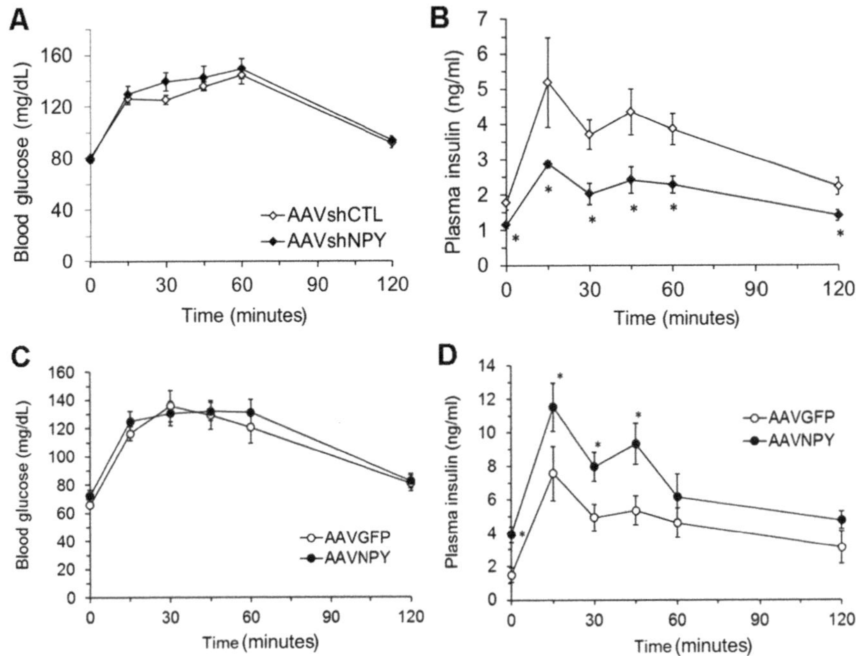

FIGURE 5.3 Effects of DMH NPY on blood glucose and insulin levels in rats in response to oral glucose administration. (**A–B**) DMH NPY knockdown affects blood glucose and insulin levels. (**C–D**) DMH NPY overexpression affects blood glucose and insulin levels. AAVNPY, rats receiving bilateral DMH injections of AAV-mediated expression of NPY; AAVGFP, rats receiving bilateral DMH injections of the control vector. Values are mean ± SEM. $^*P < 0.05$ compared to AAVshCTL or AAVGFP rats.

the liver, adipose tissue, and muscle (Li et al., 2016). Consistent with increased insulin action on HGP, DMH NPY knockdown results in increased hepatic phosphorylation of protein kinase B (Akt, the key molecule in the insulin signaling pathway) (Li et al., 2016). Neuroanatomical studies confirmed that DMH NPY neurons project to the hindbrain NTS and DMV (Figure 5.1) and this knockdown resulted in increased content of the principal vagal neurotransmitter acetylcholine (ACh) in the liver (Li et al., 2016), suggesting that DMH NPY descending signals to the DMV limit hepatic vagal efferent activity to control HGP. Consistent with this view, hepatic vagotomy abrogates the inhibitory effect of DMH NPY knockdown on HGP (Li et al., 2016). Intriguingly, hepatic vagotomy seems to reduce the potency of insulin action as the insulin infusion rate needs to increase in vagotomized rats to achieve the insulin clamp (Li et al., 2016). Hepatic vagotomy also limited the inhibitory effects of DMH NPY knockdown on Akt phosphorylation in the liver (Li et al., 2016). In contrast, the glycemic effect of DMH NPY knockdown was not affected by vagal deafferentation, indicating that vagal afferents are not required for this glycemic effect (Li et al., 2016). Together, these results demonstrate a distinct role for DMH NPY in the regulation of glucose homeostasis through hepatic vagal efferents and insulin action on HGP.

5.4 DETERMINATION OF DMH NEURONAL FUNCTIONS VIA AAV-MEDIATED GENE EXPRESSION

The recombinant vector of AAV-mediated gene expression is aimed at replenishing mutant or deficient genes to restore gene function as gene therapy or to study gene function as a "gain-of-function" approach. OLETF rats have a congenital defect in the expression of the *Cck1r* gene, resulting in a lack of CCK1Rs (Takiguchi et al., 1997). To determine a specific role for DMH CCK1Rs in the development of obesity and diabetes of OLETF rats, CCK1Rs were replenished in the DMH of OLETF rats via the delivery of AAV vector expressing CCK1Rs into the DMH (Zhu et al., 2012). Gene expression determination confirmed that this injection brought about 65% *Cck1r* mRNA expression in the DMH of OLETF rats compared to that of lean Long–Evans Tokushima Otsuka (LETO) control rats (Zhu et al., 2012). Although the exact replenishment in endogenous CCK1R neurons in the DMH of OLETF rats was unable to be determined, this replenishment did demonstrate the important role of DMH CCK1Rs in the control of meal size; meal patterns were partially normalized in OLETF rats receiving AAVCCK1R with a significant decrease in meal size during the dark (Zhu et al., 2012). This finding is consistent with an earlier report showing that DMH NPY mainly produces a nocturnal and meal size-specific feeding effect (Yang et al., 2009). Importantly, the results from CCK1R replacement revealed a novel role for DMH CCK1R signaling in glucose homeostatic regulation as this replacement lowered plasma glucose levels of OLETF rats and parenchymal microinjection of CCK into the DMH of intact rats enhanced glucose tolerance (Zhu et al., 2012). Since DMH NPY modulates hepatic insulin sensitivity to affect glucose homeostasis (Li et al., 2016), these data provide additional evidence suggesting that DMH CCK may modulate DMH NPY regulation of glucose homeostasis through interacting with CCK1Rs in the DMH.

Using AAV-mediated overexpression of NPY in the DMH of rats, researchers have confirmed the effects of DMH NPY overexpression on food intake, body weight, and glucose homeostasis as seen in OLETF rats that develop hyperphagia, obesity, and impaired glucose homeostasis (Yang et al., 2009; Zheng et al., 2013), providing additional support for the role of DMH NPY in the regulation of energy balance and glucose homeostasis. There is a caveat that AAV-mediated gene delivery may infect neurons nonspecifically, such as DMH CCK1R replenishment or DMH NPY overexpression, though this approach is still important for addressing specific questions including identifying (e.g. DMH CCK1Rs) or verifying (e.g. DMH NPY) gene function. Thus, the results from the gene expression approach will also provide critical and supportive evidence for determining gene function.

5.5 CHEMOGENETIC DETERMINATION OF DMH NEURONAL FUNCTIONS

Physical activity or exercise provides numerous health benefits and is an important lifestyle intervention in fighting metabolic diseases such as obesity and type 2 diabetes. Systemically, exercise causes increased energy expenditure, leading to increases in fuel use in muscle, lipolysis in adipose tissue, and fat catabolism in the liver (Borer, 2003). However, the effects of exercise on hypothalamic regulation of energy balance or how changes in hypothalamic signals contribute to the effects of exercise on energy balance is poorly understood. While physical exercise (e.g. voluntary access to running wheels) exerts a profound action in the control of obesity in certain obesity models, including OLETF rats (Bi et al., 2005), diet-induced obese (DIO) rats (Levin and Dunn-Meynell, 2004), and *Mc4r* knockout mice (Irani et al., 2005), exercise appears less effective in obese animals with a deficit in leptin signaling in both leptin deficient ob/ob mice (Dubuc et al., 1984) and leptin receptor deficient Zucker fatty rats (Stern and Johnson, 1977), suggesting that intact leptin signaling is important for the effects of physical exercise on body weight regulation. In support of this notion, using the immediate early gene product c-Fos as a marker of neuronal activation, c-Fos immunohistochemistry revealed that, while running activity produced c-Fos activation in both hypothalamus and extra-hypothalamic areas of intact rats including the PVN and DMH as well as the central nucleus of the amygdala (CeA), area postrema (AP), and NTS, this running activity induced significant c-Fos activation in the CeA, AP, and NTS, but not the PVN and DMH in Zucker fatty rats (Zhang et al., 2018). Within the DMH, exercise-induced c-Fos activation was widely distributed in intact rats, particularly in the ventral and caudal DMH, whereas this c-Fos activation was not observed in Zucker fatty rats (Zhang et al., 2018), suggesting that this population of DMH neurons may play an important role in mediating the feeding and body weight effects of physical exercise.

The designer receptors exclusively activated by designer drugs (DREADD)-based chemogenetic tools provide unique approaches for the *in vivo* study of neuronal functions (Roth, 2016). Among G protein-coupled DREADDs, the hM3D(Gq) DREADD contains engineered human M3 muscarinic receptors and is typically used for neuronal excitation (Roth, 2016). This receptor can be activated by the selective designer drug clozapine N-oxide (CNO, Armbruster et al., 2007). The findings of exercise-induced c-Fos activation in the DMH of intact rats, particularly in the ventral and caudal DMH where LepRb expressing-neurons are located (Bi et al., 2003; Elmquist et al., 1998) and where this c-Fos activation is not observed in Zucker fatty rats (Zhang et al., 2018), suggest that Zucker fatty rats have a deficit in exercise-induced activation of DMH neurons (likely LepRb expressing-neurons), leading to ineffectiveness of physical exercise on food intake and body weight. In support of this view, chemogenetic stimulation of neurons in these DMH subregions of Zucker fatty rats receiving AAV-mediated DREADD (AAV5-hSyn-hM3D(Gq)-mCherry) significantly increased running activity and decreased food intake and body weight of these rats (Zhang et al., 2018). Thus, these results demonstrate that ventral and caudal DMH neurons contribute to the action of the DMH in the regulation of physical activity and food intake, implying that leptin and/or other factors may act on these neurons to modulate physical activity, food intake, and body weight.

5.6 OPTOGENETIC DETERMINATION OF DMH NEURONAL FUNCTIONS

Mapping the targets of leptin in the brain using the mouse LepRb-IRES-Cre reporter line revealed large numbers of GFP-staining cells in the dorsal and ventral subregions of the DMH and very few GFP cells were found in the compact subregion of the DMH in mice (Scott et al., 2009), suggesting that LepRb-expressing neurons in the dorsal and ventral DMH may mediate leptin action in the regulation of food intake and energy expenditure. Subsequent studies provided evidence that LepRb neurons in different subregions of the DMH play distinct roles in energy balance regulation. Activation of LepRb neurons in the dorsal DMH/dorsal hypothalamic area (DHA) of mice promotes BAT thermogenesis (via innervating rostral raphe pallidus neurons) and locomotor activity, leading to increased energy expenditure and decreased body weight, but does not affect food intake (Rezai-Zadeh et al., 2014; Zhang et al., 2011), whereas LepRb neurons in the ventral DMH of mice exert a feeding inhibitory action as LepRb neurons in the ventral DMH send inhibitory GABAergic input to AgRP neurons in the ARC to modulate feeding behavior (Garfield et al., 2016). In addition, the RFamide prolactin-releasing peptide (PrRP)-expressing neurons in the caudal DMH of mice mediate the thermogenic effect of leptin; DMH PrRP neurons can be activated by leptin, and selective disruption of LepRbs in these neurons blocks the thermogenic responses to leptin and causes obesity (Dodd et al., 2014). Surprisingly, although DMH LepRb neurons mainly project to the PVN (Gautron et al., 2010), a role for this pathway in the control of food intake and energy expenditure remains undetermined.

Optogenetics is a state-of-the-art technique that creates light-sensitive ion channels in neurons to study neuronal function in the body via manipulating light-induced neuronal activity (stimulation or inhibition). This method can also be used to modulate neural activity at the axonal projections/terminals to map neural circuits. Using this approach, Otgon-Uul et al. (2016) have identified the important role of DMH GABAergic neurons in the regulation of energy balance. ChRFR-C167A is a bistable variant of chimeric channelrhodopsin that provides bimodal regulation: illumination of blue light (470 nm) induces long lasting opening which can be canceled by illumination of yellow light (592 nm). In the study, AAV-mediated ChRFR-C167A-Venus under the control of a GAD1 promoter was delivered into the DMH of mice (Otgon-Uul et al., 2016). Data showed that optogenetic activation of GABAergic neurons in the DMH promoted food intake (Otgon-Uul et al., 2016). Patch clamp recording further determined that leptin hyperpolarized and lowering glucose depolarized DMH GABAergic neurons, indicating that DMH GABAergic neurons are modulated by leptin and glucose signals (Otgon-Uul et al., 2016). Furthermore, light illumination in the PVN via optical fiber targeted in the PVN resulted in the increased food intake of mice receiving AAV-mediated ChRFR-C167A-Venus in the DMH (Otgon-Uul et al., 2016). Thus, these results provide new evidence suggesting that DMH GABAergic neurons send inhibitory signals to the PVN to limit PVN neuronal activity to modulate food intake. But whether DMH GABAergic neurons projecting to the PVN are LepRb-expressing neurons, and what the specific location of these GABAergic neurons within the DMH is, are not determined. The identity of PVN neurons innervated by these DMH GABAergic neurons is also undetermined. Nevertheless, the optogenetics allow the researchers to identify a new neural pathway of DMH GABAergic innervation on PVN neurons in the control of food intake and energy balance.

5.7 CONCLUSIONS

Using AAV-mediated manipulation of gene expression in the DMH, researchers have demonstrated distinct actions of DMH neural signaling in the regulation of energy balance and glucose homeostasis. In particular, DMH NPY serves as an important orexigenic output of the DMH to affect food intake, brown fat thermogenesis, energy expenditure, and glucose homeostasis. DMH NPY descending signals to the NTS and DMV modulate local satiety signaling and hepatic vagal efferent activity to affect food intake and hepatic glucose production. DMH NPY neural signaling is affected by DMH CCK and indirectly by DMH GLP-1, but not by leptin. While leptin receptor-expressing neurons in different DMH subregions exert distinct actions in the control of food intake and energy expenditure, the targets and neural circuits of these actions merit further investigation. Overall, growing evidence has established that the DMH plays critical roles in maintaining energy balance and glucose homeostasis. Identification of the neural mechanism of these actions will provide potential strategies for preventing and/or treating obesity, diabetes, and their associated comorbidities.

ACKNOWLEDGMENTS

The work from the authors' laboratory was supported by the US National Institute of Diabetes and Digestive and Kidney Diseases Grants DK103710 and DK104867.

REFERENCES

Anand, B.K., and Brobeck, J.R. (1951). Localization of a "feeding center" in the hypothalamus of the rat. *Proceedings of the Society for Experimental Biology and Medicine 77*, 323–324.

Andermann, M.L., and Lowell, B.B. (2017). Toward a wiring giagram understanding of appetite control. *Neuron 95*, 757–778.

Armbruster, B.N., Li, X., Pausch, M.H., Herlitze, S., and Roth, B.L. (2007). Evolving the lock to fit the key to create a family of G protein-coupled receptors potently activated by an inert ligand. *Proceedings of the National Academy of Sciences of the United States of America 104*, 5163–5168.

Beck, B. (2006). Neuropeptide Y in normal eating and in genetic and dietary-induced obesity. *Philosophical Transactions of the Royal Society of London. Series B, Biological Sciences 361*, 1159–1185.

Beiroa, D., Imbernon, M., Gallego, R., Senra, A., Herranz, D., Villarroya, F., Serrano, M., Ferno, J., Salvador, J., Escalada, J., et al. (2014). GLP-1 agonism stimulates brown adipose tissue thermogenesis and browning through hypothalamic AMPK. *Diabetes 63*, 3346–3358.

Bernardis, L.L., Box, B.M., and Stevenson, J.A. (1963). Growth following hypothalamic lesions in the weanling rat. *Endocrinology 72*, 684–692.

Bi, S. (2013). Dorsomedial hypothalamic NPY modulation of adiposity and thermogenesis. *Physiology & Behavior 121*, 56–60.

Bi, S., Kim, Y.J., and Zheng, F. (2012). Dorsomedial hypothalamic NPY and energy balance control. *Neuropeptides 46*, 309–314.

Bi, S., Ladenheim, E.E., Schwartz, G.J., and Moran, T.H. (2001). A role for NPY overexpression in the dorsomedial hypothalamus in hyperphagia and obesity of OLETF rats. *American Journal of Physiology. Regulatory, Integrative and Comparative Physiology 281*, R254–R260.

Bi, S., Robinson, B.M., and Moran, T.H. (2003). Acute food deprivation and chronic food restriction differentially affect hypothalamic NPY mRNA expression. *American Journal of Physiology. Regulatory, Integrative and Comparative Physiology 285*, R1030–R1036.

Bi, S., Scott, K.A., Hyun, J., Ladenheim, E.E., and Moran, T.H. (2005). Running wheel activity prevents hyperphagia and obesity in Otsuka long-evans Tokushima Fatty rats: role of hypothalamic signaling. *Endocrinology 146*, 1676–1685.

Bi, S., Scott, K.A., Kopin, A.S., and Moran, T.H. (2004). Differential roles for cholecystokinin a receptors in energy balance in rats and mice. *Endocrinology 145*, 3873–3880.

Billington, C.J., Briggs, J.E., Grace, M., and Levine, A.S. (1991). Effects of intracerebroventricular injection of neuropeptide Y on energy metabolism. *The American Journal of Physiology 260*, R321–R327.

Borer, K. (2003). *Exercise Endocrinology*. 2nd Edition, Human Kinetics, Champaign, IL.

Cady, G., Landeryou, T., Garratt, M., Kopchick, J.J., Qi, N., Garcia-Galiano, D., Elias, C.F., Myers, M.G., Jr., Miller, R.A., Sandoval, D.A., et al. (2017). Hypothalamic growth hormone receptor (GHR) controls hepatic glucose production in nutrient-sensing leptin receptor (LepRb) expressing neurons. *Molecular Metabolism 6*, 393–405.

Cannon, B., and Nedergaard, J. (2004). Brown adipose tissue: function and physiological significance. *Physiological Reviews 84*, 277–359.

Chao, P.T., Yang, L., Aja, S., Moran, T.H., and Bi, S. (2011). Knockdown of NPY expression in the dorsomedial hypothalamus promotes development of brown adipocytes and prevents diet-induced obesity. *Cell Metabolism 13*, 573–583.

Chen, J., Scott, K.A., Zhao, Z., Moran, T.H., and Bi, S. (2008). Characterization of the feeding inhibition and neural activation produced by dorsomedial hypothalamic cholecystokinin administration. *Neuroscience 152*, 178–188.

Chen, M., Shrestha, Y.B., Podyma, B., Cui, Z., Naglieri, B., Sun, H., Ho, T., Wilson, E.A., Li, Y.Q., Gavrilova, O., et al. (2017). Gsalpha deficiency in the dorsomedial hypothalamus underlies obesity associated with Gsalpha mutations. *The Journal of Clinical Investigation 127*, 500–510.

Cone, R.D. (2006). Studies on the physiological functions of the melanocortin system. *Endocrine Reviews 27*, 736–749.

de La Serre, C.B., Kim, Y.J., Moran, T.H., and Bi, S. (2016). Dorsomedial hypothalamic NPY affects cholecystokinin-induced satiety via modulation of brain stem catecholamine neuronal signaling. *American Journal of Physiology. Regulatory, Integrative and Comparative Physiology 311*, R930–R939.

DeFronzo, R.A., Tobin, J.D., and Andres, R. (1979). Glucose clamp technique: a method for quantifying insulin secretion and resistance. *The American Journal of Physiology 237*, E214–E223.

Dimicco, J.A., and Zaretsky, D.V. (2007). The dorsomedial hypothalamus: a new player in thermoregulation. *American Journal of Physiology. Regulatory, Integrative and Comparative Physiology 292*, R47–R63.

Dodd, G.T., Worth, A.A., Nunn, N., Korpal, A.K., Bechtold, D.A., Allison, M.B., Myers, M.G., Jr., Statnick, M.A., and Luckman, S.M. (2014). The thermogenic effect of leptin is dependent on a distinct population of prolactin-releasing peptide neurons in the dorsomedial hypothalamus. *Cell Metabolism 20*, 639–649.

Dubuc, P.U., Cahn, P.J., and Willis, P. (1984). The effects of exercise and food restriction on obesity and diabetes in young ob/ob mice. *International Journal of Obesity 8*, 271–278.

Egawa, M., Yoshimatsu, H., and Bray, G.A. (1991). Neuropeptide Y suppresses sympathetic activity to interscapular brown adipose tissue in rats. *The American Journal of Physiology 260*, R328–R334.

Elmquist, J.K., Bjorbaek, C., Ahima, R.S., Flier, J.S., and Saper, C.B. (1998). Distributions of leptin receptor mRNA isoforms in the rat brain. *The Journal of Comparative Neurology 395*, 535–547.

Elmquist, J.K., Elias, C.F., and Saper, C.B. (1999). From lesions to leptin: hypothalamic control of food intake and body weight. *Neuron 22*, 221–232.

Fire, A., Xu, S., Montgomery, M.K., Kostas, S.A., Driver, S.E., and Mello, C.C. (1998). Potent and specific genetic interference by double-stranded RNA in Caenorhabditis elegans. *Nature 391*, 806–811.

Friedman, J. (2014). 20 YEARS OF LEPTIN: Leptin at 20: an overview. *The Journal of Endocrinology 223*, T1–T8.

Garfield, A.S., Shah, B.P., Burgess, C.R., Li, M.M., Li, C., Steger, J.S., Madara, J.C., Campbell, J.N., Kroeger, D., Scammell, T.E., et al. (2016). Dynamic GABAergic afferent modulation of AgRP neurons. *Nature Neuroscience 19*, 1628–1635.

Gautron, L., and Elmquist, J.K. (2011). Sixteen years and counting: an update on leptin in energy balance. *The Journal of Clinical Investigation 121*, 2087–2093.

Gautron, L., Lazarus, M., Scott, M.M., Saper, C.B., and Elmquist, J.K. (2010). Identifying the efferent projections of leptin-responsive neurons in the dorsomedial hypothalamus using a novel conditional tracing approach. *The Journal of Comparative Neurology 518*, 2090–2108.

Guan, X.M., Yu, H., Trumbauer, M., Frazier, E., Van der Ploeg, L.H., and Chen, H. (1998a). Induction of neuropeptide Y expression in dorsomedial hypothalamus of diet-induced obese mice. *Neuroreport 9*, 3415–3419.

Guan, X.M., Yu, H., and Van der Ploeg, L.H. (1998b). Evidence of altered hypothalamic pro-opiomelanocortin/ neuropeptide Y mRNA expression in tubby mice. *Brain Research. Molecular Brain Research 59*, 273–279.

Hetherington, A.W., and Ranson, S.W. (1940). Hypothalamic lesions and adiposity in the rat. *The Anatomical Record 78*, 149–172.

Hill, D.R., Shaw, T.M., Graham, W., and Woodruff, G.N. (1990). Autoradiographical detection of cholecystokinin-A receptors in primate brain using 125I-Bolton Hunter CCK-8 and 3H-MK-329. *The Journal of Neuroscience: The Official Journal of the Society for Neuroscience 10*, 1070–1081.

Irani, B.G., Xiang, Z., Moore, M.C., Mandel, R.J., and Haskell-Luevano, C. (2005). Voluntary exercise delays monogenetic obesity and overcomes reproductive dysfunction of the melanocortin-4 receptor knockout mouse. *Biochemical and Biophysical Research Communications 326*, 638–644.

Kawaguchi, M., Scott, K.A., Moran, T.H., and Bi, S. (2005). Dorsomedial hypothalamic corticotropin-releasing factor mediation of exercise-induced anorexia. *American Journal of Physiology. Regulatory, Integrative and Comparative Physiology 288*, R1800–R1805.

Kesterson, R.A., Huszar, D., Lynch, C.A., Simerly, R.B., and Cone, R.D. (1997). Induction of neuropeptide Y gene expression in the dorsal medial hypothalamic nucleus in two models of the agouti obesity syndrome. *Molecular Endocrinology 11*, 630–637.

Kim, Y.J., and Bi, S. (2016). Knockdown of neuropeptide Y in the dorsomedial hypothalamus reverses high-fat diet-induced obesity and impaired glucose tolerance in rats. *American Journal of Physiology. Regulatory, Integrative and Comparative Physiology 310*, R134–R142.

Lee, S.J., Sanchez-Watts, G., Krieger, J.P., Pignalosa, A., Norell, P.N., Cortella, A., Pettersen, K.G., Vrdoljak, D., Hayes, M.R., Kanoski, S.E., et al. (2018). Loss of dorsomedial hypothalamic GLP-1 signaling reduces BAT thermogenesis and increases adiposity. *Molecular Metabolism 11*, 33–46.

Levin, B.E., and Dunn-Meynell, A.A. (2004). Chronic exercise lowers the defended body weight gain and adiposity in diet-induced obese rats. *American Journal of Physiology. Regulatory, Integrative and Comparative Physiology 286*, R771–R778.

Li, L., de La Serre, C.B., Zhang, N., Yang, L., Li, H., and Bi, S. (2016). Knockdown of neuropeptide y in the dorsomedial hypothalamus promotes hepatic insulin sensitivity in male rats. *Endocrinology 157*, 4842–4852.

Morrison, S.F., Madden, C.J., and Tupone, D. (2014). Central neural regulation of brown adipose tissue thermogenesis and energy expenditure. *Cell Metabolism.*

Morrison, S.F., and Nakamura, K. (2011). Central neural pathways for thermoregulation. *Frontiers in Bioscience: a Journal and Virtual Library 16*, 74–104.

Morton, G.J., Cummings, D.E., Baskin, D.G., Barsh, G.S., and Schwartz, M.W. (2006). Central nervous system control of food intake and body weight. *Nature 443*, 289–295.

Okada, T., Nomoto, T., Shimazaki, K., Lijun, W., Lu, Y., Matsushita, T., Mizukami, H., Urabe, M., Hanazono, Y., Kume, A., et al. (2002). Adeno-associated virus vectors for gene transfer to the brain. *Methods 28*, 237–247.

Otgon-Uul, Z., Suyama, S., Onodera, H., and Yada, T. (2016). Optogenetic activation of leptin- and glucose-regulated GABAergic neurons in dorsomedial hypothalamus promotes food intake via inhibitory synaptic transmission to paraventricular nucleus of hypothalamus. *Molecular Metabolism 5*, 709–715.

Passini, M.A., Watson, D.J., and Wolfe, J.H. (2004). Gene delivery to the mouse brain with adeno-associated virus. *Methods in Molecular Biology 246*, 225–236.

Picard, A., Soyer, J., Berney, X., Tarussio, D., Quenneville, S., Jan, M., Grouzmann, E., Burdet, F., Ibberson, M., and Thorens, B. (2016). A Genetic Screen Identifies Hypothalamic Fgf15 as a Regulator of Glucagon Secretion. *Cell Reports 17*, 1795–1806.

Pinol, R.A., Zahler, S.H., Li, C., Saha, A., Tan, B.K., Skop, V., Gavrilova, O., Xiao, C., Krashes, M.J., and Reitman, M.L. (2018). Brs3 neurons in the mouse dorsomedial hypothalamus regulate body temperature, energy expenditure, and heart rate, but not food intake. *Nature Neuroscience 21*, 1530–1540.

Rezai-Zadeh, K., and Munzberg, H. (2013). Integration of sensory information via central thermoregulatory leptin targets. *Physiology & Behavior 121*, 49–55.

Rezai-Zadeh, K., Yu, S., Jiang, Y., Laque, A., Schwartzenburg, C., Morrison, C.D., Derbenev, A.V., Zsombok, A., and Munzberg, H. (2014). Leptin receptor neurons in the dorsomedial hypothalamus are key regulators of energy expenditure and body weight, but not food intake. *Molecular Metabolism 3*, 681–693.

Rinaman, L. (1999). Interoceptive stress activates glucagon-like peptide-1 neurons that project to the hypothalamus. *The American Journal of Physiology 277*, R582–R590.

Roth, B.L. (2016). DREADDs for neuroscientists. *Neuron 89*, 683–694.

Sanacora, G., Kershaw, M., Finkelstein, J.A., and White, J.D. (1990). Increased hypothalamic content of preproneuropeptide Y messenger ribonucleic acid in genetically obese Zucker rats and its regulation by food deprivation. *Endocrinology 127*, 730–737.

Schroeder, M., Zagoory-Sharon, O., Shbiro, L., Marco, A., Hyun, J., Moran, T.H., Bi, S., and Weller, A. (2009). Development of obesity in the Otsuka Long-Evans Tokushima Fatty rat. *American Journal of Physiology. Regulatory, Integrative and Comparative Physiology 297*, R1749–R1760.

Scott, M.M., Lachey, J.L., Sternson, S.M., Lee, C.E., Elias, C.F., Friedman, J.M., and Elmquist, J.K. (2009). Leptin targets in the mouse brain. *The Journal of Comparative Neurology 514*, 518–532.

Smith, M.S. (1993). Lactation alters neuropeptide-Y and proopiomelanocortin gene expression in the arcuate nucleus of the rat. *Endocrinology 133*, 1258–1265.

Stellar, E. (1954). The physiology of motivation. *Psychological Review 61*, 5–22.

Stern, J.S., and Johnson, P.R. (1977). Spontaneous activity and adipose cellularity in the genetically obese Zucker rat (fafa). *Metabolism, Clinical and Experimental 26*, 371–380.

Takiguchi, S., Takata, Y., Funakoshi, A., Miyasaka, K., Kataoka, K., Fujimura, Y., Goto, T., and Kono, A. (1997). Disrupted cholecystokinin type-A receptor (CCKAR) gene in OLETF rats. *Gene 197*, 169–175.

Thompson, R.H., Canteras, N.S., and Swanson, L.W. (1996). Organization of projections from the dorsomedial nucleus of the hypothalamus: a PHA-L study in the rat. *The Journal of Comparative Neurology 376*, 143–173.

Tritos, N.A., Elmquist, J.K., Mastaitis, J.W., Flier, J.S., and Maratos-Flier, E. (1998). Characterization of expression of hypothalamic appetite-regulating peptides in obese hyperleptinemic brown adipose tissue-deficient (uncoupling protein-promoter-driven diphtheria toxin A) mice. *Endocrinology 139*, 4634–4641.

Vrang, N., Hansen, M., Larsen, P.J., and Tang-Christensen, M. (2007). Characterization of brainstem preproglucagon projections to the paraventricular and dorsomedial hypothalamic nuclei. *Brain Research 1149*, 118–126.

Waterson, M.J., and Horvath, T.L. (2015). Neuronal regulation of energy homeostasis: Beyond the hypothalamus and feeding. *Cell Metabolism 22*, 962–970.

Wilding, J.P., Gilbey, S.G., Bailey, C.J., Batt, R.A., Williams, G., Ghatei, M.A., and Bloom, S.R. (1993). Increased neuropeptide-Y messenger ribonucleic acid (mRNA) and decreased neurotensin mRNA in the hypothalamus of the obese (ob/ob) mouse. *Endocrinology 132*, 1939–1944.

Yang, L., Scott, K.A., Hyun, J., Tamashiro, K.L., Tray, N., Moran, T.H., and Bi, S. (2009). Role of dorsomedial hypothalamic neuropeptide Y in modulating food intake and energy balance. *The Journal of Neuroscience: The Official Journal of the Society for Neuroscience 29*, 179–190.

Zaretskaia, M.V., Zaretsky, D.V., Shekhar, A., and DiMicco, J.A. (2002). Chemical stimulation of the dorsomedial hypothalamus evokes non-shivering thermogenesis in anesthetized rats. *Brain Research 928*, 113–125.

Zhang, N., Yang, L., Guo, L., and Bi, S. (2018). Activation of dorsomedial hypothalamic neurons promotes physical activity and decreases food intake and body weight in zucker fatty rats. *Frontiers in Molecular Neuroscience 11*, 179.

Zhang, Y., Kerman, I.A., Laque, A., Nguyen, P., Faouzi, M., Louis, G.W., Jones, J.C., Rhodes, C., and Munzberg, H. (2011). Leptin-receptor-expressing neurons in the dorsomedial hypothalamus and median preoptic area regulate sympathetic brown adipose tissue circuits. *The Journal of Neuroscience: The Official Journal of the Society for Neuroscience 31*, 1873–1884.

Zheng, F., Kim, Y.J., Chao, P.T., and Bi, S. (2013). Overexpression of neuropeptide y in the dorsomedial hypothalamus causes hyperphagia and obesity in rats. *Obesity 21*, 1086–1092.

Zhu, G., Yan, J., Smith, W.W., Moran, T.H., and Bi, S. (2012). Roles of dorsomedial hypothalamic cholecystokinin signaling in the controls of meal patterns and glucose homeostasis. *Physiology & Behavior 105*, 234–241.

6 The Ventromedial Hypothalamic Nucleus in the Regulation of Energy Homeostasis

Le Trung Tran and Ki Woo Kim

Departments of Oral Biology and Applied Biological Science, BK21 Four, Yonsei University College of Dentistry, Seoul, 03722, Korea

CONTENTS

6.1 INTRODUCTION

In order to maintain an appropriate energy state for the body, numerous signals regarding body nutrient availability, feeding status, and the amount of heat required for maintaining body functions are processed by the central nervous system (CNS). The harmony provided by the CNS keeps the ratio of food intake and energy expenditure stable, preserving a balanced body weight. A mismatch in the intake versus expenditure would result in metabolic dysregulation and diseases, such as obesity and diabetes.

When discussing the central regulation of energy homeostasis, one of the most overlooked areas is the ventromedial nucleus of the hypothalamus (VMH). First described by the Spanish neuroscientist S. R. Cajal in the early 19th century, this brain region was identified as the center of satiety responsible for controlling food intake and body weight, converging nutrient signals, and orchestrating appetite. The VMH later stirred up controversy surrounding its role in feeding behaviors. Nowadays, a number of textbooks and review articles put aside the historic VMH when discussing neural circuits involved in the mechanism of body weight maintenance. However, new lines of evidence have demonstrated that the VMH is a central hub for the maintenance of energy homeostasis. This chapter, therefore, focuses on the VMH, its structural architecture, and its steroidogenic factor-1 (SF1) neurons – one representative subset of VMH cell populations – to shine some light on the importance of this humble hypothalamic region. We also underline the significant roles of SF1 neurons in homeostatic regulation, particularly in energy and glucose homeostasis. Novel discoveries of non-SF1 neuronal populations within the VMH will also be discussed briefly.

6.2 THE VENTROMEDIAL NUCLEUS OF THE HYPOTHALAMUS (VMH)

The term "ventromedial nucleus of the hypothalamus (VMH)," hereafter, refers only to the ventromedial hypothalamic nucleus, its capsule, and its projections. The nomenclature should be clarified to avoid any confusion between the VMH and the mediobasal hypothalamus (containing different nuclei), a rather general area of the hypothalamus including not only the VMH itself but also other surrounding hypothalamic nuclei. The abbreviation VMH follows the popular stereotaxic atlas by Paxinos and Watson [1], as well as the adult mouse brain atlas from the Allen Institute for Brain Science.

6.2.1 ANATOMY

Highly conserved across different species [2], the VMH is a distinct group of neurons in the mediobasal (also known as the intermediate) hypothalamus. This cell population is close to the base of the diencephalon and the third ventricle (Figure 6.1). This region can be seen with Cresyl Violet stain (Nissl staining) on sagittal and coronal slices as an oval, pear-shaped bilateral nucleus. Easily distinguishable from the surrounding cell-poor and dendritic processes-rich zone (usually referred to as the "shell" or "capsule") [3], the VMH, also known as the "core," is a cell-rich area with clear separation from the adjacent nuclei [4,5]. Most of the VMH axons are beaded and, along with afferent dendrites to the VMH, form a dendritic grid encircling the core [6]. This nucleus, spanning laterally through a length of around 1mm in the house mouse (*Mus musculus)* brain, is surrounded by the anterior hypothalamus and dorsomedial hypothalamus at its rostral and caudal superior, and the arcuate nucleus and median eminence at its inferior. Laterally, it is bounded by lateral hypothalamic nuclei (Figure 6.1A).

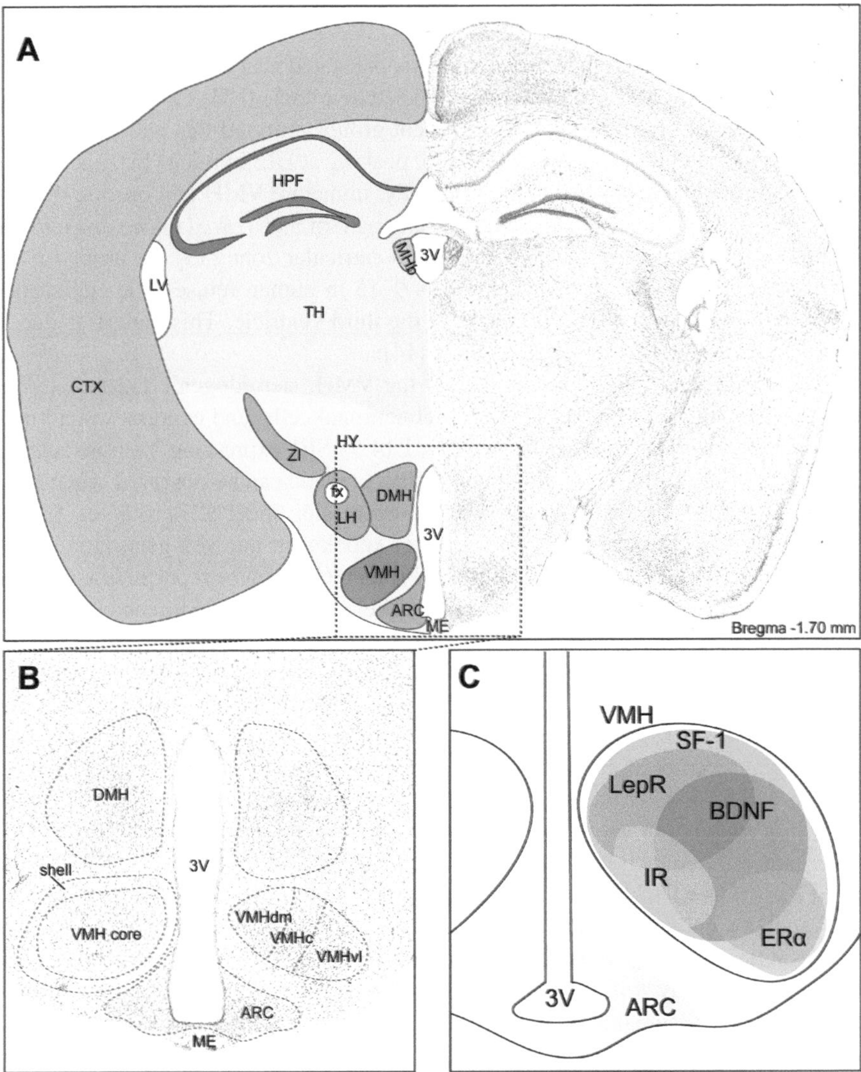

FIGURE 6.1 Anatomy and cytoarchitecture of the VMH. (**A**) Nissl-stained coronal section of a P84 mouse brain, with simplified atlas (adapted from the ***Allen Brain Atlas*** (7)) for landmarking hypothalamic nuclei. (**B**) The mediobasal hypothalamus, with clear divisions of the VMH. (**C**) Neuronal subset distribution of the VMH. Based on data from (8).

Based on the anatomical position, neuronal populations, and functions, the VMH is further divided into four subdivisions: the anterior (VMHa), two clear parts of the dorsomedial (VMHdm), the central (VMHc), and the ventrolateral (VMHvl) (9). The cell density is higher in the peripheral regions (i.e. dorsomedial and ventrolateral) than in the center of the nucleus. These subdivisions are easily distinguishable by Nissl staining on coronal brain sections, but are harder to find on sagittal planes (Figure 6.1.B).

6.2.2 Development and Cytoarchitecture

VMH cells originated from neuronal precursors located near the lower portion of the third ventricle [10]. Using radioactively labeled thymidine ([^{3}H] thymidine) to determine the time of origin of neurons, different groups reported that cell proliferation starts early on embryonic day (E) 10 to 15, peaking at E13 in mice [11], and around E30 in non-human primates [12]. Genetically, immature VMH neurons are derived from precursors with the expression pattern of *Rax*(+)/*Nkx2.1*(+)/*Six3*-high/*Otp*(−)/*Nkx2.2*(+) in the hypothalamic ventricular zone [13]. At around E16–E17 in mice, E18–E19 in rats, and weeks 9–15 in human fetuses, the egg-shaped VMH begins to surface on either side of the third ventricle. This pattern is due to neuronal migrations under the glial guide [14].

One crucial and ubiquitous marker of the VMH, steroidogenic factor 1 (SF-1; NR5A1), emerges at around E9.5 in VMH neuronal cells, and expresses in all neurons during neurogenesis. However, by E14.5, SF1-expressing neurons cluster around the VMHdm. This developmental characteristic can be observed when comparing the mouse lines with Cre recombinase expression under SF1 promoter (*Sf-Cre*) crossing with a reporter line versus reporter-knockin in the SF1 gene [15], as the Cre-driven expression of green fluorescent Protein (GFP) in the reporter line is linked to the SF1 lineage of cells during neuronal development. The SF1 gene owns a conserved VMH-specific enhancer in intron 6, which displays a high degree of tissue specificity in development [16]. SF1 shows essential roles in VMH cytoarchitecture, as knocking out SF1 showed hypocellularity in the VMH and aberrant expression of other VMH neuronal populations, such as brain-derived neurotrophic factor (Bdnf) or estrogen receptor alpha (ERα), as well as diminished or altered neuronal projections to and from other brain regions. SF1 acts as a critical transcription factor in the VMH, as its binding sites are found upstream of many different genes, including other transcription factors such as *Nkx2.2* or neuronal marker *Bdnf* [16–18]. The role of SF1 neurons will be discussed further in this chapter.

Another significant factor that affects the migration of VMH neurons is neurotransmitter signaling. Expressing γ-aminobutyric acid (GABA) A and B receptors, VMH neurons may follow GABA signaling during differentiation and movement. $GABA_A$ receptor signaling affects cell orientation [19], while activation of $GABA_B$ receptors slows down cell movement [20]. However, the interaction between these receptors still requires further study.

6.3 THE HISTORICAL VIEW ON THE ROLES OF THE VMH

Through the process of developing the technique for hypophysectomy and understanding the complications after pituitary removal, very early studies show that the concomitant extreme obesity is due to damage of adjacent hypothalamic areas, not the ablation of the pituitary [21–23]. In the 1930s, early studies using mechanical lesions, electrode implantation, or procaine injection into rats' VMH showed an increase in food intake, along with voracious eating behavior and significant weight gain. In those rats, increased appetite appears immediately after recovery from lesions or, in conscious animals, after injection. The hyperphagic phenotype in these rats is characterized by rapid weight gain (doubling in just 30 days) with an increase in both meal size and meal frequency, and some animals show an aberrant circadian pattern and remarkably high food intake even during the light phase. The size of the lesions is correlated with the degree of hyperphagia, as bilateral lesions produced maximum obesity [24]. Apart from rats, hyperphagia and obesity also occurred in other species, including other rodents [25], birds [26,27], other mammals, and non-human primates [28,29] when given VMH lesions. However, it is debatable whether the irritation from the metal stereotaxic/electroablation apparatus [30,31], the accidental damage to other proximal regions (e.g. the arcuate nucleus or the ventral noradrenergic bundle [32–34]), or the VMH lesion itself caused obesity. Also, some evidence shows that the obese phenotype is due to a metabolic and autonomic disorder, rather than feeding behavior. To highlight the role of the VMH, ample genetic studies have been performed to support its importance.

6.4 THE SF1 NEURONS

6.4.1 SF1 as a Marker of the VMH

To obtain clear insight into the functions of the VMH and to avoid any ambiguity associated with traditional methods, neuroscientists are now extensively using genetic approaches with different tools such as Cre-loxP and chemogenetic and optogenetic systems. This new toolbox helps to reveal and manipulate diverse neuronal populations in the VMH, as well as characterize new groups of neurons. Using microdissection [35], oligo microarray, and *in situ* hybridization [36] , studies reveal unique gene expression in the VMH. Of these genes, SF1 (Nr5a1) is highly enriched in the VMH, widely expressed throughout this nucleus from embryonic to postnatal stages. In mature mouse brains, SF1 is dominantly expressed in the dorsomedial part of the VMH (Figure 6.2). As *Sf1* expresses both exclusively and extensively in the VMH, genetic tools such as SF1-Cre (Cre recombinase expressing under SF1 endogenous promoter) mouse line provides access to isolate and study the function of this region.

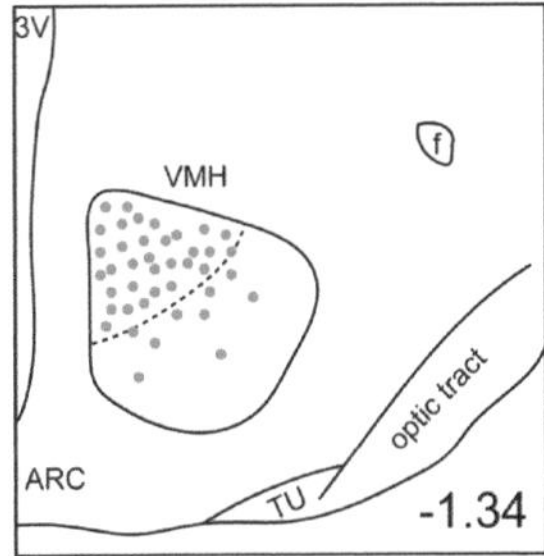

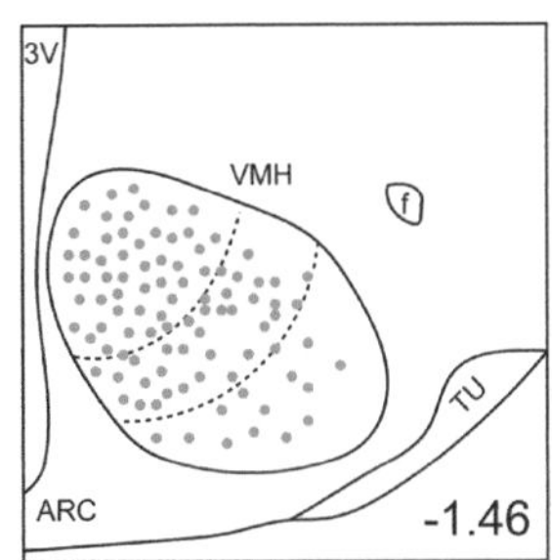

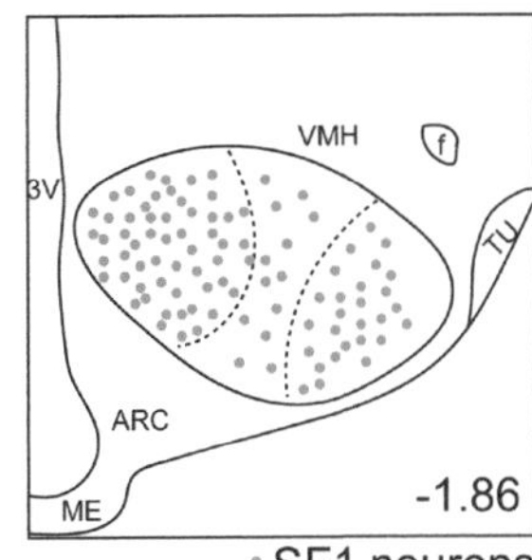

FIGURE 6.2 Steroidogenic factor 1 (SF1)-expressing neuron distribution throughout different sections of the mediobasal hypothalamus in mice. Numbers represent the relative anterior-posterior positions to Bregma (mm). ARC: arcuate nucleus; f: column of fornix; ME: median eminence; TU: tuberal nucleus; VMH: ventromedial hypothalamus; 3V: third ventricle. Based on [37] and unpublished data courtesy of Ki Woo Kim in 2020.

6.4.2 SF1 Neuronal Connections

SF1-expressing neurons in the VMH have rich afferent and efferent connections to neighboring nuclei of the hypothalamus, as well as to brain structures outside of the hypothalamus, such as the midbrain or hindbrain. The generation of SF1-Cre mouse lines [37,38], along with conditionally expressing fluorescence reporter mice, a stereotaxic fluorescence-delivering virus [39], and a retrotracing virus [40], has greatly enabled the effective tracing of the efferent projections of the SF1 neurons. Early fiber projections from SF1-expressing neurons to the ventral supraoptic commissure, epithalamus, habenular nucleus, periaqueductal gray, retrochiasmatic area, medial preoptic area, bed nucleus of stria terminalis, vertical band of Broca, and medial septum appear at around E10.5 to E17.5 in mouse embryos. The descending fiber tracts penetrate the anterior hypothalamus, amygdala, zona incerta, periventricular system, and dorsal and ventral premammillary nuclei at the postnatal stage. Fibers also penetrate the mesencephalic reticular formation, ventral tegmental area, tegmental nucleus, parabrachial nucleus, and locus coeruleus [15] (Figure 6.3).

6.4.3 The Role of SF1 in the VMH

SF1 in the VMH gained a role as an energy metabolism regulator after the study of the germline knockout of SF1, which globally deletes SF1 from the VMH, anterior pituitary gland, adrenal cortex, and sexual organs. Global knockout exhibits neonatal lethality due to adrenal insufficiency [41]. After wild-type adrenal gland transplantation into SF1-KO mice in order to rescue them, these animals exhibit massive

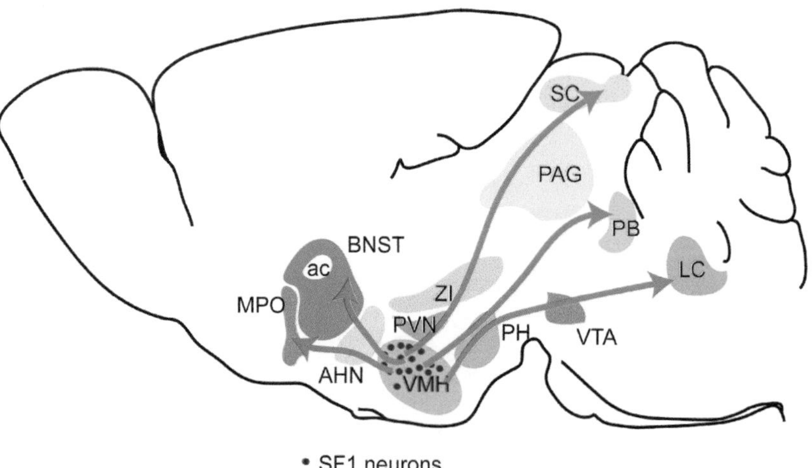

FIGURE 6.3 Sagittal diagram of SF1 neuron projections to other hypothalamic nuclei and brain regions. Red lines represent projections from SF1 neurons in the VMH. VMH: ventromedial hypothalamus; AHN: anterior hypothalamus; BNST: bed nucleus of the stria terminalis; ZI: zona incerta; PH: posterior hypothalamus; VTA: ventral tegmental area; PAG: periaqueductal gray; PB: parabrachial nucleus; SC: superior colliculus; LC: locus coeruleus. Based on data from [15] and the *Allen Brain Atlas* [7].

obesity, suggesting that SF1 in the VMH has an essential role against obesity. However, as SF1 is crucial for the development of the VMH, the phenotype could have been derived from impaired VMH formation. To address this problem, the Elmquist group has developed mouse models with specific SF1 deletion in the VMH [42]. Prenatal deletion of SF1 in the VMH using Nestin-Cre leads to late-onset obesity with increased adiposity on a standard chow diet, and fast-onset obesity in KO mice on a high fat diet. To examine whether SF1 KO in the VMH causes potential defects in the development of this nuclei, this group has also used an alternative model in which CamKII-Cre transgenic mice are used to postnatally knockout SF1 in the VMH, as Cre recombinase expresses after birth. Postnatal SF1 knockout does not cause voracious eating behavior in mice, but rather causes obesity with dysregulation of glucose, leptin, and insulin levels on an obesogenic diet. This might be due to an imbalance in energy expenditure, impaired thermogenic gene expression in brown adipose tissue, and blunted glutaminergic marker Vglut2 expression in the VMH [43]. This further supports the notion that VMH SF1 is required for the regulation of body weight homeostasis.

6.4.4 Genetic Modulation Reveals the Thermogenic Roles of SF1 Neurons

The above-mentioned SF1-Cre transgenic mouse line also enables genetic manipulation that is restricted to VMH neurons. As SF1 is expressed in around 81% of leptin-responsive neurons in the VMH [44], deletion of the leptin receptor (LepR) from the VMH using SF1-Cre mice reveals the importance of leptin signaling in SF1 neurons. SF1 neurons can be leptin-activated neurons (characterized by an increase in action potential frequency and resting membrane potential) [37,45], and deletion of LepR from these neurons abolishes the depolarizing effect of leptin. LepR-deficient neurons also show reduced phospho-STAT3 induction upon leptin injection *in vivo*, with around an 80% reduction in number in the VMH of mice with SF1-Cre-mediated leptin receptor deletion, compared to their wild-type littermate [37]. Knockout of LepR in the VMH results in obesity with the same degree as observed when knocking out the leptin receptor in proopiomelanocortin (POMC) neurons [46]. The obesity induced by the loss of leptin signaling in SF1 neurons is mainly due to decreased energy expenditure during five to nine weeks of age, which can be compensated at a later age [37].

Another important signaling pathway in the VMH is the insulin-mediated signaling pathway, as demonstrated by studies showing that insulin can activate VMH neurons [47] and that inhibition of insulin signaling causes hyperphagia [48]. Deletion of the insulin receptor (IR) specifically in SF1 neurons enhances glucose metabolism and prevents high-fat diet-induced obesity [49]. Interestingly, mice with IR deletion in SF1 neurons exhibit increased cellular activity in POMC neurons under a high-fat diet, suggesting that an increased projection from SF1 neurons to POMC might protect against diet-induced obesity.

In addition, Sohn et al. provide data supporting segregated leptin and insulin-responsive SF1 neuronal populations in the VMH. These authors have identified heterogenous subsets of SF1 neurons that respond to the acute effects of leptin

[45]. Furthermore, as leptin and insulin actions converge on the phosphoinositide 3-kinases (PI3K) pathway, electrophysiological studies have identified that leptin and insulin action on SF1 neurons requires PI3K signaling [45]. The action of leptin-mediated depolarization requires the p110β subunit in the SF1 neurons, while the ablation of p110α and p110β blocks the inhibitory effects of leptin and insulin. Indeed, ablation of PI3K through the deletion of the p110α subunit in SF1 neurons causes high sensitivity to diet-induced obesity without any alteration in glucose metabolism. Mice lacking p110α in SF1 neurons exhibit blunted autonomic nerve-mediated diet-induced thermogenesis and a basal metabolic rate, which may contribute to the obese phenotype. Similarly, deletion of the p110β subunit in SF1 neurons also results in blunted energy expenditure and obesity in mice on a high-fat diet [50]. Interestingly, deletion of the transcription factor FoxO1, a downstream effector of PI3K, in SF1 neurons shows metabolic benefits: increased heat generation through the autonomic nervous system, as well as improved insulin sensitivity [51]. Several lines of evidence support the claim that FoxO1 might transcriptionally regulate the expression of SF1: (1) the mRNA and protein levels of SF1 increase in FoxO1 KO animals, (2) the FoxO1 binding motif is found in the promoter region of SF1, and (3) chromatin immunoprecipitation and luciferase assays using the mouse SF1 promoter indicate that FoxO1 binds to and suppresses the transcription of SF1 [51].

Other genes, which are generally considered to be involved in metabolism, have also been investigated using the Cre transgenic models. For example, deletion of the metabolic sensor SIRT1 from SF1 neurons renders mice sensitive to diet-induced obesity through a decrease of adaptive thermogenesis and insulin insensitivity [52]. Viskaitis et al.'s modulation of SF1 neuronal activity using chemo- and optogenetic approaches further confirm that the activation of SF1 neurons is associated with feeding alterations and that the feeding behavior driven by SF1 neurons is also affected by anxiety and emotional stress [53]. Another novel role of the VMH in circadian regulation has also been discovered through the ablation of the clock-controlling transcription factor, BMAL1, demonstrating that SF1 neuron circadian rhythm controls the sympathetic outflow to brown adipose tissues, thus controlling heat generation [54].

6.4.5 SF1 Neurons Regulate Glucose Homeostasis

Besides the regulatory roles of SF1 neurons in energy balance, this population also plays a role as a critical hub that maintains glucose homeostasis. Oomura et al. suggest the existence of glucose sensing neurons in the VMH at a very early time [55,56]. Chemical lesions with gold thio-glucose or injection of 2-deoxyglucose (a non-metabolizing glucose analog) [57–60] indicate that a subset of VMH neurons are glucose-sensing neurons and that the lesions impair hormonal responses in hypoglycemic counter-regulation. Patch-clamp studies suggest that the VMH neurons directly respond to the level of glucose [61,62]. It is also suggested that the SF1 neurons control glucose levels through modulation of hepatic glucose output, which is dependent on hepatic sympathetic innervation [63]. Genetic modulations also provide new insights into glucose responsiveness of SF1 neurons. Disruption of glutamate release from VMH SF1 neurons, by deletion of Vglut2 using SF1-Cre, demonstrates that SF1 neurons counter-regulate against hypoglycemia [64]. Under hypoglycemic conditions, mice without Vglut2 in SF1 neurons exhibit impaired glucagon response, along with blunted epinerphrine surges that are normally seen in hypoglycemic crisis [62]. Interestingly, induction of c-Fos (a marker for neuronal activity) in the dorsal motor nucleus of the vagus (in which parasympathetic preganglionic neurons are located) by insulin injection is significantly reduced with Vglut2 deletion (64), further supporting the notion that SF1 neurons are involved in autonomic nervous response.

In addition, leptin and insulin downstream effectors have been demonstrated as regulators of glucose homeostasis in SF1 neurons. Intracerebroventricular injection of leptin into the VMH increases glucose uptake in brown adipose tissue and heart and skeletal muscle, and this effect is blunted by sympathetic denervation [65–67]. Disruption in normal glucose and insulin homeostasis by the deletion of p110β [50] or FoxO1 [51] suggests that leptin-PI3K-FoxO1 is a potential pathway for glycemic control in SF1 neurons. Moreover, SF1 is required for normal glucose homeostasis in rodents, especially at older ages [51].

Optogenetic activation of SF1 neurons in the VMH causes abrupt hyperglycemia and impairs glucose and pyruvate tolerance [68]. The sharp increase in blood glucose level is affected by a drop in the insulin level, and an increase in cortisol and glucagon levels [66]. In contrast, activation of SF1 neurons by designer receptors exclusively activated by designer drugs (DDREAD) resulted in whole body insulin sensitivity being increased without any hyperglycemic response [69]. This discrepancy suggests that there could be a diverse neuronal subpopulation among the SF1 neurons that respond to glucose differently. Further study is required to completely segregate the functions of each subset of neurons.

6.5 NON-SF1 NEURONAL CIRCUITS IN THE VMH

6.5.1 VMH and ARC Crosstalk

The roles of POMC and agouti-related protein (AgRP)/neuropeptide Y (NPY) neurons, along with the melanocortin system, in the feeding circuits are well established [70]. Interestingly, both MC3 and MC4 receptors are found in the VMH. Also, POMC and AgRP/NPY neurons project to the VMH [71]. The action of POMC and AgRP on the VMH is thought to use VMH Bdnf-expressing neurons as a downstream factor [72]. The projections from AgRP/NPY and POMC neurons to the VMH remain unclear.

VMH neurons demonstrate dense innervation into the area between the VMH shell and the dorsal ARC surface. Combining laser scanning photostimulation and whole-cell voltage patch-clamp techniques, Jeffrey Freidman's group discovered the "microcircuit" in which excitatory neurons in the medial part of the VMH connects and activates POMC neurons in the ARC, while a weaker connection from excitatory neurons in the lateral part excites AgRP/NPY neurons. These circuits are regulated by caloric statuses [73]. This model provides evidence that the VMH acts as a "satiety" hub, suppressing food intake through POMC and other neurons.

6.5.2 Estrogen Receptor Alpha (ERα)-Expressing Neurons

Contrary to SF1-neurons, estrogen receptor alpha (ERα or ESR1)-expressing neurons reside along the central and ventrolateral area of the VMH. Using a knock-in ESR1-Cre mouse, an anterograde adeno-associated virus (AAV), and a monosynaptic retrograde rabies virus, Brandon Weissbourd's group has mapped out the dense connectome of ESR1-neurons in the VMH, discovering substantial output projections to the medial preoptic area/anterior hypothalamus, and to many of the high-degree bidirectional projections called the canonical "feeding" nuclei (e.g. the arcuate nucleus (ARC), the paraventricular nucleus (PVN), the parabrachial nuclei (PB)). This means that the majority of projecting neurons also receives a feedback input, and the glutamatergic ESR1 neurons collateralize to different, but defined, targets [74].

Multiple studies have demonstrated the role of ERα-neurons in the control of energy balance. First, the application of estrogen to the VMH and the diencephalon reduces food intake in ovariectomized rats [75,76]. In addition, the deletion of ESR1 in SF1 neurons decreases the sympathetic tone with decreased thermogenesis from brown adipose tissue and increased lipid accumulation in white adipose tissue. This may be due to the PI3K pathway, the function of SF1 as a transcription factor [77], or the homeobox transcription factor Nkx2-1 [78].

Whole-brain ERα knockout using Nestin-Cre [77] or VMH-targeted ERα knockdown using RNA interference in mice [79] causes impairments in energy balance with increased food intake and fat accumulation, as well as decreased energy expenditure in female mice or rats fed a normal chow diet. ERα knockout in SF1 neurons using SF1-Cre and $ER\alpha^{lox/lox}$ mice causes an obese phenotype that is less extensive in female mice, associated with increased food intake, a marked accumulation of white adipose tissue (especially gonadal fat), blood glucose dysregulation, and decreased heat generation in brown adipose tissue, due to a drop in sympathetic nervous system outflow to the brown adipose tissue [77]. It is worth noting that the expression of leptin receptors in the VMH is also affected by the deletion of ERα in SF1 neurons [77]. Collectively, ERα in the VMH plays an important role in the regulation of energy balance, especially in female individuals.

The majority of ERα neurons in the VMHvl are glucose-sensing neurons, as detected by the change in resting membrane potential and the firing rate in fluctuating glucose concentrations during whole-cell patch-clamp experiments [80]. The ERα-glucose-excitatory neurons respond to hypoglycemia through the Abbc8-K_{ATP} channel, and the hypoglycemic condition activates the ERα-glucose-inhibitory neurons through the chloride Ano4 channel. Glucose-inhibited and excited neurons also have respective projections to the medioposterior arcuate nucleus of the hypothalamus and dorsal raphe nuclei, increasing blood glucose level and counteracting hypoglycemia.

6.5.3 Cholecystokinin Receptor B (CCKRB)-Expressing Neurons

Cholecystokinin (CCK) is a satiety hormone, synthesized by endocrine cells along the small intestinal mucosa or in the central nervous system, causing a reduction in food intake. The eight amino acids at the C terminal of CCK (CCK octapeptide – CCK8) is a bioactive fragment of CCK, efficiently reducing food intake in starved rats when injected intraperitoneally. Kulkosy et al. suggest that the anorexigenic action of CCK8 is not mandated through the VMH, as CCK8-injected VMH-lesioned rats ate the same amount of chow as the saline-injected ones [81]. However, three years later, the same group suggest that the VMH is involved in the CCK8 food intake, but only when the rats are given a highly palatable diet [82]. Other studies have also shown that when injected directly to the VMH, CCK8 can trigger gut motor changes, mimicking feeding in rats. This effect only happens when CCK8 is infused in the VMH, but not the LH [83,84].

Neurons in the VMH also express CCK receptor B (a brain-specific receptor opposed to receptor A in the peripheral). Around 55% of SF1 neurons respond to exogenous CCK, which does not elicit any response in non-SF1 neurons in the VMH. It has been proven that the CCK neurons in the lateral PB project to CCKRB neurons in the VMH, which acts as a downstream effector to drive hepatic glucose production in response to hypoglycemia [85]. This response depends on the sympathetic nervous system and adrenal function, which targets tissue under the sympathetic nervous system (SNS) output, rather than pancreatic islet hormones (i.e. insulin or glucagon) [86].

6.6 CONCLUSIONS

The hypothalamus has seen a securing role for it as the primary site for the central regulation of metabolic homeostasis. While the function of other nuclei is relatively straightforward, the VMH shows a change in the paradigm regarding its regulation of energy balance throughout research history, from gross lesioning to electrical stimulation and to extensive studies on genetic factors and micro-neural circuits. Hence, the VMH has had its role shifted from the debatable "satiety center" to a much more complex and highly intertwined hub for the maintenance of blood glucose and energy homeostasis, at least partially through the regulation of the autonomous nervous system. Throughout this chapter, we have discussed the overall structure and the importance of the VMH, mostly by SF1 neurons, which play pivotal roles in the regulation of energy balance through adaptation and responses to obesogenic and thermogenic environments. Moreover, genetic studies have demonstrated that SF1 neurons might converge and mediate the effect of various hormones, including leptin, cholecystokinin, and orexin, on glucose metabolism. However, there are still perhaps numerous other neuronal populations and circuits that remain unknown. The gap in our knowledge urges more in-depth research to fully reveal the function of other subsets of VMH neurons. To achieve this, there is a need for the development of more efficient screening tools, as well as unambiguous and accessible models.

ACKNOWLEDGMENTS

We would like to thank Jessica Hong (Brown University, Providence, RI, USA) and Ashley Giannita (Weill Cornell Medicine, New York, NY, USA) for reading this chapter. This work was supported by the National Research Foundation, Korea (2021R1A2C4002011 and 2020M3E5E2038221 for K.W.K) and the BK21 FOUR Project, Yonsei University College of Dentistry.

REFERENCES

1. Paxinos G, and Keith B.J. Franklin. *Paxinos and Franklin's the Mouse Brain in Stereotaxic Coordinates*. San Diego, Elsevier Science; 2019.
2. Löhr H, and Hammerschmidt M. Zebrafish in endocrine systems: recent advances and implications for human disease. *Annual Review of Physiology* 2011;73(1):183–211.
3. Crandall JE, Tobet SA, Fischer I, and Fox TO. Age-dependent expression of microtubule-associated protein 2 in the ventromedial nucleus of the hypothalamus. *Brain Research Bulletin* 1989;22(3):571–574.
4. Canteras NS, Simerly RB, and Swanson LW. Organization of projections from the ventromedial nucleus of the hypothalamus: A Phaseolus vulgaris-Leucoagglutinin study in the rat. *The Journal of Comparative Neurology* 1994;348(1):41–79.
5. Van Houten M, and Brawer JR. Cytology of neurons of the hypothalamic ventromedial nucleus in the adult male rat. *The Journal of Comparative Neurology* 1978;178(1):89–115.
6. Eugene Millhouse O. The organization of the ventromedial hypothalamic nucleus. *Brain Research* 1973;55(1):71–87.
7. Sunkin SM, Ng L, Lau C, Dolbeare T, Gilbert TL, Thompson CL, et al. Allen Brain Atlas: an integrated spatio-temporal portal for exploring the central nervous system. *Nucleic Acids Research* 2013;41(Database issue):D996-D1008.
8. Choi Y-H, Fujikawa T, Lee J, Reuter A, and Kim KW. Revisiting the ventral medial nucleus of the hypothalamus: the roles of SF-1 neurons in energy homeostasis. *Frontiers in Neuroscience*2013;7(71): 71–84.
9. McClellan KM, Parker KL, and Tobet S. Development of the ventromedial nucleus of the hypothalamus. *Frontiers in Neuroendocrinology* 2006;27(2):193–209.
10. Altman J, and Bayer SA. The development of the rat hypothalamus. *Advances in Anatomy, Embryology, and Cell Biology* 1986;100:1–178.
11. Shimada M, and Nakamura T. Time of neuron origin in mouse hypothalamic nuclei. *Experimental Neurology* 1973;41(1):163–173.
12. van Eerdenburg FJCM, and Rakic P. Early neurogenesis in the anterior hypothalamus of the rhesus monkey. *Developmental Brain Research* 1994;79(2):290–296.
13. Bedont JL, Newman EA, and Blackshaw S. Patterning, specification, and differentiation in the developing hypothalamus. *WIREs Developmental Biology* 2015;4(5):445–468.
14. Rakic P, Cameron RS, and Komuro H. Recognition, adhesion, transmembrane signaling and cell motility in guided neuronal migration. *Current Opinion in Neurobiology* 1994;4(1):63–69.
15. Cheung CC, Kurrasch DM, Liang JK, and Ingraham HA. Genetic labeling of steroidogenic factor-1 (SF-1) neurons in mice reveals ventromedial nucleus of the hypothalamus (VMH) circuitry beginning at neurogenesis and development of a separate non-SF-1 neuronal cluster in the ventrolateral VMH. *The Journal of Comparative Neurology* 2013;521(6):1268–1288.
16. Shima Y, Zubair M, Ishihara S, Shinohara Y, Oka S, Kimura S, et al. Ventromedial hypothalamic nucleus-specific enhancer of Ad4BP/SF-1 gene. *Molecular Endocrinology* 2005;19(11):2812–2823.
17. Lee J, Yang DJ, Lee S, Hammer GD, Kim KW, and Elmquist JK. Nutritional conditions regulate transcriptional activity of SF-1 by controlling sumoylation and ubiquitination. *Scientific Reports* 2016;6(1):19143.
18. Ikeda Y, Shen WH, Ingraham HA, and Parker KL. Developmental expression of mouse steroidogenic factor-1, an essential regulator of the steroid hydroxylases. *Molecular Endocrinology* 1994;8(5):654–662.

19. Dellovade TL, Davis AM, Ferguson C, Sieghart W, Homanics GE, and Tobet SA. GABA influences the development of the ventromedial nucleus of the hypothalamus. *Journal of Neurobiology* 2001;49(4):264–276.
20. Davis AM, Henion TR, and Tobet SA. γ-aminobutyric acidB receptors and the development of the ventromedial nucleus of the hypothalamus. *The Journal of Comparative Neurology* 2002;449(3):270–280.
21. Erdheim J. *Über hypophysenganggeschwülste und hirncholesteatome*. Gerold; 1904.
22. Smith PE. The disabilities caused by hypophysectomy and their repair: the tuberal (Hypothalamic) syndrome in the rat. *The Journal of the American Medical Association* 1927;88(3):158–161.
23. Camus J, and Roussy GJE. Experimental researches on the pituitary body diabetes insipidus, glycosuria and those dystrophies considered as hypophyseal in origin. *Endocrinology* 1920;4(4):507–522.
24. Brooks CM, and Lambert HF. A study of the effect of limitation of food intake and the method of feeding on the rate of weight gain during hypothalamic obesity in the albino rat. *The American Journal of Physiology* 1946;147(4):695–707.
25. Mrosovsky N. Hypothalamic hyperphagia without plateau in ground squirrels. *Physiology & Behavior* 1974;12(2):259–264.
26. Auffray P, and Blum JC. Hyperphagia and hepatic steatosis in the goose after lesion of the ventromedial nuclleus of the hypothalamus. *Comptes rendus hebdomadaires des seances de l'Academie des sciences Serie D: Sciences naturelles.* 1970;270(19):2362–2365.
27. Buntin JD, Hnasko RM, and Zuzick PH. Role of the ventromedial hypothalamus in prolactin-induced hyperphagia in ring doves. *Physiology and Behavior* 1999;66(2):255–261.
28. Snapir N, Ravona H, and Perek M. Effect of electrolytic lesions in various regions of the basal hypothalamus in white leghorn cockerels upon food intake, obesity, blood plasma triglycerides and proteins. *Poultry Science* 1973;52(2):629–636.
29. Baile CA, Mahoney AW, and Mayer J. Preliminary report on hypothalamic hyperphagia in ruminants. *Journal of Dairy Science* 1967;50(11):1851–1854.
30. Reynolds RW. Ventromedial hypothalamic lesions without hyperphagia. *The American Journal of Physiology*. 1963;204(1):60–62.
31. Reynolds RWJPR. An irritative hypothesis concerning the hypothalamic regulation of food intake. *Psychological Review* 1965;72(2):105.
32. Gold RM. Hypothalamic obesity: the myth of the ventromedial nucleus. *Science* 1973;182(4111):488–490.
33. Broberger C, and Hökfelt T. Hypothalamic and vagal neuropeptide circuitries regulating food intake. *Physiology & Behavior* 2001;74(4):669–682.
34. Schwartz MW, Woods SC, Porte D, Seeley RJ, and Baskin DG. Central nervous system control of food intake. *Nature* 2000;404(6778):661–671.
35. Segal JP, Stallings NR, Lee CE, Zhao L, Socci N, Viale A, et al. Use of laser-capture microdissection for the identification of marker genes for the ventromedial hypothalamic nucleus. *The Journal of Neuroscience* 2005;25(16):4181–4188.
36. Dellovade TL, Young M, Ross EP, Henderson R, Caron K, Parker K, et al. Disruption of the gene encoding SF-1 alters the distribution of hypothalamic neuronal phenotypes. *The Journal of Comparative Neurology* 2000;423(4):579–589.
37. Dhillon H, Zigman JM, Ye C, Lee CE, McGovern RA, Tang V, et al. Leptin directly activates SF1 neurons in the VMH, and this action by leptin is required for normal body-weight homeostasis. *Neuron* 2006;49(2):191–203.
38. Bingham NC, Anderson KK, Reuter AL, Stallings NR, and Parker KL. Selective loss of leptin receptors in the ventromedial hypothalamic nucleus results in increased adiposity and a metabolic syndrome. *Endocrinology* 2008;149(5):2138–2148.

39. Oh SW, Harris JA, Ng L, Winslow B, Cain N, Mihalas S, et al. A mesoscale connectome of the mouse brain. *Nature* 2014;508(7495):207–214.
40. Wang L, Chen Irene Z, and Lin D. Collateral pathways from the ventromedial hypothalamus mediate defensive behaviors. *Neuron* 2015;85(6):1344–1358.
41. Majdic G, Young M, Gomez-Sanchez E, Anderson P, Szczepaniak LS, Dobbins RL, et al. Knockout mice lacking steroidogenic factor 1 are a novel genetic model of hypothalamic obesity. *Endocrinology* 2002;143(2):607–614.
42. Kim KW, Zhao L, Donato J, Jr., Kohno D, Xu Y, Elias CF, et al. Steroidogenic factor 1 directs programs regulating diet-induced thermogenesis and leptin action in the ventral medial hypothalamic nucleus. *Proceedings of the National Academy of Sciences of the United States of America* 2011;108(26):10673–10678.
43. Kinyua AW, Yang DJ, Chang I, and Kim KW. Steroidogenic factor 1 in the ventromedial nucleus of the hypothalamus regulates age-dependent obesity. *PLoS ONE* 2016;11(9):e0162352.
44. Ramos-Lobo AM, Teixeira PDS, Furigo IC, and Donato J. SOCS3 ablation in SF1 cells causes modest metabolic effects during pregnancy and lactation. *Neuroscience* 2017;365:114–124.
45. Sohn J-W, Oh Y, Kim KW, Lee S, Williams KW, and Elmquist JK. Leptin and insulin engage specific PI3K subunits in hypothalamic SF1 neurons. *Molecular Metabolism* 2016;5(8):669–679.
46. Balthasar N, Coppari R, McMinn J, Liu SM, Lee CE, Tang V, et al. Leptin receptor signaling in pomc neurons is required for normal body weight homeostasis. *Neuron* 2004;42(6):983–991.
47. Spanswick D, Smith MA, Mirshamsi S, Routh VH, and Ashford MLJ. Insulin activates ATP-sensitive K+ channels in hypothalamic neurons of lean, but not obese rats. *Nature Neuroscience* 2000;3(8):757–758.
48. Davidowa H, and Plagemann A. Inhibition by insulin of hypothalamic VMN neurons in rats overweight due to postnatal overfeeding. *NeuroReport.* 2001;12(15): 3201–3204.
49. Klöckener T, Hess S, Belgardt BF, Paeger L, Verhagen LAW, Husch A, et al. High-fat feeding promotes obesity via insulin receptor/PI3K-dependent inhibition of SF-1 VMH neurons. *Nature Neuroscience* 2011;14(7):911–918.
50. Fujikawa T, Choi Y-H, Yang DJ, Shin DM, Donato J, Kohno D, et al. P110β in the ventromedial hypothalamus regulates glucose and energy metabolism. *Experimental & Molecular Medicine* 2019;51(4):1–9.
51. Kim KW, Donato J, Jr., Berglund ED, Choi Y-H, Kohno D, Elias CF, et al. FOXO1 in the ventromedial hypothalamus regulates energy balance. *The Journal of Clinical Investigation* 2012;122(7):2578–2589.
52. Ramadori G, Fujikawa T, Anderson J, Berglund Eric D, Frazao R, Michán S, et al. SIRT1 deacetylase in SF1 neurons protects against metabolic imbalance. *Cell Metabolism* 2011;14(3):301–312.
53. Viskaitis P, Irvine EE, Smith MA, Choudhury AI, Alvarez-Curto E, Glegola JA, et al. Modulation of SF1 neuron activity coordinately regulates both feeding behavior and associated emotional states. *Cell Reports* 2017;21(12):3559–3572.
54. Orozco-Solis R, Aguilar-Arnal L, Murakami M, Peruquetti R, Ramadori G, Coppari R, et al. The circadian clock in the ventromedial hypothalamus controls cyclic energy expenditure. *Cell Metabolism* 2016;23(3):467–478.
55. Oomura Y, Ono T, Ooyama H, and Wayner MJ. Glucose and osmosensitive neurones of the rat hypothalamus. *Nature* 1969;222(5190):282–284.
56. Oomura Y, Kimura K, Ooyama H, Maeno T, Iki M, and Kuniyoshi M. Reciprocal activities of the ventromedial and lateral hypothalamic areas of cats. *Science* 1964;143(3605):484–485.

57. Mayer J, and Marshall NB. Specificity of gold thioglucose for ventromedial hypothalamic lesions and hyperphagia. *Nature* 1956;178(4547):1399–1400.
58. Likuski H, Debons A, and Cloutier R. Inhibition of gold thioglucose-induced hypothalamic obesity by glucose analogues. *The American Journal of Physiology* 1967;212(3):669–676.
59. Borg WP, During MJ, Sherwin RS, Borg MA, Brines ML, and Shulman GI. Ventromedial hypothalamic lesions in rats suppress counterregulatory responses to hypoglycemia. *The Journal of Clinical Investigation* 1994;93(4):1677–1682.
60. Borg WP, Sherwin RS, During MJ, Borg MA, and Shulman GI. Local ventromedial hypothalamus glucopenia triggers counterregulatory hormone release. *Diabetes* 1995;44(2):180–184.
61. Song Z, and Routh VH. Recurrent hypoglycemia reduces the glucose sensitivity of glucose-inhibited neurons in the ventromedial hypothalamus nucleus. *American Journal of Physiology. Regulatory, Integrative and Comparative Physiology* 2006;291(5):R1283-R12R7.
62. Cotero VE, and Routh VH. Insulin blunts the response of glucose-excited neurons in the ventrolateral-ventromedial hypothalamic nucleus to decreased glucose. *American Journal of Physiology. Endocrinology and Metabolism* 2009;296(5):E1101-E11E9.
63. Shimazu T, and Minokoshi Y. Systemic glucoregulation by glucose-sensing neurons in the ventromedial hypothalamic nucleus (VMH). *Journal of Endocrine Society* 2017;1(5):449–459.
64. Tong Q, Ye C, McCrimmon RJ, Dhillon H, Choi B, Kramer MD, et al. Synaptic glutamate release by ventromedial hypothalamic neurons is part of the neurocircuitry that prevents hypoglycemia. *Cell Metabolism* 2007;5(5):383–393.
65. Kamohara S, Burcelin R, Halaas JL, Friedman JM, and Charron MJ. Acute stimulation of glucose metabolism in mice by leptin treatment. *Nature* 1997;389(6649):374–377.
66. Minokoshi Y, Haque MS, and Shimazu T. Microinjection of leptin into the ventromedial hypothalamus increases glucose uptake in peripheral tissues in rats. *Diabetes* 1999;48(2):287–291.
67. Haque MS, Minokoshi Y, Hamai M, Iwai M, Horiuchi M, and Shimazu T. Role of the sympathetic nervous system and insulin in enhancing glucose uptake in peripheral tissues after intrahypothalamic injection of leptin in rats. *Diabetes* 1999;48(9):1706–1712.
68. Meek TH, Nelson JT, Matsen ME, Dorfman MD, Guyenet SJ, Damian V, et al. Functional identification of a neurocircuit regulating blood glucose. *Proceedings of the National Academy of Sciences* 2016;113(14):E2073–E2E82.
69. Coutinho EA, Okamoto S, Ishikawa AW, Yokota S, Wada N, Hirabayashi T, et al. Activation of SF1 neurons in the ventromedial hypothalamus by DREADD technology increases insulin sensitivity in peripheral tissues. *Diabetes* 2017;66(9):2372–2386.
70. Sohn J-W. Network of hypothalamic neurons that control appetite. *BMB Reports* 2015;48(4):229–233.
71. King BM. The rise, fall, and resurrection of the ventromedial hypothalamus in the regulation of feeding behavior and body weight. *Physiology & Behavior* 2006;87(2):221–244.
72. Xu B, Goulding EH, Zang K, Cepoi D, Cone RD, Jones KR, et al. Brain-derived neurotrophic factor regulates energy balance downstream of melanocortin-4 receptor. *Nature Neuroscience* 2003;6(7):736–742.
73. Sternson SM, Shepherd GMG, and Friedman JM. Topographic mapping of VMH → arcuate nucleus microcircuits and their reorganization by fasting. *Nature Neuroscience* 2005;8(10):1356–1363.
74. Lo, L, Yao, S, Kim, D, Cetin, A, Harris, J, & Zeng, H, et al. Connectional architecture of a mouse hypothalamic circuit node controlling social behavior. *Proceedings Of The National Academy Of Sciences* 2019;116(15): 7503–7512. doi: 10.1073/pnas.1817503116

75. Wade GN, and Zucker I. Modulation of food intake and locomotor activity in female rats by diencephalic hormone implants. *Journal of Comparative and Physiological Psychology* 1970;72(2):328–336.
76. Jankowiak R, and Stern JJ. Food intake and body weight modifications following medial hypothalamic hormone implants in female rats. *Physiology and Behavior* 1974;12(5):875–879.
77. Xu Y, Nedungadi Thekkethil P, Zhu L, Sobhani N, Irani Boman G, Davis Kathryn E, et al. Distinct hypothalamic neurons mediate estrogenic effects on energy homeostasis and reproduction. *Cell Metabolism* 2011;14(4):453–465.
78. Krause WC, and Ingraham HA. Origins and functions of the ventrolateral VMH: a complex neuronal cluster orchestrating sex differences in metabolism and behavior. *Advances in Experimental Medicine and Biology* 2017;1043:199–213.
79. Musatov S, Chen W, Pfaff DW, Mobbs CV, Yang X-J, Clegg DJ, et al. Silencing of estrogen receptor α in the ventromedial nucleus of hypothalamus leads to metabolic syndrome. *Proceedings of the National Academy of Sciences of the United States of America* 2007;104(7):2501–2506.
80. He Y, Xu P, Wang C, Xia Y, Yu M, Yang Y, et al. Estrogen receptor-α expressing neurons in the ventrolateral VMH regulate glucose balance. *Nature Communications* 2020;11(1):2165.
81. Kulkosky PJ, Breckenridge C, Krinsky R, and Woods SC. Satiety elicited by the C-terminal octapeptide of cholecystokinin-pancreozymin in normal and VMH-lesioned rats. *Behavioral Biology* 1976;18(2):227–234.
82. Krinsky R, Lotter EC, and Woods SC. Appetite suppression caused by CCK is diet specific in VMH-lesioned rats. *Physiological Psychology* 1979;7(1):67–69.
83. Liberge M, Arruebo MP, and Bueno L. Role of hypothalamic cholecystokinin octapeptide in the colonic motor response to a meal in rats. *Gastroenterology* 1991;100(2):441–449.
84. Liberge M, Arruebo P, and Bueno L. CCK8 neurons of the ventromedial (VMH) hypothalamus mediate the upper gut motor changes associated with feeding in rats. *Brain Research* 1990;508(1):118–123.
85. Garfield AS, Shah BP, Madara JC, Burke LK, Patterson CM, Flak J, et al. A parabrachial-hypothalamic cholecystokinin neurocircuit controls counterregulatory responses to hypoglycemia. *Cell Metabolism* 2014;20(6):1030–1037.
86. Flak JN, Goforth PB, Dell'Orco J, Sabatini PV, Li C, Bozadjieva N, et al. Ventromedial hypothalamic nucleus neuronal subset regulates blood glucose independently of insulin. *The Journal of Clinical Investigation* 2020;130(6):2943–2952.

7 Current Genetic Techniques Available for Investigating Feeding Behavior and the Control of Energy Balance

Mitchell T. Harberson and Jennifer W. Hill
The University of Toledo, USA

CONTENTS

7.1 INTRODUCTION

Recent years have seen an explosion in new technologies that enable the neuroscientist to investigate neuronal circuits at a level of detail not previously possible. Building on genetic approaches to manipulating specific genes such as Cre-lox technology that were developed by an earlier generation, new techniques can closely monitor, map, and manipulate neuronal activity, calcium fluxes, and circuit function in ways that were not previously thought possible. Importantly, these approaches can be selected for their fast or slow time scales as appropriate to examine effects on single cells, physiology, or behavior. Finally, the dream of visualizing the activity of neurons in behaving mice is being achieved by a growing number of laboratories, helped by the propagation of new technology. While a full discussion of the history associated with each of these advances cannot be contained in a chapter, we will focus on several of the most impactful developments: the advent and recent progress in chemogenetics, optogenetics, and genetically encoded indicators. Finally, their specific impact on the field of the neuronal control of food intake and energy homeostasis will be discussed.

7.2 CHEMOGENETICS

Chemogenetics, also called pharmacogenetics, is the use of engineered proteins that respond to the administration of previously unrecognized small molecules. Many of these proteins are engineered G protein-coupled receptors (GPCRs) or ligand-gated ion channels (LGICs). These receptors can be expressed in transgenic animals to allow temporal control over neuronal physiology.

7.2.1 Chemogenetics: GPCRs

Chemogenetics were first developed in 1991. An adrenaline-insensitive b2-adrenergic receptor was developed using site-directed mutagenesis [1] that could be activated by 1-(3',4'-dihydroxyphenyl)-3-methyl-1-butanone (L-185,870). However, the low potency of L-185,870 at this GPCR made this first-generation chemogenetic technology an ineffective research tool. Nevertheless, it served as a proof of concept.

Second-generation chemogenetic tools called "receptors activated solely by synthetic ligands" (RASSLs) had an improved drug potency at the modified receptors. The first RASSL was a κ-opioid receptor (KOR) that was designed to be activated by synthetic spiradoline while remaining unresponsive to native ligands [2]. Generated using site-directed mutagenesis, this RASSL was still not an ideal tool because it had high levels of constitutive activity. In addition, spiradoline can act on the endogenous KOR [3].

Third-generation chemogenetic tools referred to as designer receptors exclusively activated by designer drugs (DREADDs) were designed using directed molecular evolution in yeast. (Although DREADDs and RASSLs were created using different techniques, these terms are now commonly used interchangeably.) The first DREADDs were designed by directed molecular evolution of the muscarinic acetylcholine receptors (mAChRs) [4]. This technique yielded DREADDs that are insensitive to endogenous mAChR effector molecules but sensitive to clozapine-N-oxide (CNO), an exogenous small molecule. CNO was chosen for its lack of pharmacological action and its ability to penetrate the blood–brain barrier.

DREADDs can alter neuronal physiology in a variety of ways, including through the introduction of receptors that have an excitatory or inhibitory effect on neuronal activity. Armbruster and Roth developed the first DREADD in 2007 based on the human M_3 acetylcholine (hM_3) receptor [4]. To generate this DREADD, the hM_3 receptor was randomly mutated and expressed in yeast with access to CNO. These yeasts were screened for the activation of the hM_3 receptor by CNO. Of the remaining receptors, investigators chose one DREADD based on its insensitivity to acetylcholine; this receptor was titled hM3Dq. hM3Dq increases neuronal excitability in the presence of CNO by coupling with the G protein, Gq. Gq regulates the expression of genes that facilitate presynaptic neurotransmitter release through the activation of protein lipase C and the subsequent increase in intracellular Ca2+ [5] (Figure 7.1.A). In 2009, hM3Dq was first proven to depolarize neurons *in vivo* when expressed in the hippocampus [6]. These mice saw a spike in the activity of hippocampal neurons that correlated with behavioral seizure observations after treatment with 0.1–5.0 mg/kg of CNO. Armbruster and Roth chose hM3Dq because it had two mutations (Y149C, A239G) that allowed CNO binding with a considerable decrease in ACh affinity. Since Y149C and A239G are well-conserved residues among the mammalian mAChR family, they hypothesized that inducing these mutations in the other mAChR subtypes would recapitulate the binding properties of hM3Dq.

Subsequently, more DREADDS were generated, including additional excitatory DREADDs that couple to Gq (hM1Dq, hM5Dq) and inhibitory DREADDs that couple to Gi (hM2Di, hM4Di) [4]. The most commonly used receptors today are the excitatory hM3Dq and inhibitory hM4Di. hM4Di inhibits neurotransmitter release through two pathways. First, Gi activates Gβ/γ which can directly open G protein-coupled inwardly rectifying potassium channels (GIRKs) to hyperpolarize the neuron. Second, β-arrestin separates from hM4Di and activates the mitogen-activated protein kinase pathway which regulates genes that facilitate presynaptic neurotransmitter release (Figure 7.1.B) [5]. Since its creation, hM4Di has been utilized for many high impact investigations including studies on the regulation of hunger [7], thermoregulation [8], and drug addiction [9].

In 2009, another excitatory DREADD was created that activates the G protein, Gs (GsD). GsD (aka rM3D) has an excitatory effect in neurons through the activation of adenylyl cyclase and cAMP production (Figure 7.1.C) [5]. GsD has been used for studies on a multitude of behaviors such as alcohol consumption [10] and circadian rhythms [11]. Interestingly, it has also been used to understand the role of cAMP in cells outside of the CNS such as in pancreatic beta-cells [12]. An additional DREADD was made that only signals through β-arrestin (Figure 7.1.B) [13]. This DREADD has not been extensively utilized, but shows promise for the study of β-arrestin signaling.

Recently, some methodological considerations have been raised concerning the use of CNO. CNO derives from the antipsychotic drug clozapine. Importantly, it can potentially be metabolized back to clozapine. Although clozapine can cause symptoms such as sedation, hypotension, and anticholinergic syndrome, less than 10% of CNO is converted in humans and non-human primates [14]. Recently CNO was found to convert to clozapine in mice and rats, but doses of CNO up to 5 mg/kg were effective DREADD agonists without significant behavioral effects [15]. Compound 21 is an alternative strong DREADD agonist that was reported to avoid conversion to clozapine [16]. Additional studies in mice showed that doses of Compound 21 ranging from 0.4 to 1.0 mg/kg are effective and present no noticeable changes in behavior [15]. Correct dosing and controls with CNO or the use of Compound 21 should allow DREADD use to contribute to advances in neuroscience research.

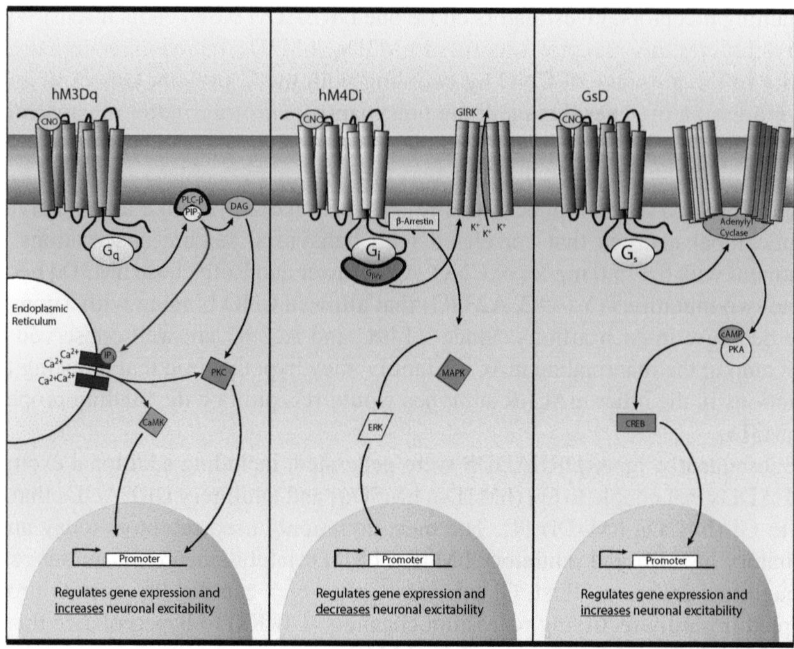

FIGURE 7.1 (**A**) Excitatory hM3Dq couples with Gq. Upon CNO activation, Gq activates protein lipase C-β (PLC-β) and converts PIP_2 into IP_3 and DAG. IP_3 binds and opens Ca^{2+} channels on the endoplasmic reticulum. Subsequently, increased cytosolic Ca^{2+} activates protein kinase C (PKC) and CaM kinase resulting in gene regulation that increases neuronal excitability. (**B**) Upon CNO binding, inhibitory hM4Di activates Gi and Gβ/γ which hyperpolarizes the neuron via opening of G protein-coupled inwardly rectifying potassium channels (GIRKs). Additionally, β-arrestin separates from hM4Di and, through the MAPK/ERK pathway, regulates gene expression to decrease neuronal excitability. (**C**) Upon CNO binding, excitatory GsD activates adenylyl cyclase through coupling with Gs. Adenylyl cyclase produces cAMP that binds and activates protein kinase A (PKA). Subsequently, PKA phosphorylates and activates many proteins, including CREB, that regulate gene expression and increase neuronal excitability.

In 2015, another inhibitory DREADD, made using the κ-opioid receptor (KORD), was designed and is activated by a pharmacologically inert compound called salvinorin B [17]. Salvinorin B activation of KORD inhibits neurotransmitter release through mechanisms similar to hM4Di (Figure 7.1.B) [5]. However, the pharmacokinetics of salvinorin B are much more rapid compared to CNO; actions of salvinorin B begin and end within one hour compared to several hours of effects following CNO administration [17]. Interestingly, because KORD has a different agonist than hM3Dq, it is possible to use both, allowing for a bidirectional investigation of neuronal circuits. For example, neurons that express both types of DREADDs can have excitatory reactions to CNO and inhibitory reactions to salvinorin B.

7.2.2 Chemogenetics: LGICs

Ligand-gated ion channels (LGICs) are another category of chemogenetic tools that provide a direct and powerful method of controlling neuronal electrophysiology. Like the GPCRs discussed above, these channels are designed to be unresponsive to endogenous effectors while capable of being activated by an otherwise unrecognized small molecule. LGICs mainly differ from GPCRs in that they provide control over membrane conductance for many ions including chloride, calcium, and potassium. Activation or inhibition of action potential firing is often secondary to these ion-selective changes in membrane conductance.

Early attempts at remote control of ion conductance involved the expression of invertebrate receptors in mammals. In 2002, glutamate-gated chloride channels (GluCl) from the roundworm *Caenorhabditis elegans* were used to silence neurons *in vitro* [18]. When the antiparasitic drug ivermectin (IVM) activates GluCl, neuronal activity is inhibited as a result of the close proximity of chloride's equilibrium potential (~–65 mV) to the resting membrane potential (~–70 mV) typically found in mammalian neurons. When these chloride channels open, the likelihood that the membrane potential will drop below the threshold for an action potential (~–50 mV) decreases. GluCl is composed of two subunits, GluClα and GluClβ, which are both necessary for operation [18]. To allow usage of GluCl *in vivo*, a single point mutation (Y182F) was made to the binding site of GluClβ to dramatically reduce the potency of endogenous glutamate [19]. This mutation did not affect the binding of IVM because it is a positive allosteric modulator with a separate binding site [19]. IVM has been used previously as an antiparasitic drug in mammals; no overt effects on neuronal physiology have been seen. However, IVM can still activate GABA receptors, glycine receptors, and α7 nAChRs at a lower potency than GluCl. These additional effects have been associated with toxicity in the central nervous system [20]. For this reason, GluCl has been further modified to have an increase in affinity for IVM [21], allowing the use of smaller doses of IVM with lower toxicity. Another problem arises with IVM's slow pharmacokinetics. IVM is typically given as an intraperitoneal injection one day before the start of a study with effects reported to last over a week [22,23]. These prolonged effects are due to the lipophilicity of IVM which causes its accumulation in fat depots and slow recirculation back into the bloodstream. A few studies have been completed using GluCl, including silencing neurons in the striatum [22] and the hypothalamus [23].

Other IVM-sensitive receptors have been developed based on the glycine receptor (GlyR). Similar to GluCl, the first GlyR was an inhibitory chloride channel [24]. In 2016, another GlyR was made with three mutations that changed the selectivity from chloride to calcium [25]. This change to a cation channel allows control over depolarization and subsequent firing of action potentials. Overall, IVM-based technologies have been proven effective, despite the need to express two subunits (GluCl), slow pharmacokinetics, and low-grade toxicity.

Newer strategies for controlling ion conductance use engineered Cys-loop ion channels that selectively bind to a synthetic agonist. The creation of these tools was made possible by the independence of the ligand-binding domain (LBD) of the α7 nAChR [26]. A chimeric LGIC is created by transplanting the extracellular LBD of the α7 nAChR on to the transmembrane ion pore domain (IPD) of the 5-HT_3 receptor. Interestingly, this chimeric receptor has the pharmacology of the α7 nAChR with the ion conductance properties of the 5-HT_3 receptor. The usefulness of these receptors was limited because they are responsive to endogenous α7 nAChR agonists, but they provided proof of concept.

In 2011, different combinations of amino acids were mutated to create alternative α7 nAChR LBDs [27]. These LBDs, called pharmacologically selective actuator modules (PSAMs), were fused to the IPD of the 5-HT_{3a} receptor to generate 76 mutant channels. These channels were screened for the ability to be activated by 71 synthetic analogs of quinuclidinyl benzamide. During the screening, many PSAMs were found to have cognate agonists, or pharmacologically selective effector molecules (PSEMs). Three combinations of PSAMs/PSEMs were chosen and further engineered for higher potency, insensitivity to ACh, and powerful and prolonged conductance. Next, the PSAMs were fused to the IPDs of various Cys-loop ion channels to generate excitatory, inhibitory, and calcium-promoting LGICs. $PSAM^{141F, Y115F}$ was attached to the 5-HT_{3a} receptor to generate PSAM-5HT3, an excitatory LGIC that is both sodium and potassium permeable (Figure 7.2.A) [27]. The usefulness of PSAM-5HT3 has been demonstrated by a few studies. For example, intraperitoneal administration of $PSEM^{89S}$ penetrated the brain to activate pro-opiomelanocortin neurons in the hindbrain. This treatment reduced thermal pain for roughly 45 minutes [28].

Another LGIC was made by combining $PSAM^{L141F, Y115F}$ with the glycine receptor IPD (PSAM-GlyR) (Figure 7.2.B) [27]. When activated, this channel increases chloride permeability and strongly inhibits action potentials in a similar manner to GluCl. PSAM-GlyR has proven to be a powerful inhibitor of neuronal firing. It has been utilized for experiments on a variety of topics including fear conditioning [29,30], amyotrophic lateral sclerosis [31], and pain response [32]. Optogenetic activation of agouti-related peptide neurons in the hypothalamus immediately increased feeding; however, this behavior was completely blocked by $PSEM^{89S}$ administration and activation of PSAM-GlyR [27]. Additionally, PSAM-GlyR has been frequently used alongside PSAM-5HT3 to give bidirectional control of neuronal electrophysiology [31–33]. One issue with this approach is that both LGICs often use the same agonist, $PSEM^{89S}$; therefore, activation and inhibition experiments need to be conducted in different mice.

A final LGIC was created by transplanting $PSAM^{Q79G, L141S}$ on to the α7 nAChR IPD to create a calcium-permeable channel that is selectively activated by $PSEM^{9S}$ (Figure 7.2.C). This channel has the potential to control calcium conductance and to promote calmodulin signaling [27], though it has not been further studied.

7.2.3 Use of Chemogenetics

The chemogenetic tools described above provide a variety of non-invasive ways to perturb neuronal physiology. DREADDs can be used to indirectly increase or decrease neuronal excitability, to investigate the effects of β-arrestin, or to study the function of the various G-proteins. Alternatively, the use of PSAM receptors gives

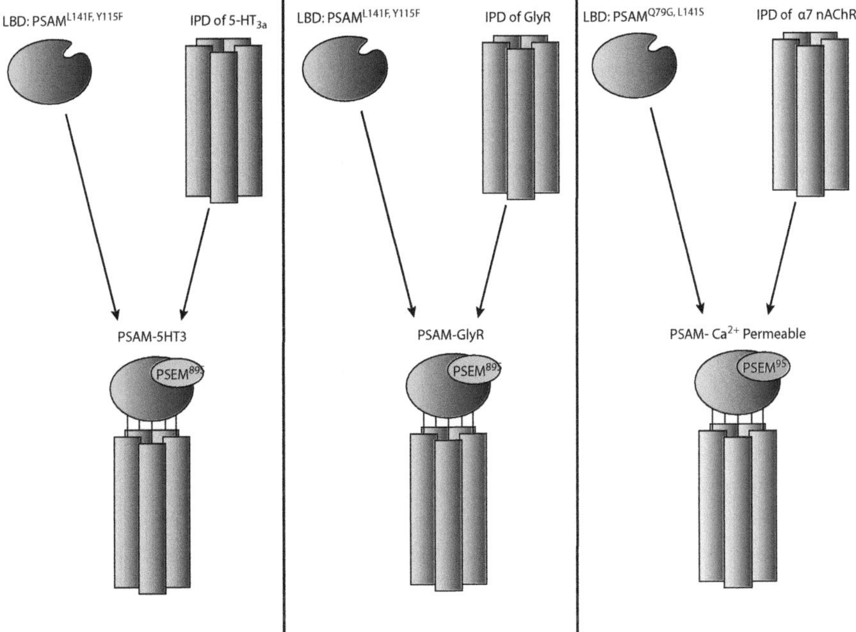

FIGURE 7.2 (**A**) The ligand-binding domain (LBD) PSAM$^{L141F, Y115F}$ was fused with the ion pore domain (IPD) of the 5-HT$_{3a}$ receptor to create PSAM-5HT3, a receptor that increases sodium and potassium permeability and increases neuronal excitability when bound to PSEM^{89S}. (**B**) The LBD PSAM$^{L141F, Y115F}$ was fused with the IPD of the glycine receptor (GlyR) to create PSAM-GlyR, a receptor that increases chloride permeability and decreases neuronal excitability when bound to PSEM^{89S}. (**C**) The LPD PSAM$^{Q79G, L141S}$ was fused with the IPD of the α7 nAChR to create a PSAM that is Ca2+ permeable. This receptor promotes Ca2+ calmodulin signaling when bound to PSEM^{9S}.

remote control over neuronal electrophysiology. Additionally, more than one receptor can be expressed in the same neuronal population assuming they have a different agonist. For example, hM3Dq and KORD can be expressed in the same neurons to allow excitation under CNO treatment and inhibition under salvinorin B treatment.

Administration of DREADD and PSAM receptor genes using adeno-associated viruses (AAVs) is an effective technique to get spatial and temporal control over receptor expression. Stereotaxic administration of one or more Cre-dependent AAVs into an animal line with a promoter-driven Cre gene can allow chemogenetic receptor expression limited to a specific neuronal population in the target brain region. This approach requires successful stereotaxic administration. In addition, investigators usually must wait to administer the agonist at least two weeks after viral administration to allow sufficient receptor expression to develop.

Alternatively, one can breed animals to generate an animal line with a promoter-driven Cre gene and a Cre-dependent chemogenetic receptor gene. For example, you could use mice that express either hM3Dq (#026220) or hM4Di (#026219) in the presence of Cre due to a loxP-flanked stop cassette found at Jackson Labs [34]. Crossing this mouse with another mouse that expresses Cre under the control of an energy-regulating gene promoter such as agouti-related peptide [35], pro-opiomelanocortin [36], or corticotropin releasing hormone [37] allows DREADD expression to be restricted to the target neuronal population. This technique does not restrict receptor expression to a targeted brain region. While breeding animals can be time-consuming, it circumvents the use of stereotaxic surgery. Using this approach, the receptor agonist can be given at any time or animal age; however, CNO administration during gestation or lactation phases has never been attempted. In comparison to optogenetics, described below, chemogenetics is often less invasive and better suited to prolonged experiments since optogenetics requires a permanent intracranial implant for light administration and prolonged light exposure is cytotoxic. Nevertheless, optogenetics has its own advantages.

7.3 OPTOGENETICS

Optogenetics is a research technique that employs the use of light-sensing proteins, often rhodopsins, to control neuronal physiology. Rhodopsins are a class of retinal-bound light-stimulated receptors that are found in both animals and microbes. Animal rhodopsins (also called type-I rhodopsins) are a class of GPCRs strictly used for phototransduction pathways. They allow the sensing of visual stimuli and the maintenance of circadian rhythms. Microbial rhodopsins (also called type-II rhodopsins) are predominantly used as research tools and include light-gated ion channels and light-activated ion pumps, and generate signal transduction pathways [38].

7.3.1 Microbial Rhodopsins

Microbial rhodopsins used in optogenetics involve engineered forms of channelrhodopsins, halorhodopsins, and archaerhodopsins. The first examples of optogenetics employed channelrhodopsins (ChRs), which are a class of excitatory channels discovered in green algae in 2002 [39]. Researchers suspect that these channels exist to guide algae toward a light source. When stimulated by blue light (470 nm), ChRs are a non-specific cation channel that increases the conductance of both sodium and potassium leading to depolarization in about 1–2 ms [40]. Two types exist, channelrhodopsin-1 (ChR1) and channelrhodopsin-2 (ChR2). Although ChR1 [39] was discovered before ChR2 [41], ChR2 is more commonly used because it has a higher initial depolarization in mammalian cells. A truncated version of ChR2 was used for the first optogenetics studies including excitation of the retina [42], hippocampus [43], and brain explants [44] from mice. Before long, a now widely used ChR2 variant was made with a single point mutation (H134) that gives a larger photocurrent [44].

Halorhodopsin is another microbial rhodopsin found in the archaeon *Natronomonas pharaonis* that is now used as an optogenetic tool. Upon yellow light stimulation (580 nm), these pumps inhibit neural activity within 10–15 ms by actively pumping chloride ions into the neuron, leading to hyperpolarization [45]. The first halorhodopsin was altered because it would aggregate in the endoplasmic reticulum rather than cell membrane. These problems were fixed in the third generation halorhodopsin (eNpHR3.0) that has export and trafficking signals added to the C-terminus [46]. eNpHR3.0 is a powerful tool for optogenetic studies that is still commonly used [47].

Lastly, the microbial archaerhodopsin is an outward proton pump found in the archaeon *Halorubrum sodomense*. ArchT is a variant of this archaerhodopsin with more than a three-fold increase in light-sensitivity [48]. When ArchT is activated by yellow or green light (566 nm), positively charged protons are pumped out of the neuron leading to hyperpolarization [49]. ArchT has been used in a variety of research studies in mice involving narcolepsy [50], regulation of pain [51], and food-seeking behavior [52]. In the next section, we will discuss how channelrhodopsins have been further engineered to acquire different types of functionality.

7.3.2 Engineered Channelrhodopsins and Other Optogenetic Tools

Channelrhodopsins have been engineered to alter the speed of their kinetics, activation wavelength, and conductance affinity. Many channelrhodopsins have been generated to promote fast kinetics. One commonly used excitatory channel called ChETA was created with a point mutation (E123T) that allows a spiking frequency of up to 200 Hz, reduced plateau potentials, and faster recovery from inactivation compared to ChR2 [53]. ChIEF (aka oChIEF) is a ChR1 and ChR2 chimeric receptor that was designed to reduce auto-inactivation and improve the rate of channel closure in the absence of light compared to ChR2 [54]. ChIEF is a valuable tool for experiments involving prolonged stimulation. Some of the fastest channel kinetics and highest light sensitivity are found in Chronos, an excitatory channelrhodopsin that turns on in 2.3 ms and turns off in 3.6 ms [55]. Overall, faster channel kinetics ensure strong temporal control and help to mimic natural action potential propagation.

Another class of channelrhodopsins called bi-stable or step function opsins (SFOs) have a stable conducting state to allow prolonged excitation after a 10-ms burst of blue light (445–470 nm). Subsequently, these channels can be inactivated by a burst of yellow light (560–590 nm) [56]. The first SFO was a ChR2 with a point mutation (C128S) that stayed active for 1–2 minutes after light activation [57]. A separate point mutation in ChR2 (D156A) led to prolonged activation of seven minutes [58]. The stabilized step function opsin, known as SSFO, contains both of these mutations to allow an almost 30-minute activation time [59]. These receptors, also called hChR2(C128S/D156A), allow longer experiments without the harmful effects of long-term light exposure. Additionally, a 30-minute activation time allows for the optic fiber to be removed after activation to give the mouse complete mobility.

Many channelrhodopsins have been developed, shifting the blue activation wavelengths (450–495 nm) in the direction of a red wavelength (620–750 nm). Red light is less phototoxic, absorbed less by blood, and scatters less in the brain. Red light's superior penetration has even allowed some experiments to administer light transcranially [60]. One of the first effective red-shifted channelrhodopsins was called C1V1. C1V1 is optimally stimulated by light at 540 nm and can generate a high photocurrent [59]. However, one issue with C1V1 is that it cannot be used alongside a blue-stimulated opsin without cross-activation. Red-shifted ChrimsonR (aka Chrimson) was designed to be used alongside blue-stimulated Chronos to allow independent excitation of two neuronal populations [55]. These two channelrhodopsins make an effective pair, since ChrimsonR's optimal stimulation at 590 nm wavelength has no effect on Chronos while the low amount of light needed to activate Chronos has no effect on Chrimson.

Although eNpHR3.0 and ArchT are the most frequently used inhibitory optogenetic tools, these pumps are less sensitive and have slower kinetics than channel-based technology. GtACR1 and GtACR2 are anion channel rhodopsins that inhibit neurons with faster kinetics and higher light sensitivity [61]. Furthermore, the development of these anion channelrhodopsins allows step function variants to be generated such as SwiChRca [62] and the next-generation version Swi++ [63]. Overall, these engineered channelrhodopsins allow excellent control over neuronal physiology.

The optogenetic toolbox has been expanded further through the creation of light-sensitive GPCRs. Opto-XRs are chimeric light-activatable GPCRs made by replacing the intracellular loop of mammalian rhodopsin with residues from various GPCRs. The X in opto-XR refers to the GPCR used. Opto-XR is an extensive family of receptors including opto-D1R (dopamine type 1 receptor) [64], opto-μOR (μ-opioid receptor) [65], opto-mGluR6 (metabotropic glutamate receptor 6) [66], opto-A2AR (adenosine 2A receptor) [67], opto-α1AR (α_{1a}-adrenergic receptor), and opto-β2AR (β_2-adrenergic receptor). Although an extensive family of receptors exists, the two primary receptors used are opto-α1AR that couples to Gq and opto-β2AR that couples to Gs. When utilized in the nucleus accumbens, opto-α1AR increased neuronal spiking and opto-β2AR decreased neuronal spiking [68]. Overall, opto-XRs are another helpful tool for understanding receptor function and neural circuits.

7.3.3 Uses of Optogenetics

The various channelrhodopsin, halorhodopsin, and archaerhodopsin variants give extensive control of excitation or inhibition of single or multiple neuronal populations. Due to the difference in activating wavelengths between opsins, it is possible to use two rhodopsins in the same brain region. For example, if both ChR2 and eNpHR3.0 are expressed in the same neurons or same brain region, depolarization can be induced by blue light and hyperpolarization can be induced by yellow light. Overall, several helpful optogenetic tools exist for neuroscience studies. These tools can be viewed in Table 7.1

Optogenetic genes can be delivered using similar methods to chemogenetics. However, additional stereotaxic surgery needs to be done to add a cannula or implant for administering the light via an optical fiber, a filament that radiates light from its tip. A 200-μm optical fiber can be placed on top of the skull or fed through a cannula into the brain. These optical fibers are coupled to either a laser or light-emitting diode. A multiplex laser can rapidly switch between activating and inhibiting wavelengths with millisecond precision; this setup is ideal when using both stimulatory and inhibitory opsins. However, to simultaneously activate two rhodopsins, two LEDs would need to be mounted on the optical fiber for simultaneous administration of two different lights [69]. It is also possible to stimulate rhodopsins in two different brain regions with the use of two separate optical fibers.

Optogenetic manipulations *in vivo* are often accompanied by simultaneous electrophysiological recordings with an electrode, which may be separate from the LED light. An optrode (aka optode) is a neural probe that combines the electrode with the optic fiber containing the light source. Additionally, voltage-sensitive dyes (VSDs) can be used as a less invasive alternative to patch-clamp and electrode monitoring of many

TABLE 7.1
List of optogenetic receptors

Name	Rhodopsin Type	Excitatory or Inhibitory	Activation Wavelength (nm)	Kinetics	Affinity
ChR2(H134R)	Channelrhodopsin	Excitatory	470, Blue	Normal	Na^+/K^+ Channel
eNpHR3.0	Halorhodopsin	Inhibitory	580, Yellow	Normal	Cl^- Pump
ArchT	Archaerhodopsin	Inhibitory	566, Green	Normal	H^+ Pump
ChETA	Channelrhodopsin	Excitatory	490, Blue	Fast	Na^+/K^+ Channel
ChIEF	Channelrhodopsin	Excitatory	460, Blue	Fast	Na^+/K^+ Channel
Chronos	Channelrhodopsin	Excitatory	500, Green	Fast	Na^+/K^+ Channel
hChR2(C128S/ D156A)	Channelrhodopsin	Excitatory	470 (active), 590 (inactive)	Slow (SSFO)	Na^+/K^+ Channel
C1V1	Channelrhodopsin	Excitatory	540, Green	Normal	Na^+/K^+ Channel
ChrimsonR	Channelrhodopsin	Excitatory	590, Yellow	Normal	Na^+/K^+ Channel
GtACR1	Channelrhodopsin	Inhibitory	515, Green	Normal	Cl^- Channel
SwiChRca	Channelrhodopsin	Inhibitory	475, Blue	Slow (SSFO)	Cl^- Channel

electrophysiological characteristics. VSDs can be directly administered or genetically encoded in the neurons. The use of genetically encoded indicators can show changes in activity caused by chemogenetics and optogenetics as discussed below.

7.4 GENETICALLY ENCODED INDICATORS

Genetically encoded indicators allow large-scale neuronal activity recordings and have become invaluable tools for understanding how neurons function individually and in circuits. Compared to externally administered dyes, genetic encoding gives promoter-specific spatial control of gene expression and the ability to analyze changes in neuronal activity over time. The latter is of particular interest, since researchers can record neuronal activity during learning, aging, or disease development such as during obesity and diabetes. The major advantage of genetically encoded indicators over electrode recording is that they allow many neurons and ensemble activity to be easily observed in living tissue. Other advantages include the capability to easily record voltage from subcellular areas like the axons or dendritic spines and being less invasive than electrodes [70].

One class of these dyes is genetically encoded pH indicators (GEPIs) that help label vesicle fusion events at the synapse. Ecliptic pHluorin is a pH-sensitive GFP molecule; it is protonated and non-fluorescent at ~5.5 pH but becomes (partly) unprotonated and fluorescent at ~7.1 pH [71]. This molecule was further improved with the creation of fluorescent super ecliptic pHluorin (SEP) which is completely deprotonated at neutral pH [72]. SEP was attached to transmembrane proteins such as Vglut2, synaptophysin, and vesicle-associated membrane protein (VAMP). It is normally localized on vesicles in the intraluminal space at a pH of ~5.5, but when a vesicle fuses at a synapse, SEP is exposed to a neutral pH and fluoresces (Figure 7.3.A). GEPIs utilizing SEP can help record neuronal activity, but autofluorescence and the scattering of 488 nm light prevent single action potential resolution *in vivo* [70].

Another small class of indicators allows optical detection of glutamate release. The primary member of this family, iGluSnFR, is an extracellular peripheral membrane protein that becomes fluorescent when bound to secreted glutamate in the synapse [73]. Although this protein is not specifically localized to any region of the neuron, it only responds to the high concentrations of glutamate found in the synapse (Figure 7.3.B). The fast kinetics of glutamate removal means that iGluSnFR is responsive to single action potentials. iGluSnFR is a helpful tool for neurotransmitter-specific detection of neuronal activity; however, similar indicators have not yet been developed for other transmitters [70].

One of the most popular classes of optical indicators is genetically encoded calcium indicators (GECIs). An increase in intracellular calcium is a sign of neuronal activation, whether calcium enters through glutamate LGICs in the dendrites or through voltage-gated calcium channels at axon terminals. All GECIs derive from calmodulin (CaM), localize to the cytosol, and fluoresce when bound to calcium (Figure 7.3.C–D); however, they are broken into two classes based on whether they contain one or two fluorophores. GECIs with two fluorophores are called Cameleons and detect intracellular calcium through fluorescence resonance energy transfer (FRET). For example, D3cpv contains CaM for calcium binding and ECFP and EYFP to generate FRET [74]. Without calcium, the activation wavelength will cause ECFP in D3cpv to fluoresce cyan. However, calcium binding changes protein conformation, bringing the two fluorophores closer together and causing energy transfer from ECFP to EYFP resulting in D3cpv fluorescing yellow.

Single-fluorophore GECIs are called GCaMPs and are bound to circularly permutated GFP (cpGFP). GCaMPs have been improved over many generations with the GCaMP6 series being the most common [75]; however, it appears that the new jGCaMP7 series is quickly being adopted [76]. jGCaMP7f sensors were designed with fast kinetics to decrease signal decay time and are useful for detecting action potentials at higher frequencies. In contrast, jGCaMP7s with slow kinetics could detect several active neurons at once. jGCaMP7c is known for low deactivated fluorescence levels, which provides greater contrast in larger neuronal populations with wide-field fluorescence imaging. By comparison, jGCaMP7b has high deactivated fluorescence levels which help detect samples and subcellular areas with small amounts of labeling or localization to structures like dendritic spines [76].

Overall, GECIs are an excellent tool for detecting neuronal activity due to the slow kinetics of calcium. In most neurons, it takes roughly 10 ms for intracellular calcium concentration to reach 150 nM and has a half decay time of 50–70 ms. This event is ten times slower than an action potential and much more efficiently detected; however, this amplification means that GECIs, in general, cannot discriminate high-frequency action potential firing.

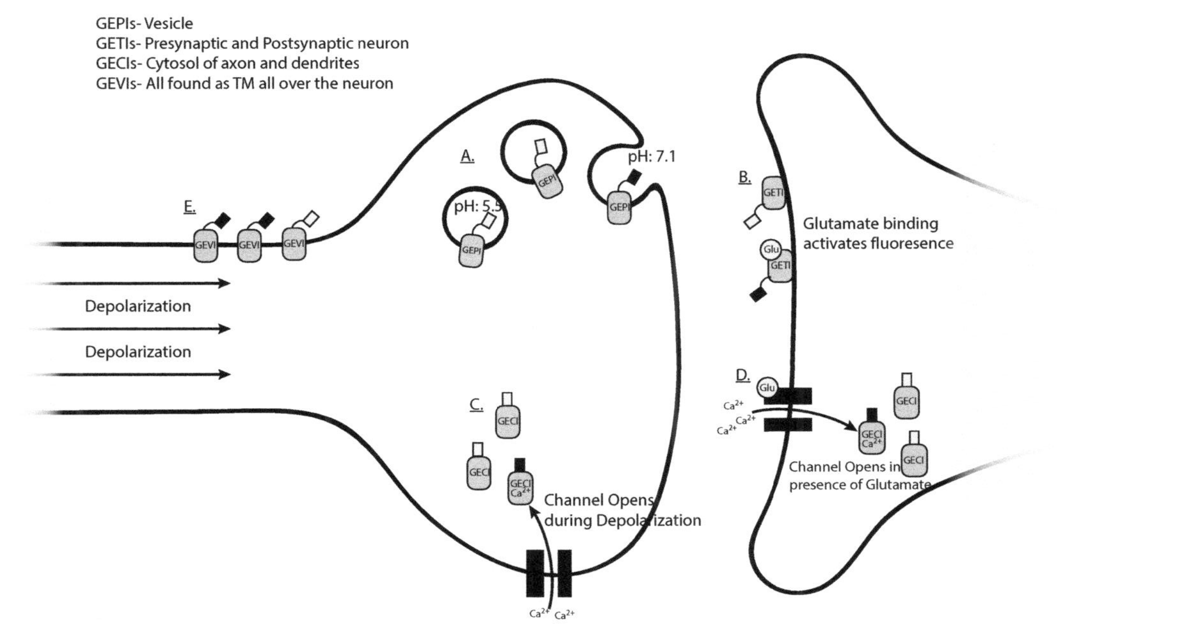

FIGURE 7.3 (**A**) Genetically encoded pH indicators (GEPIs) are found on vesicles with the GFP molecule at a 5.5 pH within the intraluminal space. When the vesicle fuses with the synapse, the GFP is exposed to a 7.1 pH and fluoresces. (**B**) Genetically encoded transmitter indicators (GETIs) are found on the cell membrane of the post-synaptic cell and will fluoresce when bound to glutamate. (**C**) Genetically encoded Ca2+ indicators (GECIs) are found in the cytosol and fluoresce when bound to Ca2+. GECIs can be activated when Ca2+ enters the axon terminal via a voltage-gated channel. (**D**) Additionally, GECIs can be activated when neurotransmitters (such as glutamate) bind and open Ca2+ channels in the post-synaptic neuron. (**E**) Genetically encoded voltage indicators (GEVIs) are voltage sensitive and will fluoresce when the neuron is depolarized.

The ongoing development of genetically encoded voltage indicators (GEVIs) takes advantage of the speed permitted by detecting voltage directly (Figure 7.3.E). GEVIs can detect certain parameters that GECIs cannot, including high-frequency firing, membrane hyperpolarizations, and subthreshold voltage changes. However, since 1997, when both GECIs and GEVIs were developed, GECIs have outmatched GEVIs with a much larger and more easily detectable response. Although GEVIs exist in many different forms with a fluorescent protein FRET pair (e.g. VSFP-CR) [77], an opsin (e.g. QuasAr3) [78], or an opsin-fluorescent protein FRET pair (e.g. Mac GEVIs) [79], it was not until the development of Arclight that responses were large enough to detect single action potentials in HEK 293 cells. Arclight combined the voltage-sensitive domain from a phosphatase found in *Ciona intestinalis* (Ci-VSD) with SEP; it decreases fluorescence by ~35% during 100 mV depolarization *in vitro* [80]. However, the slow kinetics of Arclight prevents it from detecting action potentials at frequencies of 100 Hz or higher.

Accelerated Sensor of Action Potentials 1 (ASAP1) is another GEVI designed to solve these problems. Instead of using Ci-VSD, ASAP1 combines the voltage-sensitive domain from the phosphatase found in *Gallus gallus* with cpGFP. This technology allows improved brightness up to ~45% and detects action potential trains at 200 Hz *in vitro* [81]. ASAP2f was developed to have similar response kinetics to ASAP1, but showed bigger responses to depolarization and hyperpolarization when tested in Drosophila [82]. Finally, an ASAP3 variant was recently developed with the promise of 51% variation in fluorescence, submillisecond activation kinetics, and responsiveness to two-photon excitation in deep tissue on awake mice [83].

Overall, GECIs still present much larger responses than GEVIs, which makes them more easily detectable. However, GEVIs remain an attractive subject of ongoing research with the capability to detect high-frequency action potentials, membrane hyperpolarizations, and subthreshold changes in voltage.

7.5 GENETIC TECHNIQUES IN THE STUDY OF ENERGY HOMEOSTASIS

Many of these genetic tools are used widely today in a variety of neuroscience fields. Several have been adopted for use in studying how the brain controls energy homeostasis. Chemogenetic experiments can analyze feeding [84–86] and levels of activity [87,88] for several hours during neural activation or inhibition in the hypothalamus. For example, one paper that was published in *Cell Metabolism* detailed the use of hM3Dq in glucose-dependent insulinotropic polypeptide receptor (GIPR) and glucose-like peptide 1 receptor (GLP1R) neurons in the hypothalamus. When measuring the first two hours of the dark cycle, food intake was decreased during GIPR neuronal activation and there was no additive effect from co-activation with GLP1R neurons [86]. Chemogenetics have also proven useful for the study of locomotion. One study expressed excitatory and inhibitory DREADDs in orexin neurons in the lateral hypothalamus to see their effects on physical activity. Activation of orexin neurons using hM3Dq led to increases in spontaneous physical activity while inhibition with hM4Di led to a decrease in spontaneous physical activity when recorded for two hours [87]. Chemogenetics have also been used to understand the role of hypothalamic populations in glucose homeostasis. For example, inhibiting POMC neurons has a detectable effect on blood glucose levels [89,90].

In contrast to chemogenetics, optogenetics allows remote control over neuronal physiology with millisecond precision. Optogenetics can demonstrate powerful behavioral effects following neuronal manipulation. One paper published in *Science* expressed ChR2 in GABA neurons in the zona incerta. These mice demonstrated induction of binge-like feeding within two to three seconds of light activation [91]. The rapid mechanisms of optogenetics also couple well with *ex vivo* electrophysiology experiments [92,93]. For example, the presence of inhibitory postsynaptic currents (IPSCs) was recorded from POMC neurons in brain slices. When upstream AgRP neurons were activated using ChR2, the blockage of GABA release in these neurons had no effect on the frequency of IPSCs in POMC neurons [94]. Optogenetics can also help analyze non-behavioral homeostatic parameters such as changes in body temperature [95], blood glucose [96], energy expenditure, and heart rate [97].

One method called channelrhodopsin-2-assisted circuit mapping (CRACM) repurposes optogenetic tools for anterograde neuronal tracing. Brain slices are optogenetically stimulated and action potentials are detected to indicate the presence of ChR2 in the axons of the target projection. CRACM works on the assumption that ChR2 is effectively trafficked down the axon. Recently it was shown that CRACM also works with the fast-kinetic Chronos receptor and the red-shifted ChrimsonR. These results open the door to studying two circuits using different wavelengths and to seeing how projections from two cell types converge in the same brain region. Additionally, this technique has been used extensively in the energy homeostasis literature. For example, CRACM was utilized to find the projections of a population of glucose-sensing estrogen receptor-α expressing neurons in the ventromedial hypothalamus [98].

Some concerns exist over the ability of optogenetics to emulate natural activity patterns with many optogenetic studies achieving firing rates near or above the maximal rate possible under spontaneous conditions. For example, striatal neurons were stimulated from a range of 0.1–3.0 mW with 1 mW reaching maximal firing rates [99]. Many animal studies have stimulated striatal neurons far above 1 mW [100]. Chemogenetics, which increases the likelihood of firing but does not directly initiate action potentials, avoids these issues. For this reason and to compare short and long-term effects of neuronal manipulation, optogenetics is frequently used alongside chemogenetics [101–104]. This approach can also help show the timescale of behavioral onset and provide evidence that the study's results were not caused by CNO, clozapine, or light administration. For example, a recent paper published in *Cell* characterized key afferent vagal neurons that detect food intake using mechanoreceptors in the intestines. These vagal neurons that project to the nucleus tractus solitarius blocked food intake in hungry mice when stimulated by ChR2 or hM3Dq. Furthermore, AgRP neurons, expressing GCamp6m, were fluorescent during optogenetic or chemogenetic activation of this vagal neuron population [105]. Lastly, genetically encoded indicators have also begun to be adopted by the field. GEVIs and GECIs are often used to see the level of activity in neurons that are targeted by or downstream of optogenetic or chemogenetic modifications [105].

7.6 CONCLUSION

The field of the CNS control of energy homeostasis and food intake has at times been accused of seeing itself as separate from the wider discipline of neuroscience. This perception perhaps had some validity when study in the field was limited to the hypothalamus, standing as it does between the brain and endocrine axes and its extensive interaction with systems outside of the CNS. However, in the past decade attention has turned to the integration of feeding-related circuits with areas of the brain controlling general decision making and motivation, motor control, sensory perception, social behavior, and the autonomic nervous system. Likewise, it is unsurprising that technologies employed in other neuroscience fields over this time frame have been quickly adopted for the study of energy homeostasis. That trend is likely to continue.

In conjunction with new techniques for manipulating genes, characterizing neurons, and visualizing neuron circuits, the revolutionary technologies we have described will no doubt continue to provide a powerful means for learning about the neural control of metabolism. As they are refined, they will bring us closer to an in depth understanding of the complex workings of the relevant nuclei. Ultimately, such advances will benefit our overall understanding of the integrated function of life-sustaining neural pathways.

REFERENCES

1 Strader, C. D. et al. Allele-specific activation of genetically engineered receptors. *J Biol Chem* 266, 5–8 (1991).

2 Coward, P. et al. Controlling signaling with a specifically designed Gi-coupled receptor. *Proc Natl Acad Sci U S A* 95, 352–357, doi:10.1073/pnas.95.1.352 (1998).

3 Sternson, S. M. & Roth, B. L. Chemogenetic tools to interrogate brain functions. *Annu Rev Neurosci* 37, 387–407, doi:10.1146/annurev-neuro-071013-014048 (2014).

4 Armbruster, B. N., Li, X., Pausch, M. H., Herlitze, S. & Roth, B. L. Evolving the lock to fit the key to create a family of G protein-coupled receptors potently activated by an inert ligand. *Proc Natl Acad Sci U S A* 104, 5163–5168, doi:10.1073/pnas.0700293104 (2007).

5 Runegaard, A. H. et al. Modulating Dopamine Signaling and Behavior with Chemogenetics: Concepts, Progress, and Challenges. *Pharmacol Rev* 71, 123–156, doi:10.1124/pr.117.013995 (2019).

6 Alexander, G. M. et al. Remote control of neuronal activity in transgenic mice expressing evolved G protein-coupled receptors. *Neuron* 63, 27–39, doi:10.1016/j.neuron.2009.06.014 (2009).

7 Atasoy, D., Betley, J. N., Su, H. H. & Sternson, S. M. Deconstruction of a neural circuit for hunger. *Nature* 488, 172–177, doi:10.1038/nature11270 (2012).

8 Ray, R. S. et al. Impaired respiratory and body temperature control upon acute serotonergic neuron inhibition. *Science* 333, 637–642, doi:10.1126/science.1205295 (2011).

9 Ferguson, S. M. et al. Transient neuronal inhibition reveals opposing roles of indirect and direct pathways in sensitization. *Nat Neurosci* 14, 22–24, doi:10.1038/nn.2703 (2011).

10 Pleil, K. E.. et al. NPY signaling inhibits extended amygdala CRF neurons to suppress binge alcohol drinking. *Nat Neurosci* 18, 545–552, doi:10.1038/nn.3972 (2015).

11 Brancaccio, M., Maywood, E. S., Chesham, J. E., Loudon, A. S. & Hastings, M. H. A Gq-Ca2+ axis controls circuit-level encoding of circadian time in the suprachiasmatic nucleus. *Neuron* 78, 714–728, doi:10.1016/j.neuron.2013.03.011 (2013).

12 Guettier, J. M. et al. A chemical-genetic approach to study G protein regulation of beta cell function in vivo. *Proc Natl Acad Sci U S A* 106, 19197–19202, doi:10.1073/pnas.0906593106 (2009).
13 Nakajima, K. & Wess, J. Design and functional characterization of a novel, arrestin-biased designer G protein-coupled receptor. *Mol Pharmacol* 82, 575–582, doi:10.1124/mol.112.080358 (2012).
14 Jann, M. W., Lam, Y. W. & Chang, W. H. Rapid formation of clozapine in guinea-pigs and man following clozapine-N-oxide administration. *Arch Int Pharmacodyn Ther* 328, 243–250 (1994).
15 Jendryka, M. et al. Pharmacokinetic and pharmacodynamic actions of clozapine-N-oxide, clozapine, and compound 21 in DREADD-based chemogenetics in mice. *Sci Rep* 9, 4522, doi:10.1038/s41598-019-41088-2 (2019).
16 Chen, X. et al. The first structure-activity relationship studies for designer receptors exclusively activated by designer drugs. *ACS Chem Neurosci* 6, 476–484, doi:10.1021/cn500325v (2015).
17 Vardy, E. et al. A new DREADD facilitates the multiplexed chemogenetic interrogation of behavior. *Neuron* 86, 936–946, doi:10.1016/j.neuron.2015.03.065 (2015).
18 Slimko, E. M., McKinney, S., Anderson, D. J., Davidson, N. & Lester, H. A. Selective electrical silencing of mammalian neurons in vitro by the use of invertebrate ligand-gated chloride channels. *J Neurosci* 22, 7373–7379 (2002).
19 Li, P., Slimko, E. M. & Lester, H. A. Selective elimination of glutamate activation and introduction of fluorescent proteins into a Caenorhabditis elegans chloride channel. *FEBS Lett* 528, 77–82, doi:10.1016/s0014-5793(02)03245-3 (2002).
20 Zemkova, H., Tvrdonova, V., Bhattacharya, A. & Jindrichova, M. Allosteric modulation of ligand gated ion channels by ivermectin. *Physiol Res* 63 Suppl 1, S215–S224 (2014).
21 Frazier, S. J., Cohen, B. N. & Lester, H. A. An engineered glutamate-gated chloride (GluCl) channel for sensitive, consistent neuronal silencing by ivermectin. *J Biol Chem* 288, 21029–21042, doi:10.1074/jbc.M112.423921 (2013).
22 Lerchner, W. et al. Reversible silencing of neuronal excitability in behaving mice by a genetically targeted, ivermectin-gated Cl- channel. *Neuron* 54, 35–49, doi:10.1016/j.neuron.2007.02.030 (2007).
23 Lin, D. et al. Functional identification of an aggression locus in the mouse hypothalamus. *Nature* 470, 221–226, doi:10.1038/nature09736 (2011).
24 Lynagh, T. & Lynch, J. W. An improved ivermectin-activated chloride channel receptor for inhibiting electrical activity in defined neuronal populations. *J Biol Chem* 285, 14890–14897, doi:10.1074/jbc.M110.107789 (2010).
25 Islam, R. et al. Ivermectin-activated, cation-permeable glycine receptors for the chemogenetic control of neuronal excitation. *ACS Chem Neurosci* 7, 1647–1657, doi:10.1021/acschemneuro.6b00168 (2016).
26 Eisele, J. L. et al. Chimaeric nicotinic-serotonergic receptor combines distinct ligand binding and channel specificities. *Nature* 366, 479–483, doi:10.1038/366479a0 (1993).
27 Magnus, C. J. et al. Chemical and genetic engineering of selective ion channel-ligand interactions. *Science* 333, 1292–1296, doi:10.1126/science.1206606 (2011).
28 Cerritelli, S., Hirschberg, S., Hill, R., Balthasar, N. & Pickering, A. E. Activation of brainstem pro-opiomelanocortin neurons produces opioidergic analgesia, Bradycardia and Bradypnoea. *PLoS One* 11, e0153187, doi:10.1371/journal.pone.0153187 (2016).
29 Lovett-Barron, M. et al. Dendritic inhibition in the hippocampus supports fear learning. *Science* 343, 857–863, doi:10.1126/science.1247485 (2014).
30 Basu, J. et al. Gating of hippocampal activity, plasticity, and memory by entorhinal cortex long-range inhibition. *Science* 351, aaa5694, doi:10.1126/science.aaa5694 (2016).

31 Saxena, S. et al. Neuroprotection through excitability and mTOR required in ALS motoneurons to delay disease and extend survival. *Neuron* 80, 80–96, doi:10.1016/j.neuron.2013.07.027 (2013).

32 Ren, W. et al. The indirect pathway of the nucleus accumbens shell amplifies neuropathic pain. *Nat Neurosci* 19, 220–222, doi:10.1038/nn.4199 (2016).

33 Donato, F., Chowdhury, A., Lahr, M. & Caroni, P. Early- and late-born parvalbumin basket cell subpopulations exhibiting distinct regulation and roles in learning. *Neuron* 85, 770–786, doi:10.1016/j.neuron.2015.01.011 (2015).

34 Zhu, H. et al. Cre-dependent DREADD (Designer Receptors Exclusively Activated by Designer Drugs) mice. *Genesis* 54, 439–446, doi:10.1002/dvg.22949 (2016).

35 Tong, Q., Ye, C. P., Jones, J. E., Elmquist, J. K. & Lowell, B. B. Synaptic release of GABA by AgRP neurons is required for normal regulation of energy balance. *Nat Neurosci* 11, 998–1000, doi:10.1038/nn.2167 (2008).

36 Balthasar, N. et al. Leptin receptor signaling in POMC neurons is required for normal body weight homeostasis. *Neuron* 42, 983–991, doi:10.1016/j.neuron.2004.06.004 (2004).

37 Taniguchi, H. et al. A resource of Cre driver lines for genetic targeting of GABAergic neurons in cerebral cortex. *Neuron* 71, 995–1013, doi:10.1016/j.neuron.2011.07.026 (2011).

38 Ernst, O. P. et al. Microbial and animal rhodopsins: structures, functions, and molecular mechanisms. *Chem Rev* 114, 126–163, doi:10.1021/cr4003769 (2014).

39 Nagel, G. et al. Channelrhodopsin-1: a light-gated proton channel in green algae. *Science* 296, 2395–2398, doi:10.1126/science.1072068 (2002).

40 Bamann, C., Kirsch, T., Nagel, G. & Bamberg, E. Spectral characteristics of the photocycle of channelrhodopsin-2 and its implication for channel function. *J Mol Biol* 375, 686–694, doi:10.1016/j.jmb.2007.10.072 (2008).

41 Nagel, G. et al. Channelrhodopsin-2, a directly light-gated cation-selective membrane channel. *Proc Natl Acad Sci U S A* 100, 13940–13945, doi:10.1073/pnas.1936192100 (2003).

42 Bi, A. et al. Ectopic expression of a microbial-type rhodopsin restores visual responses in mice with photoreceptor degeneration. *Neuron* 50, 23–33, doi:10.1016/j.neuron.2006.02.026 (2006).

43 Boyden, E. S., Zhang, F., Bamberg, E., Nagel, G. & Deisseroth, K. Millisecond-timescale, genetically targeted optical control of neural activity. *Nat Neurosci* 8, 1263–1268, doi:10.1038/nn1525 (2005).

44 Nagel, G. et al. Light activation of channelrhodopsin-2 in excitable cells of Caenorhabditis elegans triggers rapid behavioral responses. *Curr Biol* 15, 2279–2284, doi:10.1016/j.cub.2005.11.032 (2005).

45 Han, X. & Boyden, E. S. Multiple-color optical activation, silencing, and desynchronization of neural activity, with single-spike temporal resolution. *PLoS One* 2, e299, doi:10.1371/journal.pone.0000299 (2007).

46 Gradinaru, V. et al. Molecular and cellular approaches for diversifying and extending optogenetics. *Cell* 141, 154–165, doi:10.1016/j.cell.2010.02.037 (2010).

47 Vecchia, D. et al. Temporal Sharpening of Sensory Responses by Layer V in the Mouse Primary Somatosensory Cortex. *Curr Biol* 30, 1589–1599, doi:10.1016/j.cub.2020.02.004 (2020).

48 Han, X. et al. A high-light sensitivity optical neural silencer: development and application to optogenetic control of non-human primate cortex. *Front Syst Neurosci* 5, 18, doi:10.3389/fnsys.2011.00018 (2011).

49 Chow, B. Y. et al. High-performance genetically targetable optical neural silencing by light-driven proton pumps. *Nature* 463, 98–102, doi:10.1038/nature08652 (2010).

50 Williams, R. H. et al. Transgenic archaerhodopsin-3 expression in hypocretin/orexin neurons engenders cellular dysfunction and features of type 2 narcolepsy. *J Neurosci* 39, 9435–9452, doi:10.1523/JNEUROSCI.0311-19.2019 (2019).

51 Siemian, J. N., Borja, C. B., Sarsfield, S., Kisner, A. & Aponte, Y. Lateral hypothalamic fast-spiking parvalbumin neurons modulate nociception through connections in the periaqueductal gray area. *Sci Rep* 9, 12026, doi:10.1038/s41598-019-48537-y (2019).
52 Schiffino, F. L. et al. Activation of a lateral hypothalamic-ventral tegmental circuit gates motivation. *PLoS One* 14, e0219522, doi:10.1371/journal.pone.0219522 (2019).
53 Gunaydin, L. A. et al. Ultrafast optogenetic control. *Nat Neurosci* 13, 387–392, doi:10.1038/nn.2495 (2010).
54 Lin, J. Y., Lin, M. Z., Steinbach, P. & Tsien, R. Y. Characterization of engineered channelrhodopsin variants with improved properties and kinetics. *Biophys J* 96, 1803–1814, doi:10.1016/j.bpj.2008.11.034 (2009).
55 Klapoetke, N. C. et al. Independent optical excitation of distinct neural populations. *Nat Methods* 11, 338–346, doi:10.1038/nmeth.2836 (2014).
56 Fenno, L., Yizhar, O. & Deisseroth, K. The development and application of optogenetics. *Annu Rev Neurosci* 34, 389–412, doi:10.1146/annurev-neuro-061010-113817 (2011).
57 Berndt, A., Yizhar, O., Gunaydin, L. A., Hegemann, P. & Deisseroth, K. Bi-stable neural state switches. *Nat Neurosci* 12, 229–234, doi:10.1038/nn.2247 (2009).
58 Bamann, C., Gueta, R., Kleinlogel, S., Nagel, G. & Bamberg, E. Structural guidance of the photocycle of channelrhodopsin-2 by an interhelical hydrogen bond. *Biochemistry* 49, 267–278, doi:10.1021/bi901634p (2010).
59 Yizhar, O. et al. Neocortical excitation/inhibition balance in information processing and social dysfunction. *Nature* 477, 171–178, doi:10.1038/nature10360 (2011).
60 Lin, J. Y., Knutsen, P. M., Muller, A., Kleinfeld, D. & Tsien, R. Y. ReaChR: a red-shifted variant of channelrhodopsin enables deep transcranial optogenetic excitation. *Nat Neurosci* 16, 1499–1508, doi:10.1038/nn.3502 (2013).
61 Govorunova, E. G., Sineshchekov, O. A., Janz, R., Liu, X. & Spudich, J. L. NEUROSCIENCE. Natural light-gated anion channels: A family of microbial rhodopsins for advanced optogenetics. *Science* 349, 647–650, doi:10.1126/science.aaa7484 (2015).
62 Berndt, A., Lee, S. Y., Ramakrishnan, C. & Deisseroth, K. Structure-guided transformation of channelrhodopsin into a light-activated chloride channel. *Science* 344, 420–424, doi:10.1126/science.1252367 (2014).
63 Berndt, A. et al. Structural foundations of optogenetics: determinants of channelrhodopsin ion selectivity. *Proc Natl Acad Sci U S A* 113, 822–829, doi:10.1073/pnas.1523341113 (2016).
64 Gunaydin, L. A. et al. Natural neural projection dynamics underlying social behavior. *Cell* 157, 1535–1551, doi:10.1016/j.cell.2014.05.017 (2014).
65 Siuda, E. R. et al. Spatiotemporal control of opioid signaling and behavior. *Neuron* 86, 923–935, doi:10.1016/j.neuron.2015.03.066 (2015).
66 van Wyk, M., Pielecka-Fortuna, J., Lowel, S. & Kleinlogel, S. Restoring the on switch in blind retinas: opto-mglur6, a next-generation, cell-tailored optogenetic tool. *PLoS Biol* 13, e1002143, doi:10.1371/journal.pbio.1002143 (2015).
67 Li, P. et al. Optogenetic activation of intracellular adenosine A2A receptor signaling in the hippocampus is sufficient to trigger CREB phosphorylation and impair memory. *Mol Psychiatry* 20, 1481, doi:10.1038/mp.2015.43 (2015).
68 Airan, R. D., Thompson, K. R., Fenno, L. E., Bernstein, H. & Deisseroth, K. Temporally precise in vivo control of intracellular signalling. *Nature* 458, 1025–1029, doi:10.1038/nature07926 (2009).
69 Mohanty, S. K. & Lakshminarayananan, V. Optical techniques in optogenetics. *J Mod Opt* 62, 949–970, doi:10.1080/09500340.2015.1010620 (2015).
70 Lin, M. Z. & Schnitzer, M. J. Genetically encoded indicators of neuronal activity. *Nat Neurosci* 19, 1142–1153, doi:10.1038/nn.4359 (2016).

71 Miesenbock, G., De Angelis, D. A. & Rothman, J. E. Visualizing secretion and synaptic transmission with pH-sensitive green fluorescent proteins. *Nature* 394, 192–195, doi:10.1038/28190 (1998).

72 Sankaranarayanan, S., De Angelis, D., Rothman, J. E. & Ryan, T. A. The use of pHluorins for optical measurements of presynaptic activity. *Biophys J* 79, 2199–2208, doi:10.1016/S0006-3495(00)76468-X (2000).

73 Marvin, J. S. et al. An optimized fluorescent probe for visualizing glutamate neurotransmission. *Nat Methods* 10, 162–170, doi:10.1038/nmeth.2333 (2013).

74 Palmer, A. E. et al. Ca2+ indicators based on computationally redesigned calmodulin-peptide pairs. *Chem Biol* 13, 521–530, doi:10.1016/j.chembiol.2006.03.007 (2006).

75 Chen, T. W. et al. Ultrasensitive fluorescent proteins for imaging neuronal activity. *Nature* 499, 295–300, doi:10.1038/nature12354 (2013).

76 Dana, H. et al. High-performance calcium sensors for imaging activity in neuronal populations and microcompartments. *Nat Methods* 16, 649–657, doi:10.1038/s41592-019-0435-6 (2019).

77 Lam, A. J. et al. Improving FRET dynamic range with bright green and red fluorescent proteins. *Nat Methods* 9, 1005–1012, doi:10.1038/nmeth.2171 (2012).

78 Adam, Y. et al. Voltage imaging and optogenetics reveal behaviour-dependent changes in hippocampal dynamics. *Nature* 569, 413–417, doi:10.1038/s41586-019-1166-7 (2019).

79 Gong, Y., Wagner, M. J., Zhong Li, J. & Schnitzer, M. J. Imaging neural spiking in brain tissue using FRET-opsin protein voltage sensors. *Nat Commun* 5, 3674, doi:10.1038/ncomms4674 (2014).

80 Jin, L. et al. Single action potentials and subthreshold electrical events imaged in neurons with a fluorescent protein voltage probe. *Neuron* 75, 779–785, doi:10.1016/j.neuron.2012.06.040 (2012).

81 St-Pierre, F. et al. High-fidelity optical reporting of neuronal electrical activity with an ultrafast fluorescent voltage sensor. *Nat Neurosci* 17, 884–889, doi:10.1038/nn.3709 (2014).

82 Yang, H. H. et al. Subcellular imaging of voltage and calcium signals reveals neural processing in vivo. *Cell* 166, 245–257, doi:10.1016/j.cell.2016.05.031 (2016).

83 Villette, V. et al. Ultrafast two-photon imaging of a high-gain voltage indicator in awake behaving mice. *Cell* 179, 1590–1608, doi:10.1016/j.cell.2019.11.004 (2019).

84 Viskaitis, P. et al. Modulation of sf1 neuron activity coordinately regulates both feeding behavior and associated emotional states. *Cell Rep* 21, 3559–3572, doi:10.1016/j.celrep.2017.11.089 (2017).

85 Fu, O. et al. Hypothalamic neuronal circuits regulating hunger-induced taste modification. *Nat Commun* 10, 4560, doi:10.1038/s41467-019-12478-x (2019).

86 Adriaenssens, A. E. et al. Glucose-dependent insulinotropic polypeptide receptor-expressing cells in the hypothalamus regulate food intake. *Cell Metab* 30, 987–996, doi:10.1016/j.cmet.2019.07.013 (2019).

87 Zink, A. N., Bunney, P. E., Holm, A. A., Billington, C. J. & Kotz, C. M. Neuromodulation of orexin neurons reduces diet-induced adiposity. *Int J Obes* 42, 737–745, doi:10.1038/ijo.2017.276 (2018).

88 Zhang, N., Yang, L., Guo, L. & Bi, S. Activation of dorsomedial hypothalamic neurons promotes physical activity and decreases food intake and body weight in zucker fatty rats. *Front Mol Neurosci* 11, 179, doi:10.3389/fnmol.2018.00179 (2018).

89 Uner, A. G. et al. Role of POMC and AgRP neuronal activities on glycaemia in mice. *Sci Rep* 9, 13068, doi:10.1038/s41598-019-49295-7 (2019).

90 Dodd, G. T. et al. Insulin regulates POMC neuronal plasticity to control glucose metabolism. *elife* 7, doi:10.7554/eLife.38704 (2018).

91 Zhang, X. & van den Pol, A. N. Rapid binge-like eating and body weight gain driven by zona incerta GABA neuron activation. *Science* 356, 853–859, doi:10.1126/science.aam7100 (2017).
92 Rau, A. R. & Hentges, S. T. GABAergic inputs to POMC neurons originating from the dorsomedial hypothalamus are regulated by energy state. *J Neurosci* 39, 6449–6459, doi:10.1523/JNEUROSCI.3193-18.2019 (2019).
93 Mangieri, L. R. et al. Defensive behaviors driven by a hypothalamic-ventral midbrain circuit. *eNeuro* 6, doi:10.1523/ENEURO.0156-19.2019 (2019).
94 Rau, A. R. & Hentges, S. T. The relevance of AgRP neuron-derived GABA inputs to POMC neurons differs for spontaneous and evoked release. *J Neurosci* 37, 7362–7372, doi:10.1523/JNEUROSCI.0647-17.2017 (2017).
95 Zhao, Z. D. et al. A hypothalamic circuit that controls body temperature. *Proc Natl Acad Sci U S A* 114, 2042–2047, doi:10.1073/pnas.1616255114 (2017).
96 Faber, C. L. et al. Distinct neuronal projections from the hypothalamic ventromedial nucleus mediate glycemic and behavioral effects. *Diabetes* 67, 2518–2529, doi:10.2337/db18-0380 (2018).
97 Pinol, R. A. et al. Brs3 neurons in the mouse dorsomedial hypothalamus regulate body temperature, energy expenditure, and heart rate, but not food intake. *Nat Neurosci* 21, 1530–1540, doi:10.1038/s41593-018-0249-3 (2018).
98 He, Y. et al. Estrogen receptor-alpha expressing neurons in the ventrolateral VMH regulate glucose balance. *Nat Commun* 11, 2165, doi:10.1038/s41467-020-15982-7 (2020).
99 Kravitz, A. V., Tye, L. D. & Kreitzer, A. C. Distinct roles for direct and indirect pathway striatal neurons in reinforcement. *Nat Neurosci* 15, 816–818, doi:10.1038/nn.3100 (2012).
100 Kravitz, A. V. & Bonci, A. Optogenetics, physiology, and emotions. *Front Behav Neurosci* 7, 169, doi:10.3389/fnbeh.2013.00169 (2013).
101 Jeong, J. H., Lee, D. K. & Jo, Y. H. Cholinergic neurons in the dorsomedial hypothalamus regulate food intake. *Mol Metab* 6, 306–312, doi:10.1016/j.molmet.2017.01.001 (2017).
102 Fenselau, H. et al. A rapidly acting glutamatergic ARC-->PVH satiety circuit postsynaptically regulated by alpha-MSH. *Nat Neurosci* 20, 42–51, doi:10.1038/nn.4442 (2017).
103 Li, X. Y. et al. AGRP neurons project to the medial preoptic area and modulate maternal nest-building. *J Neurosci* 39, 456–471, doi:10.1523/JNEUROSCI.0958-18.2018 (2019).
104 Engstrom Ruud, L., Pereira, M. M. A., de Solis, A. J., Fenselau, H. & Bruning, J. C. NPY mediates the rapid feeding and glucose metabolism regulatory functions of AgRP neurons. *Nat Commun* 11, 442, doi:10.1038/s41467-020-14291-3 (2020).
105 Bai, L. et al. Genetic identification of vagal sensory neurons that control feeding. *Cell* 179, 1129–1143, doi:10.1016/j.cell.2019.10.031 (2019).

8 The Central Action of Thyroid Hormone on Energy Metabolism

Siyi Shen

Chinese Academy of Sciences, China

Yan Li

Jiangnan University, China

Shengnan Liu

Chinese Academy of Sciences, China

Ying Yan

Chinese Academy of Sciences, China

Jingjing Jiang

Zhongshan Hospital Fudan University, China

Hao Ying

Chinese Academy of Sciences, China; Ministry of health, China

CONTENTS

8.1 INTRODUCTION

8.1.1 Thyroid Hormone and Thyroid Hormone Receptor

Thyroid hormone (TH) plays an essential role in metabolic pathways, including growth, differentiation, development, physiological function of all organs or tissues, and maintenance of metabolic homeostasis (Anyetei-Anum, Roggero, and Allison 2018, Brent 2012, Hollenberg and Forrest 2008, Song, Yao, and Ying 2011, Yao et al. 2014). TH consists of two principal forms, namely triiodothyronine (T3, L-3,5,3'-triiodothyronine) and thyroxine (T4, L-3,5,3',5'-tetraiodothyronine). T3, the considerably more active form of TH, can be converted by type 1 (DIO1) or type 2 deiodinase (DIO2) from T4 in the tissues, which is the most abundant TH in the blood. Type 3 deiodinase (DIO3) deactivates TH via inner ring deiodination, converting T3 into diiodothyronine (T2, 3,5-diiodo-L-thyronine) or T4 into reverse triiodothyronine (reverse T3, or rT3, 3,3',5'-triiodothyronine). Circulating TH levels are maintained by a feedback loop commonly referred to as the hypothalamic–pituitary–thyroid (HPT) axis (Lopez et al. 2013, Martinez-Sanchez et al. 2014, Song, Yao, and Ying 2011).

The actions of TH are mainly mediated by a thyroid hormone receptor (TR). A range of transcription factors, such as retinoid X receptor (RXR), liver X receptor (LXR), and peroxisome proliferator-activated receptor (PPAR) are also implicated in TH action (Yao et al. 2014). TR belongs to the nuclear receptor superfamily with α and β subtypes, of which TRα is highly expressed in tissues including heart, bone, muscle, and fat, whereas TRβ is mainly expressed in tissues such as liver, kidney, and pituitary (Anyetei-Anum, Roggero, and Allison 2018). Due to the different expression of TR in different tissues, TH effects are regulated temporally and spatially. Once transported into cells, TH works in a genomic or non-genomic mode (Davis, Goglia, and Leonard 2016, Kublaoui and Levine 2014, Moeller and Broecker-Preuss 2011). The genomic signaling pathway directly influences gene transcription and translation. TR binds to short, repeated sequences of DNA called thyroid response elements (TREs), which are composed of two (A/G) GGT(C/A/G)A "half-sites" separated by 4 bps. The ability of TR to recognize TREs enables TH to positively regulate the expression of many target genes by recruiting coactivators, while in the absence of T3, unliganded TR interacts with corepressors to suppress target gene transcription (Song, Yao, and Ying 2011). As for the non-genomic signaling pathway, it involves more rapid cellular changes or indirect signaling without transcription or translation. For instance, though there is no specific molecular mechanism proposed, it is speculated that TH will bind to TRα1 in the cytoplasm, upregulate cGMP concentration, and activate PKG correspondingly (Kublaoui and Levine 2014). Other non-genomic effects referring to modulation of mitochondrial metabolism, glucose uptake, and cytoskeletal organization can also be observed in past research (Davis, Goglia, and Leonard 2016, Martin et al. 2014, Moeller and Broecker-Preuss 2011).

8.1.2 Thyroid Dysfunction

Hypothyroidism and hyperthyroidism are clinical syndromes in which the circulating TH level is disturbed due to thyroid dysfunction. Hypothyroidism results from any condition that leads to TH deficiency. Accompanied by reduced hepatic glucose production, hypothyroid rodents show insulin resistance supposedly resulting from reduced glucose utilization and turnover in both skeletal muscle and adipose tissue (Cettour-Rose et al.

2005). The manifestations of hypothyroidism in humans are always a decreased metabolic rate and sometimes gained weight despite reduced food intake. Conversely, hyperthyroidism is characterized by excessive production of TH as well as enhanced β-adrenergic activity (Song, Yao, and Ying 2011). Increased appetite and weight loss are common symptoms in patients with hyperthyroidism (MayoClinic 2018).

Resistance to thyroid hormone (RTH) is a syndrome in which patients may have features of both hypothyroidism and hyperthyroidism, mainly caused by mutations of the TRβ gene (Beato-Vibora, Arroyo-Diez, and Rodriguez-Lopez 2013). It is characterized by impaired sensitivity to TH, excessive circulating T3 and T4 levels, and elevated or non-suppressed thyroid-stimulating hormone (TSH) levels (Persani and Campi 2019).

8.1.3 Central Nervous System and Metabolism

The central nervous system (CNS) integrates nutrition and hormone signals and monitors metabolism in the body through neural activity. Neurons supervise and respond to metabolic intermediates that reflect the circulating energy status, such as those in fatty acid biosynthetic pathways, which are considered as hypothalamic signaling mediators because of their ability to sense and respond to changes in circulating fuels (Wolfgang and Lane 2006).

The hypothalamus is key in the central integration of inputs. It is divided into several parts, such as the ventromedial nucleus (VMN), the paraventricular nucleus (PVN), the anterior hypothalamic area (AHA), the arcuate nucleus (ARC), and the dorsomedial nucleus (DMN), which conduct different regulatory functions. In detail, for example, the VMN is a critical region involved in energy homeostasis, while the ARC is known for feeding control (Gao and Horvath 2007). Hypothalamic output depends on the sympathetic and parasympathetic nerves, which are two parts of the autonomic nervous system (ANS). The sympathetic nervous system (SNS) and parasympathetic nervous system (PSNS) are mutually opposed and coordinated. They govern the activities of organs and blood vessels, participate in the endocrine regulation of glucose and lipid metabolism, and control body temperature and sleep.

8.1.4 TH Action on Metabolism Via the Central Nervous System

For more than a century, researchers have been studying how TH locally exerts its critical function in target tissues including the liver, white adipose tissue (WAT), brown adipose tissue (BAT), skeletal muscle, and the heart. Although much evidence has been cited regarding the role of TH in peripheral metabolic regulation, growing evidence demonstrates the potential roles of TH in the brain (Figure 8.1 and Table 8.1). Moreover, colocalization imaging has shown that TRα and TRβ are expressed in several areas of the hypothalamus, such as the VMN and PVN (Barrett et al. 2007, Lopez et al. 2010).

Due to limited technologies applied to explore the TH action in the brain at this time, the relationship between TH and its role via the CNS is still not completely understood. This chapter summarizes the current evidence on central actions of TH on global energy balance. Both consistent and controversial reports with possible mechanism are presented. Furthermore, it will discuss some advanced technologies that will be applied to this area in the future.

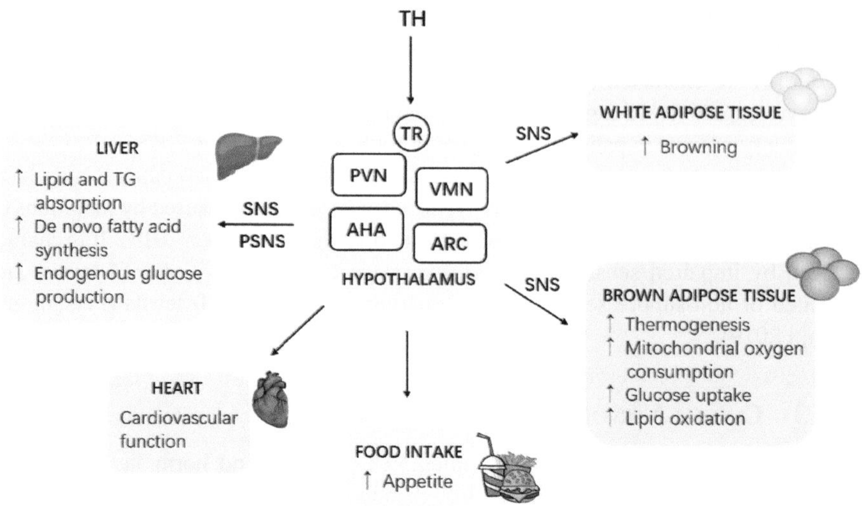

FIGURE 8.1 Thyroid hormone affects diverse functions of adipose tissues, the liver, the heart, as well as food intake via the central nervous system.

8.2 CENTRAL ACTION OF TH ON ENERGY EXPENDITURE AND THERMOGENESIS

It has long been recognized that thyroid status and energy expenditure are intimately connected in rodents and humans (Li et al. 2019, Nedergaard, Dicker, and Cannon 1997, Weiner et al. 2017, Zhang et al. 2014). Homeotherm species must control core body temperature to maintain normal physiological processes. Generally, the heat production program is composed of obligatory and facultative thermogenesis, while the latter includes shivering thermogenesis and non-shivering thermogenesis, which is also known as adaptive thermogenesis. In a thermoneutral environment, it is sufficient to maintain body temperature based on obligatory thermogenesis – that is, the heat production is generated by the metabolic rate. Facultative heat generation is defined as a resistance to heat loss due to the skin's response to cold-sensitive thermoreceptors below thermoneutrality. Involuntary skeletal muscle activity is a major way of shivering thermogenesis. On the other hand, the heat production activities of brown adipose tissue and the browning of white adipose tissue are the two key constituents of non-shivering thermogenesis (Iwen, Oelkrug, and Brabant 2018). TH is of vital importance to both types of thermogenesis, especially facultative thermogenesis. Evidence suggests that plasma TH participates in thermoregulation during shivering and non-shivering cold adaptation (Zhang et al. 2014). At the same time, a growing number of studies have reported that as the main central integrator of metabolic signals, the hypothalamus governs the activity of adipocytes through its sympathetic output. This process requires the β-adrenoceptors (β-ARs) to promote brown adipocyte thermogenesis and mature white adipocyte browning (Bartness et al. 2010, Bartness and Song, 2007a, 2007b, Perkins et al. 1981).

The first evidence suggesting a link between central TH action and thermogenesis of adipose tissue appeared in mice with a mutant TRα1 heterozygote, in which increased

TABLE 8.1
Evidence of the central regulatory role of thyroid hormone on energy metabolism

Animal Model	Treatment	Major Findings	Interpretation	Reference
Mice (heterozygous for a mutant TRα1 with low affinity to T3)	–	↓body weight and fat depots ↑food intake ↑glucose handling and fatty acid metabolism in liver and adipose tissues ↑lipid mobilization and β-oxidation in adipose tissues	The phenotype of these mice resembles a state of hyperthyroidism.	(Sjogren et al. 2007)
	Blockage of sympathetic signaling to BAT	Normalizes the metabolic phenotype	Hypermetabolism in these mice is the result of increased sympathetic signaling.	
Rats	T3 (i.c.v. or VMN injection for 1–3 h)	↑BAT sympathetic nerve activity	–	(Lopez et al. 2010)
	T3 (chronic i.c.v. injection for 4 d)	↓body weight ↑thermogenic markers (such as UCP1, UCP3, DIO2) expression in BAT	–	
	T3 (chronic i.c.v. injection for 4 d) + β3-AR antagonist SR59230A	Prevents the reduction in body weight and blocks the thermogenic program in BAT	Central T3 increases BAT thermogenesis through β3-ARs.	
Rats	T3 (chronic i.c.v. injection)	↓body weight ↑thermogenic markers (such as UCP1, UCP3, PGC1α, FGF21) expression in BAT ↑BAT glucose uptake, lipid oxidation, and mitochondrial oxygen consumption ↑BAT sympathetic nerve activity	–	(Martinez-Sanchez, et al. 2017b)
	T3 (chronic i.c.v. injection) + β3-ARs antagonist SR59230A	Prevents the effect on body weight and blocks the T3-mediated activation of the AMPK pathway in BAT	Central T3 regulates lipid oxidation in BAT via the SNS.	
	T3 (chronic VMN injection)	↑BAT sympathetic tone and thermogenesis ↑*de novo* fatty acid synthesis and triglyceride content in the liver	–	
	T3 (chronic VMN injection) + vagotomy	Completely clears away the phenotype in the liver	Central T3 regulates lipogenesis in the liver via the PSNS.	
Rats	T3 (chronic i.c.v. or VMN injection)	↑browning of WAT	–	(Martinez-Sanchez, et al. 2017a)

(Continued)

TABLE 8.1 (CONTINUED)

Animal Model	Treatment	Major Findings	Interpretation	Reference
Ucp1$^{-/-}$ mice	T3 (chronic i.c.v. injection)	Fails to induce any change in feeding, BAT thermogenesis, energy expenditure, and browning of WAT	UCP1 is essential for mediation of the central actions of TH on energy balance.	(Alvarez-Crespo et al. 2016)
Dio3$^{-/-}$ mice	–	↑TH levels in the brain ↓adipocyte size in BAT and WAT ↑fat loss, ameliorative adiposity ↑energy expenditure ↑locomotor activity ↑mRNA levels of AgRP, NPY ↓mRNA levels of POMC	–	(Wu et al. 2017)
Rats	T4 (in drinking water)	↑EGP ↓insulin sensitivity in liver	–	(Klieverik et al. 2008)
	T4 (in drinking water) + sympathetic denervation	Attenuates the increase in EGP	–	
	T4 (in drinking water) + parasympathetic denervation	↑plasma insulin	–	
Rats	T3 (PVN injection for 2 h)	↑EGP ↑plasma glucose	Central T3 regulates EGP via a sympathetic pathway to the liver.	(Klieverik et al. 2009)
	T3 (PVN injection for 2 h) + selective hepatic sympathetic denervation	Completely prevents the effect of T3 on EGP		
Mice (heterozygous for a mutant TRα1 with low affinity to T3)	T3 (in drinking water)	↓population of parvalbuminergic neurons in the AHA ↑blood pressure	The parvalbuminergic neurons depend on TH signaling to regulate cardiovascular function via modulation of central autonomic outflow.	(Mittag et al. 2013)
Rats	T3 (intraperitoneal injection for 7 d)	↑mRNA levels of NPY ↓mRNA levels of POMC ↑food intake	–	(Ishii et al. 2003)
Rats	T3 (a single VMN injection for 1 h)	↑food intake	–	(Kong et al. 2004)
Mice (selective knockdown of TRβ in the VMN)	–	↑body weight ↑food intake ↓energy expenditure	–	(Hameed et al. 2017)
	T3 (subcutaneous injection for 24 h)	Fails to mount an orexigenic response		
Rats	Fasting	↑hypothalamic DIO2 activity ↑local T3 production in the ARC ↓TRH mRNA levels ↑food intake	–	(Coppola et al. 2005)

Animal Model	Treatment	Major Findings	Interpretation	Reference
Mice	Fasting	↑hypothalamic DIO2 activity ↑local T3 production in the ARC ↑UCP2 expression in NPY/AgRP neurons ↑proliferation in NPY/AgRP neurons ↑food intake	–	(Coppola et al. 2007)
Rats	TH (Chronic ARC injection)	↑mTOR signaling ↑mRNA levels of NPY/AgRP ↓mRNA levels of POMC ↑food intake	–	(Varela et al. 2012)

BAT activity and thermogenesis were blunted by a blockade of sympathetic signaling to BAT (Sjogren et al. 2007). Through a standard norepinephrine test, Golozoubova et al. found that mice lacking all hormone-binding TRs had impaired ability to induce thermogenesis adrenergically. Even though TRs per se were not necessary for uncoupling protein 1 (UCP1) expression in BAT, the basal metabolic rate of these mice was obviously reduced and cold tolerance was damaged (Golozoubova et al. 2004). It is foreseeable and undisputed that hyperthyroid rats exhibit hypermetabolism. As chronic intracerebroventricular (i.c.v.) administrated T3 for four days, both euthyroid and hypothyroid rats had increased expression of representative thermogenic markers such as UCP1, UCP3, and DIO2 in BAT without altering serum T3 or T4 concentration. Pharmacological blockage of β3-AR by SR59230A prevented the thermogenic program, implying that activated sympathetic nerve flow was involved in central T3 action. The same phenotype was obtained when T3 was specifically injected into the VMN (Lopez et al. 2010). AMP-activated protein kinase (AMPK), as a key factor regulating nutrient metabolism, has a significant effect on energy balance and responds to a host of hormones not only in the periphery but also in the brain (Martinez de Morentin et al. 2016, Minokoshi et al. 2004). Further studies then revealed the underlying molecular mechanisms by which T3 inhibited AMPK activity and facilitated *de novo* lipogenesis in the hypothalamus, specifically in the VMN, resulting in the activation of the sympathetic nerve signal (Lopez et al. 2010). Furthermore, the decreased AMPK level, caused by T3, reduced ceramide-induced endoplasmic reticulum (ER) stress, which contributed to the improved sympathetic tone and BAT thermogenesis as well (Martinez-Sanchez et al. 2017b).

The significance of T3 acting on the hypothalamus is also reflected in WAT. This showed remarkable browning of WAT as proved by overtly upregulated expression of UCP1. In consideration of the role of AMPK in the SNS–BAT axis, a hypothesis was proposed that AMPK in the hypothalamus was essential to the central regulation of WAT browning. Activation of AMPK in the VMN of i.c.v. T3-treated rats blunted weight loss as well as reversed stimulation of browning markers in gonadal white adipose tissue (gWAT), evidenced by an increased adipocyte area and a decreased UCP1 stained area (Martinez-Sanchez et al. 2017a). Prolonged central T3 treatment delivered by osmotic minipumps induced oxygen consumption and elevated body temperature, which was compatible with BAT recruitment and inguinal white adipose tissue (iWAT) beiging. Intriguingly, this chronic T3 fusion had no significant effects in the absence of UCP1 (Alvarez-Crespo et al. 2016). *Dio3*$^{-/-}$ mice manifested a hypothyroid state in circulating (Hernandez et al. 2007), whereas in the CNS, they displayed increased T3 availability. Morphologically, these mice showed decreased adipocyte size in BAT and WAT, increased fat loss, and ameliorative adiposity. Though their UCP1 mRNA expression did not change, elevated locomotor activity was enhanced, compatible with an increase in energy expenditure (Wu et al. 2017).

A contradictory finding was proposed by Zhang et al. that mRNA expression of genes involved in thermogenesis remained unchanged after administrating T3 into the PVN or VMN of rats for 7 or 28 days. This discrepancy probably was due to the divergence of the duration of treatment, dose of T3, or the route of administration (Zhang et al. 2016a, Zhang et al. 2016b).

Discouragingly, the role of intrahypothalamic T3 in modulating adipose tissue in humans has not been firmly established yet. It is not even clear what the function of TH is on BAT activity in humans. A case report showed that, in a small group of hyperthyroid patients, active BAT was present only in one patient with normalized thyroid function after therapy (Zhang et al. 2014, Zhang et al. 2017). Although the above techniques cannot be used clinically, the pathways revealed by these animal experiments provide an understanding of the effects between TH and energy expenditure.

8.3 CENTRAL ACTION OF TH ON HEPATIC GLUCOSE AND LIPID METABOLISM

An important effect of TH is to modulate glucose and lipid metabolism in the liver. Recent evidence suggests that the SNS and PSNS are major regulators of hepatic metabolism. Robust data from Klieverik et al. show the relationship between central neuron activities and hepatic glucose metabolism (Klieverik et al. 2008, Klieverik et al. 2009). Selective hepatic sympathectomy or parasympathectomy were performed in euthyroid and thyrotoxic rats. As a result, thyrotoxicosis showed elevation of endogenous glucose production (EGP) and inhibition of insulin sensitivity in the liver, which was attenuated by sympathetic denervation and rescued by parasympathetic denervation respectively (Klieverik et al. 2008). Specifically, when T3 stimulated PVN neurons of euthyroid rats, EGP was facilitated through a sympathetic pathway to the liver, in which circulating glucoregulatory hormones did not take part, further verifying the role of the ANS (Klieverik et al. 2009). In contrast, according to the conclusions of Zhang et al., none of the genes involved in glucose metabolism were altered in the liver after intrahypothalamic T3 delivered during either 7 or 28 days to the PVN or VMN of rats (Zhang et al. 2016a, Zhang et al. 2016b).

Lipid metabolism in the liver can also be regulated by TH at the central level. Chronic injection of T3 in the VMN decreased the hepatic pAMPK and phosphorylated acetyl-CoA carboxylase (pACC) protein level via the hypothalamic AMPK-JNK1 axis, thus increasing *de novo* fatty acid synthesis and triglyceride content in the liver. As these alterations were completely cleared away by vagotomy, it was concluded that this central regulation of hepatic lipid metabolism was mediated by parasympathetic nerves (Martinez-Sanchez et al. 2017b).

8.4 CENTRAL ACTION OF TH ON CARDIOVASCULAR FUNCTION

The earliest definition of hyperthyroidism clearly described the close relationship between the thyroid and heart. The crucial impacts of TH on cardiovascular function have been widely known, mainly including rapid heartbeat, palpitations, cardiac enlargement, enhancing overall protein synthesis, decreasing systemic vascular resistance, and increasing blood volume (Kahaly and Dillmann 2005).

Mittag et al. have noted that TH could influence heart function and metabolism through the ANS. In the AHA, there is a previously unknown population of parvalbuminergic neurons sensitive to intrinsic temperature. The neurons depend on TH signaling to integrate temperature information and modulate cardiovascular parameters. Transgenic mice with these cells ablated exhibited hypertension and temperature-dependent tachycardia, supporting the role of autonomic regulation in blood pressure and heart rate. In fact, this regulation was impaired after a point mutation in TRα1 (Mittag et al. 2013). The discovery subverts the view that TH can only regulate cardiovascular function through the systemic circulation.

8.5 CENTRAL ACTION OF TH ON FOOD INTAKE

Extensive research in both humans and animals over recent decades has revealed that the CNS plays a crucial role in feeding regulation, and therefore energy homeostasis (Gao and Horvath 2007, Sohn 2015, Timper and Bruning 2017). Elegant data has suggested that the hypothalamus can integrate hormonal signals, thereby altering fatty acid metabolism which is related to feeding (Lopez, Lelliott, and Vidal-Puig 2007). There are two groups of neurons in the ARC of the hypothalamus which produce peptides for regulating appetite: agouti-related peptide (AgRP) and neuropeptide Y (NPY) are appetite-stimulating, while pro-opiomelanocortin (POMC) and amphetamine-regulated transcript (CART) are appetite-suppressing (Coll et al. 2008). These neurons project to other regions of the hypothalamus such as the PVN, POA, VMN, and DMN, through which a variety of hormones regulate energy metabolism (Coll et al. 2008, Kalra et al. 1999).

Clinically, hyperthyroid patients show hyperphagia. In keeping with that, thyrotoxicosis rats show increased hypothalamic NPY and decreased hypothalamic POMC mRNA levels with declining circulating leptin levels (Ishii et al. 2003). Seven days of intrahypothalamic T3 treatment to the PVN or VMN did not change food intake in rats (Zhang et al. 2016a, Zhang et al. 2016b). However, it made them considerably orexigenic in one hour after being given a single injection of T3 into the VMN (Kong et al. 2004). Furthermore, the VMN specific knockdown of TRβ in the mice resulted in obesity which was a direct consequence of hyperphagia (Hameed et al. 2017). TH triggers downstream transcriptional factors UCPs which mediate food intake as well. In UCP1 KO mice, central T3 treatment failed to induce any change in feeding, implying the positive effect of UCP1 being involved in the central actions of T3 (Alvarez-Crespo et al. 2016).

Thyrotropin-releasing hormone (TRH) neurons are symmetrically contacted by nerve terminals containing NPY/AgRP (Legradi and Lechan 1999). In rats, food deprivation-induced elevation in hypothalamic DIO2 activity catalyzed local T3 production in the ARC with decreased TRH mRNA levels. This might indicate that the elevated T3 concentration could alter the expression of neuropeptides in leptin-responsive arcuate neurons, which strongly project to the PVN TRH neurons, thereby affecting appetite (Coppola et al. 2005). Moreover, in adult mice, the elevated hypothalamic DIO2 activity increased UCP2-dependent mitochondrial proliferation in NPY/AgRP neurons, which was also mediated through local T3 in the ARC. The mitochondrial uncoupling improved nerve excitability and ultimately stimulated appetite (Coppola et al. 2007). Besides, mice devoid of DIO3 manifested abnormal expression of AgRP, NPY, and POMC, which was regarded as a result of an excessive TH level in the brain (Wu et al. 2017).

Investigations focusing on the link between the mammalian target of the rapamycin (mTOR) pathway and energy balance have found that the mTOR pathway also works as a mediator in the central control of food intake (Catania, Binder, and Cota 2011, Lopez et al. 2006). High colocalization of mTOR signaling and NPY/AgRP neurons was displayed by immunohistochemistry (Cota et al. 2006). Recent experiments discovered that increased feeding, manifesting as upregulation in mRNA levels of NPY/AgRP as well as downregulation in mRNA levels of POMC, was related to advanced mTOR signaling evoked by TH administration to the ARC of rats (Varela et al. 2012). There is another feeding-controlling neuropeptide called neuropeptide S (NPS), found not only in the DMN of the hypothalamus and the amygdala but also in the brainstem area close to the locus coeruleus (LC) and Barrington's nucleus. Early experiments addressed the possible connection between food intake patterns observed in hyperthyroid rats and the expression of NPS and its receptor NPS-R, which is ubiquitously expressed in the brain. Hyperthyroidism declined mRNA and protein levels of NPS and NPS-R in the hypothalamus but appreciably increased NPS-R expression in the brainstem. No significant change was observed in NPS and NPS-R expression in the amygdala (Gonzalez et al. 2012).

8.6 CONCLUSION

8.6.1 Peripheral Role or Central Role?

The balance of energy metabolism guarantees the body will adapt to the changes of environment inside and outside. TH is an indispensable determinant of a variety of physiologic processes and exerts functions not merely via circulation but also at the central level. Furthermore, there are still many unknown pathways to be studied. It has been reported that the ARC may have a potential role in hepatic metabolism via central TH signaling in light of its capability to express TRs and modulate hepatic glucose production (Bartness and Song 2007a, Koenner, Klockener, and Bruning 2009).

A question is whether neuromodulation plays a major role in acute TH concentration alterations, and whether endocrine regulation is more important when faced with long-term changes. Nevertheless, the purpose of this chapter is to offer a more comprehensive understanding and an unbiased look at TH signal pathways rather than to weigh which mode is dominant. Indeed, the two modes do not conflict with each other. It has been widely known that TH activates the thermogenic gene in adipose tissues and affects the hepatic glycolipid signaling pathway via a genomic or nongenomic mechanism. It is now believed that these changes can also be triggered by sympathetic or parasympathetic output, respectively.

8.6.2 Prospects

8.6.2.1 Targeted Drug Development

Studies aimed at assessing how organs and organisms respond to central TH have furthered our understanding of the physiological effects of TH. Given that TH has diverse effects on various tissues, especially its negative impact on the heart, TH analogs are often used clinically instead of directly using TH to treat metabolic syndromes. In actuality, most of the existing drugs are designed according to the peripheral effects of TH (Baxter and Webb 2009, Pearce 2012). Uncovering the new mechanisms involved in TH actions provides new ideas for the treatment of atherosclerosis, obesity, and type 2 diabetes. New TH targets and the correlation between TH-dependent central effects and these diseases in humans may be the focus in designing new molecular analogs to treat abnormal energy balances.

8.6.2.2 Novel Techniques Applied to Explore the Central Action of TH

In 1977, the Nobel Prize in Physiology and Medicine was awarded to Rosalyn Sussman Yalow, an American endocrinologist, in recognition of her establishment of a radioimmunoassay for hormones. Radioisotope labeling, combined with molecular biology techniques, makes it possible to track TH and study its functions in cells (Wheeler 2013). However, it is difficult to distinguish the impact of TH on a single tissue because of the complex crosstalk between organizations. Based on the fact that thyroid dysfunction leads to changes in local TH concentration in the hypothalamus, the researchers realized that it would be possible to dive deeper into the function of TH from the center rather than the periphery.

Thanks to the development of neurobiology, specific groups of neurons in the brain and even the hypothalamus, as well as specific energy sensors, have been identified in recent decades. Sophisticated neurobiological approaches have been used to monitor the scope and targets of TH. To be specific: stereotactic microinjection rules out peripheral effects, allowing researchers to focus on neural networks; sympathectomy, parasympathectomy, and vagotomy make it possible to distinguish which tissues sense nerve signals; measurement of sympathetic nerve activity can detect the extent to which the tissue responds to neural signal flow. Challenging and exciting work would involve excellent technologies assisted with suitable animal models to be applied in further studies. Nowadays neurobiology is entering the era of optogenetics, featuring a combination of genetic engineering and light to manipulate the activity of individual nerve cells. This emerging technology, combined with the rapid development of neuroimaging, may help us detect the molecular mechanisms that underlie the central actions of TH intuitively and accurately. This may also help us to better characterize and distinguish the peripheral and central roles of TH in space and time.

ACKNOWLEDGMENTS

This work was supported by MOST of China (2016YFA0500102, 2016YFC1304905) and National Natural Science Foundation of China (91957205, 31525012, 31871195, 82070821).

REFERENCES

Alvarez-Crespo, M., R. I. Csikasz, N. Martinez-Sanchez, C. Dieguez, B. Cannon, J. Nedergaard, and M. Lopez. 2016. "Essential role of UCP1 modulating the central effects of thyroid hormones on energy balance." *Mol Metab* 5 (4):271–282. doi: 10.1016/j.molmet.2016.01.008.

Anyetei-Anum, C. S., V. R. Roggero, and L. A. Allison. 2018. "Thyroid hormone receptor localization in target tissues." *J Endocrinol* 237 (1):R19–R34. doi: 10.1530/JOE-17-0708.

Barrett, P., F. J. Ebling, S. Schuhler, D. Wilson, A. W. Ross, A. Warner, P. Jethwa, A. Boelen, T. J. Visser, D. M. Ozanne, et al. 2007. "Hypothalamic thyroid hormone catabolism acts as a gatekeeper for the seasonal control of body weight and reproduction." *Endocrinology* 148 (8):3608–3617. doi: 10.1210/en.2007-0316.

Bartness, T. J., Y. B. Shrestha, C. H. Vaughan, G. J. Schwartz, and C. K. Song. 2010. "Sensory and sympathetic nervous system control of white adipose tissue lipolysis." *Mol Cell Endocrinol* 318 (1–2):34–43. doi: 10.1016/j.mce.2009.08.031.

Bartness, T. J., and C. K. Song. 2007a. "Brain-adipose tissue neural crosstalk." *Physiol Behav* 91 (4):343–351. doi: 10.1016/j.physbeh.2007.04.002.

Bartness, T. J.. 2007b. "Thematic review series: adipocyte biology. Sympathetic and sensory innervation of white adipose tissue." *J Lipid Res* 48 (8):1655–1672. doi: 10.1194/jlr.R700006-JLR200.

Baxter, J. D., and P. Webb. 2009. "Thyroid hormone mimetics: potential applications in atherosclerosis, obesity and type 2 diabetes." *Nat Rev Drug Discov* 8 (4):308–320. doi: 10.1038/nrd2830.

Beato-Vibora, P., J. Arroyo-Diez, and R. Rodriguez-Lopez. 2013. "Thyroid hormone resistance caused by a novel deleterious variant of the thyroid hormone receptor beta gene." *Eur J Obstet Gynecol Reprod Biol* 167 (1):118–119. doi: 10.1016/j.ejogrb.2012.11.001.

Brent, G. A. 2012. "Mechanisms of thyroid hormone action." *J Clin Invest* 122 (9):3035–3043. doi: 10.1172/JCI60047.

Catania, C., E. Binder, and D. Cota. 2011. "mTORC1 signaling in energy balance and metabolic disease." *Int J Obes* 35 (6):751–761. doi: 10.1038/ijo.2010.208.

Cettour-Rose, P., C. Theander-Carrillo, C. Asensio, M. Klein, T. J. Visser, A. G. Burger, C. A. Meier, and F. Rohner-Jeanrenaud. 2005. "Hypothyroidism in rats decreases peripheral glucose utilisation, a defect partially corrected by central leptin infusion." *Diabetologia* 48 (4):624–633. doi: 10.1007/s00125-005-1696-4.

Coll, A. P., G. S. H. Yeo, I. S. Farooqi, and S. O'Rahilly. 2008. "SnapShot: The hormonal control of food intake." *Cell* 135 (3). doi: 10.1016/j.cell.2008.10.014.

Coppola, A., J. Hughes, E. Esposito, L. Schiavo, R. Meli, and S. Diano. 2005. "Suppression of hypothalamic deiodinase type II activity blunts TRH mRNA decline during fasting." *FEBS Lett* 579 (21):4654–4658. doi: 10.1016/j.febslet.2005.07.035.

Coppola, A., Z. W. Liu, Z. B. Andrews, E. Paradis, M. C. Roy, J. M. Friedman, D. Ricquier, D. Richard, T. L. Horvath, X. B. Gao, et al.2007. "A central thermogenic-like mechanism in feeding regulation: an interplay between arcuate nucleus T3 and UCP2." *Cell Metab* 5 (1):21–33. doi: 10.1016/j.cmet.2006.12.002.

Cota, D., K. Proulx, K. A. B. Smith, S. C. Kozma, G. Thomas, S. C. Woods, and R. J. Seeley. 2006. "Hypothalamic mTOR signaling regulates food intake." *Science* 312 (5775):927–930. doi: 10.1126/science.1124147.

Davis, P. J., F. Goglia, and J. L. Leonard. 2016. "Nongenomic actions of thyroid hormone." *Nat Rev Endocrinol* 12 (2):111–121. doi: 10.1038/nrendo.2015.205.

Gao, Q., and T. L. Horvath. 2007. "Neurobiology of feeding and energy expenditure." *Annu Rev Neurosci* 30:367–398. doi: 10.1146/annurev.neuro.30.051606.094324.

Golozoubova, V., H. Gullberg, A. Matthias, B. Cannon, B. Vennstrom, and J. Nedergaard. 2004. "Depressed thermogenesis but competent brown adipose tissue recruitment in mice devoid of all hormone-binding thyroid hormone receptors." *Mol Endocrinol* 18 (2):384–401. doi: 10.1210/me.2003-0267.

Gonzalez, C. R., P. B. M. de Morentin, N. Martinez-Sanchez, C. Gomez-Diaz, R. Lage, L. Varela, C. Dieguez, R. Nogueiras, J. P. Castano, and M. Lopez. 2012. "Hyperthyroidism differentially regulates neuropeptide S system in the rat brain." *Brain Res* 1450:40–48. doi: 10.1016/j.brainres.2012.02.024.

Hameed, S., M. Patterson, W. S. Dhillo, S. A. Rahman, Y. Ma, C. Holton, A. Gogakos, G. S. H. Yeo, B. Y. H. Lam, J. Polex-Wolf, et al.2017. "Thyroid hormone receptor beta in the ventromedial hypothalamus is essential for the physiological regulation of food intake and body weight." *Cell Rep* 19 (11):2202–2209. doi: 10.1016/j.celrep.2017.05.066.

Hernandez, A., M. E. Martinez, X. H. Liao, J. Van Sande, S. Refetoff, V. A. Galton, and D. L. St Germain. 2007. "Type 3 deiodinase deficiency results in functional abnormalities at multiple levels of the thyroid axis." *Endocrinology* 148 (12):5680–5687. doi: 10.1210/en.2007-0652.

Hollenberg, A. N., and D. Forrest. 2008. "The thyroid and metabolism: the action continues." *Cell Metab* 8 (1):10–12. doi: 10.1016/j.cmet.2008.06.008.

Ishii, S., J. Kamegai, H. Tamura, T. Shimizu, H. Sugihara, and S. Oikawa. 2003. "Hypothalamic neuropeptide Y/Y1 receptor pathway activated by a reduction in circulating leptin, but not by an increase in circulating ghrelin, contributes to hyperphagia associated with triiodothyronine-induced thyrotoxicosis." *Neuroendocrinology* 78 (6):321–330. doi: 10.1159/000074885.

Iwen, K. A., R. Oelkrug, and G. Brabant. 2018. "Effects of thyroid hormones on thermogenesis and energy partitioning." *J Mol Endocrinol* 60 (3):R157–R170. doi: 10.1530/Jme-17-0319.

Kahaly, G. J., and W. H. Dillmann. 2005. "Thyroid hormone action in the heart." *Endocr Rev* 26 (5):704–728. doi: 10.1210/er.2003-0033.

Kalra, S. P., M. G. Dube, S. Y. Pu, B. Xu, T. L. Horvath, and P. S. Kalra. 1999. "Interacting appetite-regulating pathways in the hypothalamic regulation of body weight." *Endocr Rev* 20 (1):68–100. doi: 10.1210/er.20.1.68.

Klieverik, L. P., S. F. Janssen, A. van Riel, E. Foppen, P. H. Bisschop, M. J. Serlie, A. Boelen, M. T. Ackermans, H. P. Sauerwein, E. Fliers, et al. 2009. "Thyroid hormone modulates glucose production via a sympathetic pathway from the hypothalamic paraventricular nucleus to the liver." *Proc Natl Acad Sci U S A* 106 (14):5966–5971. doi: 10.1073/pnas.0805355106.

Klieverik, L. P., H. P. Sauerwein, M. T. Ackermans, A. Boelen, A. Kalsbeek, and E. Fliers. 2008. "Effects of thyrotoxicosis and selective hepatic autonomic denervation on hepatic glucose metabolism in rats." *Am J Physiol Endocrinol Metab* 294 (3):E513–E520. doi: 10.1152/ajpendo.00659.2007.

Koenner, A. C., T. Klockener, and J. C. Bruning. 2009. "Control of energy homeostasis by insulin and leptin: Targeting the arcuate nucleus and beyond." *Physiol Behav* 97 (5):632–638. doi: 10.1016/j.physbeh.2009.03.027.

Kong, W. M., N. M. Martin, K. L. Smith, J. V. Gardiner, I. P. Connoley, D. A. Stephens, W. S. Dhillo, M. A. Ghatei, C. J. Small, and S. R. Bloom. 2004. "Triiodothyronine stimulates food intake via the hypothalamic ventromedial nucleus independent of changes in energy expenditure." *Endocrinology* 145 (11):5252–5258. doi: 10.1210/en.2004-0545.

Kublaoui, B., and M. Levine. 2014. *Pediatric Endocrinology* (Fourth ed.). Philadelphia, PA: Saunders.

Legradi, G., and R. M. Lechan. 1999. "Agouti-related protein containing nerve terminals innervate thyrotropin-releasing hormone neurons in the hypothalamic paraventricular nucleus." *Endocrinology* 140 (8):3643–3652. doi: 10.1210/endo.140.8.6935.

Li, L., B. Li, M. Li, and J. R. Speakman. 2019. "Switching on the furnace: Regulation of heat production in brown adipose tissue." *Mol Asp Med* 68:60–73. doi: 10.1016/j.mam.2019.07.005.

Lopez, M., C. V. Alvarez, R. Nogueiras, and C. Dieguez. 2013. "Energy balance regulation by thyroid hormones at central level." *Trends Mol Med* 19 (7):418–427. doi: 10.1016/j.molmed.2013.04.004.

Lopez, M., C. J. Lelliott, S. Tovar, W. Kimber, R. Gallego, S. Virtue, M. Blount, M. J. Vazquez, N. Finer, T. J. Powles, et al. 2006. "Tamoxifen-induced anorexia is associated with fatty acid synthase inhibition in the ventromedial nucleus of the hypothalamus and accumulation of malonyl-CoA." *Diabetes* 55 (5):1327–1336. doi: 10.2337/db05-1356.

Lopez, M., C. J. Lelliott, and A. Vidal-Puig. 2007. "Hypothalamic fatty acid metabolism: a housekeeping pathway that regulates food intake." *BioEssays* 29 (3):248–261. doi: 10.1002/bies.20539.

Lopez, M., L. Varela, M. J. Vazquez, S. Rodriguez-Cuenca, C. R. Gonzalez, V. R. Velagapudi, D. A. Morgan, E. Schoenmakers, K. Agassandian, R. Lage, et al. 2010. "Hypothalamic AMPK and fatty acid metabolism mediate thyroid regulation of energy balance." *Nat Med* 16 (9):1001–1008. doi: 10.1038/nm.2207.

Martin, N. P., E. Marron Fernandez de Velasco, F. Mizuno, E. L. Scappini, B. Gloss, C. Erxleben, J. G. Williams, H. M. Stapleton, S. Gentile, and D. L. Armstrong. 2014. "A rapid cytoplasmic mechanism for PI3 kinase regulation by the nuclear thyroid hormone receptor, TRbeta, and genetic evidence for its role in the maturation of mouse hippocampal synapses in vivo." *Endocrinology* 155 (9):3713–3724. doi: 10.1210/en.2013-2058.

Martinez de Morentin, P. B., A. Urisarri, M. L. Couce, and M. Lopez. 2016. "Molecular mechanisms of appetite and obesity: a role for brain AMPK." *Clin Sci (Lond)* 130 (19):1697–1709. doi: 10.1042/CS20160048.

Martinez-Sanchez, N., C. V. Alvarez, J. Ferno, R. Nogueiras, C. Dieguez, and M. Lopez. 2014. "Hypothalamic effects of thyroid hormones on metabolism." *Best Pract Res Clin Endocrinol Metab* 28 (5):703–712. doi: 10.1016/j.beem.2014.04.004.

Martinez-Sanchez, N., J. M. Moreno-Navarrete, C. Contreras, E. Rial-Pensado, J. Ferno, R. Nogueiras, C. Dieguez, J. M. Fernandez-Real, and M. Lopez. 2017a. "Thyroid hormones induce browning of white fat." *J Endocrinol* 232 (2):351–362. doi: 10.1530/JOE-16-0425.

Martinez-Sanchez, N., P. Seoane-Collazo, C. Contreras, L. Varela, J. Villarroya, E. Rial-Pensado, X. Buque, I. Aurrekoetxea, T. C. Delgado, R. Vazquez-Martinez, et al.. 2017b. "Hypothalamic AMPK-ER Stress-JNK1 Axis mediates the central actions of thyroid hormones on energy balance." *Cell Metab* 26 (1):212–229e12. doi: 10.1016/j.cmet.2017.06.014.

MayoClinic. 2018. *Hyperthyroidism*. Rochester, Minn.: Mayo Foundation for Medical Education and Research. https://www.mayoclinic.org/diseases-conditions/hyperthyroidism/diagnosis-treatment/drc-20373665

Minokoshi, Y., T. Alquier, N. Furukawa, Y. B. Kim, A. Lee, B. Xue, J. Mu, F. Foufelle, P. Ferre, et al. 2004. "AMP-kinase regulates food intake by responding to hormonal and nutrient signals in the hypothalamus." *Nature* 428 (6982):569–574. doi: 10.1038/nature02440.

Mittag, J., D. J. Lyons, J. Sallstrom, M. Vujovic, S. Dudazy-Gralla, A. Warner, K. Wallis, A. Alkemade, K. Nordstrom, H. Monyer, et al. 2013. "Thyroid hormone is required for hypothalamic neurons regulating cardiovascular functions." *J Clin Investig* 123 (1):509–516. doi: 10.1172/Jci65252.

Moeller, L. C., and M. Broecker-Preuss. 2011. "Transcriptional regulation by nonclassical action of thyroid hormone." *Thyroid Res* 4 Suppl 1:S6. doi: 10.1186/1756-6614-4-S1-S6.

Nedergaard, J., A. Dicker, and B. Cannon. 1997. "The interaction between thyroid and brown-fat thermogenesis - Central or peripheral effects?" *Thermoregulation* 813:712–717. doi: 10.1111/j.1749-6632.1997.tb51772.x.

Pearce, E. N. 2012. "Thyroid hormone and obesity." *Cur Opin Endocrinol Diab Obes* 19 (5):408–413. doi: 10.1097/MED.0b013e328355cd6c.

Perkins, M. N., N. J. Rothwell, M. J. Stock, and T. W. Stone. 1981. "Activation of brown adipose tissue thermogenesis by the ventromedial hypothalamus." *Nature* 289 (5796):401–402. doi: 10.1038/289401a0.

Persani, L., and I. Campi. 2019. "Syndromes of Resistance to Thyroid Hormone Action." *Exp Suppl* 111:55–84. doi: 10.1007/978-3-030-25905-1_5.

Sjogren, M., A. Alkemade, J. Mittag, K. Nordstrom, A. Katz, B. Rozell, H. Westerblad, A. Arner, and B. Vennstrom. 2007. "Hypermetabolism in mice caused by the central action of an unliganded thyroid hormone receptor alpha1." *EMBO J* 26 (21):4535–4545. doi: 10.1038/sj.emboj.7601882.

Sohn, J. W. 2015. "Network of hypothalamic neurons that control appetite." *BMB Rep* 48 (4):229–233. doi: 10.5483/BMBRep.2015.48.4.272.

Song, Y., X. Yao, and H. Ying. 2011. "Thyroid hormone action in metabolic regulation." *Protein Cell* 2 (5):358–368. doi: 10.1007/s13238-011-1046-x.

Timper, K., and J. C. Bruning. 2017. "Hypothalamic circuits regulating appetite and energy homeostasis: pathways to obesity." *Dis Model Mech* 10 (6):679–689. doi: 10.1242/dmm.026609.

Varela, L., N. Martinez-Sanchez, R. Gallego, M. J. Vazquez, J. Roa, M. Gandara, E. Schoenmakers, R. Nogueiras, K. Chatterjee, M. Tena-Sempere, et al.. 2012. "Hypothalamic mTOR pathway mediates thyroid hormone-induced hyperphagia in hyperthyroidism." *J Pathol* 227 (2):209–222. doi: 10.1002/path.3984.

Weiner, J., M. Hankir, J. T. Heiker, W. Fenske, and K. Krause. 2017. "Thyroid hormones and browning of adipose tissue." *Mol Cell Endocrinol* 458:156–159. doi: 10.1016/j.mce.2017.01.011.

Wheeler, M. J. 2013. "A short history of hormone measurement." *Methods Mol Biol* 1065:1–6. doi: 10.1007/978-1-62703-616-0_1.

Wolfgang, M. J., and M. D. Lane. 2006. "Control of energy homeostasis: role of enzymes and intermediates of fatty acid metabolism in the central nervous system." *Annu Rev Nutr* 26:23–44. doi: 10.1146/annurev.nutr.25.050304.092532.

Wu, Z., M. E. Martinez, D. L. St Germain, and A. Hernandez. 2017. "Type 3 Deiodinase Role on Central Thyroid Hormone Action Affects the Leptin-Melanocortin System and Circadian Activity." *Endocrinology* 158 (2):419–430. doi: 10.1210/en.2016-1680.

Yao, X., H. Xia, Y. C. Wang, and H. Ying. 2014. "Thyroid hormone receptor coregulators in metabolic regulation." *J Endocrinol Diabetes Obes* 2 (3):1051.

Zhang, Z., P. H. Bisschop, E. Foppen, H. C. van Beeren, A. Kalsbeek, A. Boelen, and E. Fliers. 2016a. "A model for chronic, intrahypothalamic thyroid hormone administration in rats." *J Endocrinol* 229 (1):37–45. doi: 10.1530/JOE-15-0501.

Zhang, Z., A. Boelen, P. H. Bisschop, A. Kalsbeek, and E. Fliers. 2017. "Hypothalamic effects of thyroid hormone." *Mol Cell Endocrinol* 458:143–148. doi: 10.1016/j.mce.2017.01.018.

Zhang, Z., E. Foppen, Y. Su, P. H. Bisschop, A. Kalsbeek, E. Fliers, and A. Boelen. 2016b. "Metabolic effects of chronic T3 Administration in the Hypothalamic Paraventricular and Ventromedial Nucleus in Male Rats." *Endocrinology* 157 (10):4076–4085. doi: 10.1210/en.2016-1397.

Zhang, Q., Q. Miao, H. Ye, Z. Zhang, C. Zuo, F. Hua, Y. Guan, and Y. Li. 2014. "The effects of thyroid hormones on brown adipose tissue in humans: a PET-CT study." *Diabetes Metab Res Rev* 30 (6):513–520. doi: 10.1002/dmrr.2556.

9 Oxytocinergic Regulation of Energy Balance

Tooru M. Mizuno
University of Manitoba, Canada

CONTENTS

9.1 INTRODUCTION

The central nervous system (CNS) plays a major role in the regulation of energy homeostasis by integrating the input from long-term energy stores such as adipocyte hormones and short-term meal-related signals such as nutrients and gut hormones. Sub-populations of hypothalamic neurons mediate CNS regulation of metabolism. Oxytocin is produced by a subset of hypothalamic neurons and is a multifunctional peptide that is integrated in parturition and milk ejection as a neurohypophyseal hormone and in social behavior and food intake as a neuropeptide. Impairments in the hypothalamic oxytocin system are related to a certain type of hyperphagia-associated obesity, emphasizing that neural circuitry involving hypothalamic oxytocin neurons plays a major role in the regulation of food intake and whole body metabolism and is a possible target for anti-hyperphagia/anti-obesity drugs. Pharmacological, histological, electrophysiological, and more advanced genetic approaches have been used to determine the physiological function of oxytocin and neuronal pathways involving oxytocin neurons as well as the role of the oxytocin system in the pathogenesis of obesity.

9.2 OXYTOCIN AND THE OXYTOCIN RECEPTOR

Oxytocin was discovered in the early 20th century. Dale found that extracts from the human posterior pituitary gland stimulated contractions of the uterine muscles of a pregnant cat (Dale 1906). Ott and Scott then found that posterior pituitary gland extracts stimulated milk secretion in a goat in the early nursing period (Ott and Scott 1910). Oxytocin is a nonapeptide consisting of a cyclic six-amino-acid structure and a tail of three amino acids (Du Vigneaud, Ressler, and Trippett 1953). The gene structure of oxytocin is similar to that of arginine vasopressin; these genes are located on the same chromosome and separated by a short intergenic region, and are in opposite transcriptional orientations (Gimpl and Fahrenholz 2001). The protein structure is also similar between these two hormones, with two different amino acids at positions 3 and 8. Mature oxytocin is produced from its precursor which consists of a signal peptide domain followed by oxytocin and neurophysin through proteolytic cleavage.

Oxytocin is synthesized mainly in the CNS, within both the magnocellular and parvocellular neurons of the paraventricular nucleus (PVN), as well as by the magnocellular neurons of the supraoptic nucleus (SON) in the hypothalamus (Swanson and Sawchenko 1983). Magnocellular oxytocin neurons project a single axon to the posterior pituitary gland, forming the classic hypothalamic-neurohypophyseal system (Brownstein, Russell, and Gainer 1980). Oxytocin is released from the posterior pituitary into the systemic circulation and acts on target organs as a hormone, exerting uterine contraction and milk ejection from the mammary glands. Oxytocin is also synthesized in PVN parvocellular neurons that project to diverse CNS regions such as the brainstem, the spinal cord, the midbrain, and the hypothalamus (Gimpl and Fahrenholz 2001, McEwen 2004, Beier et al. 2015, Xiao et al. 2017, Maejima et al. 2014). Although oxytocin neurons are predominantly present in PVN and SON, oxytocin is also produced by the parvocellular neurons of other brain regions. Magnocellular oxytocin neurons are also a source of oxytocin in the CNS. Some of these neurons project axon collaterals to brain regions such as the forebrain and midbrain (Ross et al. 2009, Knobloch et al. 2012). Oxytocin is also released locally from dendrites and cell bodies within the PVN and SON and acts locally in an autocrine fashion (Douglas, Johnstone, and Leng 2007, Ludwig and Leng 2006, Russell, Leng, and Douglas 2003).

Many different oxytocin actions are mediated by the activation of a unique oxytocin receptor. This oxytocin receptor belongs to the superfamily of G protein-coupled receptors (Gimpl and Fahrenholz 2001, Gould and Zingg 2003). Together with the three vasopressin receptor subtypes, V1a, V1b, and V2, the oxytocin receptor forms a subfamily of structurally related receptors. The oxytocin receptor is coupled mainly to $G_{q/11}$ and activates phospholipase C (Ku et al. 1995). Oxytocin may interact with not only the oxytocin receptor but also the structurally related V1a receptor, though with a lower binding affinity (Chini and Manning 2007, Song and Albers 2018). The oxytocin receptor is widely distributed within the brain, as well as in various peripheral tissues, consistent with its large variety of physiological actions (Gimpl and Fahrenholz 2001).

9.3 REGULATION OF ENERGY BALANCE BY OXYTOCIN

In addition to its classical role in the reproductive function, oxytocin participates in the regulation of energy balance, which is mainly mediated by its action in the CNS. The anorexigenic effect of oxytocin was first reported by Arletti et al. in 1989. A single intraperitoneal (i.p.) and intracerebroventricular (i.c.v.) injection of oxytocin reduced food intake in fasted rats, while i.c.v. administration of the oxytocin receptor antagonist increased food intake (Arletti, Benelli, and Bertolini 1989). These findings have been replicated in rodents fed a standard chow or low-fat diet in multiple studies (Maejima et al. 2018). Nasal treatment of oxytocin is also effective in reducing food intake in mice (Maejima et al. 2015). Oxytocin-induced anorexia has also been found in both high-fat diet-induced obese (DIO) and genetically obese rodent models (Maejima et al. 2018). These effects have been extended to DIO nonhuman primates and obese humans (Blevins et al. 2015, Lawson et al. 2015, Thienel et al. 2016).

Oxytocin affects not only feeding but also body weight and adiposity. Oxytocin treatment reduces body weight and fat mass in lean and obese rodents, while treatment with the oxytocin receptor antagonist increases body weight (Zhang et al. 2011, Maejima et al. 2018). Additionally, nasal oxytocin treatment causes a reduction of body weight in overweight/obese humans (Zhang et al. 2013).

Previous studies, however, have reported inconsistent effects of oxytocin on energy expenditure (Zhang and Cai 2011, Zhang et al. 2011, Maejima et al. 2011, Blevins et al. 2016). There is evidence to support the role of oxytocin in the mobilization of energy substrates. Oxytocin treatment reduces the respiratory quotient (RQ) and increases levels of lipolysis- and fatty acid oxidation-related genes in white adipose tissue in DIO rodents, though these changes are not observed in pair-fed animals (Maejima et al. 2011, Deblon et al. 2011, Blevins et al. 2016). Similarly, the intranasal administration of oxytocin reduces RQ and causes a shift from carbohydrate to fat utilization in men (Lawson et al. 2015). These findings in pharmacological studies suggest that CNS oxytocin signaling plays an important role in the regulation of acute food intake and long-term energy homeostasis and that impairments in the oxytocin system contribute to the development of obesity.

9.4 THE NEURAL PATHWAY OF FEEDING-REGULATING OXYTOCINERGIC NEURONS

9.4.1 The Site of Oxytocin Action

PVN oxytocin neurons project to many CNS regions, where oxytocin is released so as to act as a neuromodulator, promoting a variety of biological effects (Sofroniew 1983, Swanson and Sawchenko 1983). Oxytocin receptors are widely distributed in the CNS, suggesting that widespread brain regions mediate the biological effects of oxytocin (Gimpl and Fahrenholz 2001, Gould and Zingg 2003). Induction of c-Fos following oxytocin treatment has been widely used to identify specific sites of oxytocin action. I.p. and intranasal injection of oxytocin induces c-Fos in the PVN, the arcuate nucleus (ARC), the ventromedial nucleus (VMN) of the hypothalamus, the nucleus of the solitary tract (NTS), the dorsal motor nucleus of the vagus (DMV), and the area postrema (AP) of the brainstem (Zhang and Cai 2011, Maejima et al. 2011, Morton et al. 2012, Maejima et al. 2015). Consistent with oxytocin-induced c-Fos expression in these brain regions, microinjection of oxytocin into some of these sites reduces food intake (Maejima et al. 2014, Noble et al. 2014, Klockars et al. 2017, Ong, Alhadeff, and Grill 2015). Thus, the anorexigenic effect of oxytocin is mediated by cells in specific hypothalamic and brainstem regions.

9.4.2 The ARC POMC-to-PVN Oxytocin Pathway

Melanocortin neurons in the ARC are the major mediator of the metabolic action of the adipocyte hormone leptin. Leptin increases anorexigenic pro-opiomelanocortin (POMC) expression and stimulates release of α-melanocyte stimulating hormone (α-MSH) by ARC neurons that project to the PVN (Cone 2005). Leptin inhibits the activity of orexigenic agouti-related peptide (AgRP) neurons in the ARC that also project to the PVN (Cone 2005). The melanocortin 4 receptor (MC4R) is expressed in oxytocin neurons and i.c.v. injection of α-MSH or a melanocortin agonist induces c-Fos in oxytocin neurons in PVN and SON (Caquineau et al. 2006, Kublaoui et al. 2008, Liu et al. 2003, Olszewski et al. 2001). Moreover, α-MSH depolarizes PVN oxytocin neurons and stimulates oxytocin secretion from rat brain slices containing PVN (Maejima et al. 2017). Taken together, PVN oxytocin neurons mediate the effect of leptin-α-MSH signaling on food intake and metabolism.

9.4.3 The PVN Oxytocin-to-Hindbrain/Spinal Cord Pathway

PVN oxytocin neurons project to the brainstem, such as the NTS, AP, and DMV, and preganglionic, sympathetic output neurons of the thoracic spinal cord regions (Sofroniew 1980, Sawchenko and Swanson 1982, Rinaman 1998, Sutton et al. 2014). Oxytocin terminals are closely associated with anorexigenic POMC neurons in the NTS, with tyrosine hydroxylase-immunoreactive neurons in the NTS and DMV, and with choline acetyltransferase (ChAT)-expressing neurons in the intermediolateral column of the spinal cord (IML) (Maejima et al. 2009, Llewellyn-Smith et al. 2012, Sutton et al. 2014). Oxytocin receptors are present in the NTS and DMV (Gimpl and

Fahrenholz 2001, Gould and Zingg 2003). Additionally, oxytocin induces large increases in cytosolic calcium concentration in isolated NTS POMC neurons (Maejima et al. 2009). Administration of oxytocin into the fourth ventricle or the NTS reduces food intake, while fourth ventricle administration of the oxytocin receptor antagonist increases food intake and meal size (Blouet et al. 2009, Ong, Alhadeff, and Grill 2015). These data collectively suggest that the PVN-hindbrain/spinal cord oxytocinergic pathway regulates food intake and metabolism by modulating the activity of NTS POMC neurons and their sympathetic output. This regulation may also be mediated by the potentiation of the effects of satiety-inducing gut signals such as cholecystokinin (CCK) through oxytocin release in the NTS (Blevins et al. 2003).

9.4.4 The PVN Oxytocin-to-ARC POMC Pathway

A subset of PVN and SON oxytocin neurons projects to the ARC (Csiffary et al. 1992, Maejima et al. 2014). Microinjection of oxytocin into the ARC decreases food intake. Oxytocin receptors are expressed in ARC POMC neurons where the axon terminals of oxytocin neurons are found. Oxytocin induces an increase in cytosolic calcium concentration in isolated ARC POMC neurons (Maejima et al. 2014). Thus, ARC POMC neurons are the direct target of PVN oxytocin neurons. Since ARC POMC neurons affect the activity of PVN oxytocin neurons, a bidirectional interaction between these two anorectic systems may play a significant role in fine-tuning food intake.

9.4.5 The PVN Oxytocin-to-VTA Dopamine Pathway

While the involvement of oxytocin in the homeostatic regulation of food intake has been well established, CNS oxytocin is implicated in another aspect of feeding: reward-associated feeding. The mesolimbic dopamine system plays a critical role in mediating the rewarding effects of food ingestion. PVN oxytocin neurons project to midbrain regions such as the ventral tegmental area (VTA) where oxytocin receptors and dopamine neurons are present (Sofroniew 1980, Gimpl and Fahrenholz 2001, Gould and Zingg 2003, Otero-Garcia et al. 2016, Xiao et al. 2017). Electrophysiology studies reveal that oxytocin increases the firing rate of a subset of VTA neurons (Tang et al. 2014). Subcutaneous oxytocin treatment reduces the intake of fructose-sweetened beverages in monkeys (Blevins et al. 2015). Similarly, intranasal oxytocin also reduces the reward-driven food intake in humans (Ott et al. 2013). Microinjection of oxytocin into the VTA decreases sucrose consumption in rats, while an oxytocin receptor antagonist increases sugar intake (Olszewski et al. 2010, Mullis, Kay, and Williams 2013, Herisson et al. 2016). These data support the possibility that oxytocin action in VTA reduces the reward value of palatable food, possibly by modulating the activity of VTA dopamine neurons.

9.4.6 The Hindbrain-to-PVN Oxytocin Pathway

There is a reciprocal neural connection between the hypothalamic PVN and the hindbrain. The vagal afferent senses gut-secreted hormones and inputs this information into the NTS neurons, which receive projections from PVN oxytocin neurons.

Peripheral administration of CCK activates hypothalamic oxytocin neurons (Verbalis et al. 1986, Renaud et al. 1987, Ueta et al. 1993). Noradrenergic neurons of the NTS are activated by gastric distension and by peripheral CCK, and some of these neurons project directly to magnocellular oxytocin neurons of the PVN and SON (Monnikes et al. 1997, Onaka et al. 1995, Ueta et al. 1993). NTS glucagon-like peptide-1 (GLP-1) neurons also project to the PVN; GLP-1 increases cytosolic calcium concentration in isolated PVN neurons including oxytocin neurons (Katsurada et al. 2014). Taken together, the vagal afferent-NTS-PVN oxytocin neuron pathway mediates the effect of postprandial gastric distension and the secretion of gut hormones on feeding suppression.

9.5 APPLICATION OF GENETIC TECHNIQUES TO DETERMINE THE PHYSIOLOGICAL EFFECTS OF OXYTOCIN AND NEURAL CIRCUITRY INVOLVING OXYTOCIN NEURONS

9.5.1 Gene Knockout and Knockdown

To determine the role of oxytocin in whole body metabolism, oxytocin-deficient and oxytocin-receptor-deficient mice were generated by conventional gene targeting through homologous recombination. Mice deficient in either oxytocin or an oxytocin receptor develop late-onset obesity under normal chow-fed conditions without alterations in food intake (Takayanagi et al. 2008, Camerino 2009). Moreover, sucrose intake was increased in the absence of oxytocin in mice (Amico et al. 2005, Miedlar et al. 2007). These findings are consistent with the results of pharmacological studies and support the critical role of oxytocin in the regulation of energy balance as well as reward-driven eating behavior. Although the cell bodies of oxytocin neurons are mainly present in the PVN and SON, oxytocin is also expressed in other brain regions. Oxytocin receptors are distributed throughout the brain as well as in peripheral tissues. Consequently, these global knockout mouse models cannot determine the site-specific role of oxytocin or its action. Conditional knockout mouse models would be useful to better understand the physiological roles of the target gene in specific sites at defined times. It has not been tested whether or not deletion of oxytocin or an oxytocin receptor from metabolism-related brain regions or cells affects energy balance.

As an alternative approach, site-specific gene knockdown can be used. Reduction of oxytocin expression was targeted specifically to the PVN by injecting oxytocin shRNA lentiviruses into the PVN. PVN-specific oxytocin knockdown caused an increase in food intake and body weight gain in both control lean and high-fat diet-fed mice (Zhang et al. 2011). To determine the CNS sites of oxytocin's effect on metabolism, site-specific oxytocin receptor knockdown rats were generated by injecting an oxytocin receptor shRNA adeno-associated virus (AAV) into the NTS. NTS-specific reduction of the oxytocin receptor caused an increase in meal size and food intake and augmented fasting-induced hyperphagia. High-fat diet-induced thermogenesis was attenuated in NTS-specific oxytocin receptor knockdown rats (Ong et al. 2017). These data are consistent with findings of pharmacological studies and support the concept that oxytocin produced in the PVN and its action in the NTS play a critical role in the regulation of energy balance.

9.5.2 Reporter Lines

Reporter rodent lines are useful for mapping the distribution of target gene expression and the assessment of neurochemical and electrophysiological responses to stimuli. They also enable the detection of single neurons and small neuron clusters expressing the target gene that would have remained undetected by conventional approaches such as *in situ* hybridization, immunohistochemistry, and receptor autoradiography.

Transgenic mice expressing green fluorescent protein (GFP) in oxytocin neurons have been generated by fusing enhanced GFP to the end of the neurophysin at the C-terminus of the pre-pro-oxytocin. The resulting transgenic mice express GFP specifically in magnocellular oxytocin neurons in the PVN and SON (Young et al. 1999). GFP fluorescence is observed in the neural lobe of the pituitary and undergoes depolarization-induced calcium-dependent secretion (Zhang et al. 2002). Thus, an oxytocin-GFP transgenic mouse serves as a valuable tool for the detailed characterization of magnocellular oxytocin neurons projecting to the posterior pituitary.

Oxytocin reporter rats were also generated by expressing the monomeric red fluorescent protein 1 (mRFP1) fusion gene under the control of the oxytocin promoter. In these rats, mRFP1 fluorescence is present throughout the SON and in the magnocellular division of the PVN with scattered mRFP1 expression in the parvocellular division of the PVN (Katoh et al. 2011). This rat model has been successfully used to determine the activation of PVN oxytocin neurons following i.p. injection of the CCK by assessing c-Fos expression in mRFP1-positive oxytocin neurons (Katoh et al. 2014, Motojima et al. 2016).

An oxytocin receptor reporter mouse line was created by targeting the lacZ reporter gene to the oxytocin receptor gene locus, downstream of the endogenous regulatory elements (Gould and Zingg 2003). Another reporter mouse was generated by replacing part of the oxytocin receptor gene with Venus, a variant of yellow fluorescent protein (YFP) (Yoshida et al. 2009). These mouse lines enabled the identification of novel CNS sites of oxytocin receptor gene expression as well as the neurochemical characterization of oxytocin receptor-expressing cells.

A combination of the injection of a cre-dependent virus, expressing fluorescent protein and knock-in mice expressing cre recombinase in a cell-type-specific manner, has become more common. For example, the AAV with a double-floxed inverse open reading frame flanking eGFP was injected into the PVN of knock-in mice expressing cre recombinase in oxytocin neurons (Hung et al. 2017). Similarly, cre-inducible AAV coding for eYFP was delivered into the specific brain site of mice in which cre recombinase is expressed by oxytocin receptor-expressing cells (Peris et al. 2017). These mice were used to determine the distribution and neural connection of oxytocin- and oxytocin-receptor-expressing neurons in specific brain regions (e.g. the VTA).

9.5.3 Ablation of Oxytocin Neurons

Pharmacological studies have demonstrated the feeding-suppressing effect of oxytocin, whereas oxytocin-deficient mice displayed an obese phenotype with normal food intake (Camerino 2009). This discrepancy could be due to compensatory changes in response to the germline deletion of the oxytocin gene. To avoid this problem and directly address the role of oxytocin neurons, these neurons were ablated in an inducible manner in adult mice. Two independent oxytocin neuron-ablated mouse models were created. Transgenic mice expressing cre recombinase under the control of the oxytocin promoter were mated with inducible diphtheria toxin receptor (DTR) mice in which a loxP-flanked STOP sequence was placed upstream of the DTR. In the resultant double mutant mice, the DTR is expressed selectively in oxytocin neurons, thus leading to ablation of the oxytocin neurons following the administration of the diphtheria toxin (Wu et al. 2012, Xi et al. 2017). In the first study by Wu et al., ablation of the oxytocin neurons in adult mice did not cause alterations in body weight under normal chow-fed conditions. When male, but not female, mice were placed on a high fat diet for 12 weeks, the lack of oxytocin neurons resulted in an increase in body weight and a decrease in energy expenditure without a significant change in food intake. Additionally, leptin-induced anorexia was attenuated in these mice (Wu et al. 2012).

In the second study by Xi et al., ablation of oxytocin neurons did not alter body weight, food intake, and energy expenditure under regular chow-fed conditions in both male and female mice. Food intake and body weight were not changed during the one-week high-fat diet feeding period in male oxytocin neuron-ablated mice. However, CCK-induced anorexia and the activation of PVN was abolished in these mice. A lack of oxytocin neurons also attenuated cold-induced thermogenesis (Xi et al. 2017). Together, these data suggest that oxytocin neurons are dispensable for body weight regulation on a standard chow diet, while they are required for normal body weight regulation in response to high-fat-diet feeding in a sex-dependent manner. Reduced energy expenditure and impaired thermogenesis may contribute to increased body weight in oxytocin neuron-ablated mice. Oxytocin neurons also mediate the anorexigenic actions of leptin and CCK. The selective effect of oxytocin neurons on energy expenditure is consistent with the metabolic phenotype of oxytocin-deficient mice, which also exhibit selective reduction in energy expenditure without increased food intake.

9.5.4 Manipulation of Oxytocin Release

Findings in mice deficient in either oxytocin or its receptor support the role of oxytocin production and/or action in the regulation of energy balance. However, these mouse models cannot address the question of whether or not hypothalamic oxytocin release is critical in the regulation of metabolism and the pathogenesis of obesity. To address this question, the synaptotagmin-4 (Syt4) gene was ablated in mice. Syt4 is an atypical modulator of synaptic exocytosis and negatively regulates oxytocin exocytosis. Syt4 deficiency caused an increase in oxytocin release and prevented high-fat diet-induced obesity in mice. To further investigate the role of PVN Syt4 in the regulation of metabolism, the Syt4 expression level in the PVN was either reduced or increased by injecting Syt4 hsRNA lentiviruses or oxytocin promoter-driven Syt4 lentiviruses into the PVN. PVN-specific Syt4 knockdown prevented high-fat diet-induced obesity, while enhanced Syt4 expression in PVN oxytocin neurons resulted in increases in food intake and body weight (Zhang et al. 2011). These findings suggest that oxytocin exocytosis is an important step in the regulation of food intake and body weight.

9.5.5 Manipulation of Specific Oxytocin Neuron Activity

There has been an explosion of studies utilizing optogenetics and chemogenetics to selectively manipulate and investigate both structural and functional neural connections. Optogenetics uses a combination of light and genetic manipulation in order to control a biological system. One of the proteins that have been widely used is channelrhodopsin-2 (ChR2), a photoexcitable cation channel. In combination with the cre-loxP system, expression of ChR2 enables cell-type-specific temporal photostimulation of neurons. ChR2-assisted circuit mapping (CRACM) combines photostimulation of presumptive presynaptic neurons expressing ChR2 with electrophysiological assessment of light-evoked postsynaptic currents in candidate downstream neurons.

Designer receptors exclusively activated by designer drugs (DREADDs) is a widely used chemogenetic technique. The activity of subsets of neurons can be acutely altered using DREADD technology. Modified human muscarinic receptors hM3Dq and hM4Di have been frequently used as activating and silencing DREADDs, respectively. The binding of an otherwise physiologically inert synthetic ligand, clozapine-*N*-oxide (CNO), activates neurons expressing hM3Dq or inhibits the activity of hM4Di-expressing neurons. Cre-dependent DREADD expression allows remote and temporal activation of neurons that express cre recombinase.

9.5.5.1 The ARC AgRP-to-PVN Oxytocin Pathway

Anorexigenic POMC and orexigenic AgRP neurons in the hypothalamic ARC project to the PVN. Pharmacological and electrophysiology studies suggest that PVN oxytocin neurons are the direct target of ARC POMC neurons. PVN oxytocin neurons express MC4R and may also receive monosynaptic inputs from ARC AgRP neurons.

The connectivity of ARC AgRP neurons and PVN oxytocin neurons was investigated using optogenetics. Photostimulation of AgRP axons in the PVN increased food intake with a magnitude similar to stimulating AgRP-expressing somata in the ARC. CRACM showed that photostimulation of AgRP axons induced inhibitory postsynaptic currents (IPSCs) in PVN neurons. There was a co-localization of the presynaptic marker synapsin-1 with AgRP in close proximity to oxytocin neuron somata in the PVN. Concomitant stimulation of ARC AgRP neuron axons and oxytocin neuron somata in the PVN occluded the feeding evoked by PVN-projecting ARC AgRP neurons (Atasoy et al. 2012). These findings suggest that PVN oxytocin neurons are postsynaptic targets of ARC AgRP neurons and mediate AgRP-evoked eating.

In a separate study using similar techniques, CRACM revealed light-evoked IPSCs in the majority of postsynaptic PVN MC4R-expressing neurons, but failed to detect light-evoked IPSCs in PVN oxytocin neurons. Optogenetic activation of ARC AgRP nerve terminals in the PVN acutely increased food intake. Simultaneous activation of somata of PVN MC4R-expressing neurons abolished ARC AgRP-evoked feeding, while activation of PVN oxytocin neuron somata did not affect it (Garfield et al. 2015). Taken together, PVN oxytocin neurons are the direct target of ARC POMC neurons and mediate the anorexigenic effect of α-MSH, while it remains a matter of debate whether or not PVN oxytocin neurons are postsynaptic targets of ARC AgRP neurons.

9.5.5.2 The PVN Oxytocin-to-Hindbrain/Spinal Cord Pathway

The PVN consists of heterogeneous cell types including oxytocin neurons. The transcription factor single minded-1 (Sim1) is expressed in nearly all PVN neurons. Oxytocin neurons are a small subpopulation of PVN neurons. To map the projection terminals of PVN oxytocin neurons, a cre-dependent adenoviral synaptophysin-mCherry terminal tracer was injected into the PVN of knock-in mice expressing cre recombinase in oxytocin neurons. PVN oxytocin neuron-derived mCherry was found in the NTS and parabrachial nucleus (PBN), but the number of mCherry-positive cells was much less compared to that of cells expressing Sim1 neuron-derived mCherry. This is consistent with the fact that oxytocin neurons are a subset (approximately 20%) of Sim1 neurons in the PVN. A robust synaptophysin-mCherry tracer was observed in thoracic spinal cord regions originating from PVN Sim1 and oxytocin neurons. mCherry immunoreactivity was localized in close proximity to neurons expressing ChAT in the IML, suggesting potential Sim1 and oxytocin neuronal connections to IML preganglionic sympathetic neurons. When retrobeads were injected into the NTS of mice expressing GFP in PVN Sim1 neurons, all retrobead-labeled PVN neurons co-expressed GFP, suggesting that all PVN-NTS projections originate from PVN Sim1 neurons. When a similar protocol was used for oxytocin neurons, a subset of PVN retrobead-labeled neurons was positive for oxytocin. However, NTS-injected retrobeads predominantly labeled PVN neurons that do not express oxytocin (Sutton et al. 2014). These findings suggest that PVN oxytocin neurons project to both the NTS and IML, though oxytocin neurons represent only a small fraction of NTS-projecting PVN neurons.

To further determine the role of PVN oxytocin neurons in the regulation of metabolism, the activity of these neurons was acutely manipulated using DREADD technology. AAV-hM3Dq-mCherry or AAV-hM4Di-mCherry was injected into the PVN of knock-in mice expressing cre recombinase in oxytocin neurons. Chemogenetic activation of PVN oxytocin neurons resulted in an increase in energy expenditure without a change in food intake, while activation of the larger population of PVN neurons (i.e. PVN Sim1 neurons) increased energy expenditure and reduced food intake (Sutton et al. 2014). Chemogenetic silencing of PVN oxytocin neurons did not affect feeding behavior (Garfield et al. 2015). Activation of PVN oxytocin neurons led to an increase in c-Fos expression in IML ChAT-expressing neurons (Sutton et al. 2014). Overall, these findings suggest that specific subsets of PVN neurons play distinct roles in the regulation of energy homeostasis. PVN oxytocin neurons project to sympathetic output areas of the thoracic spinal cord and participate in the regulation of energy expenditure, but they do not play a major role in feeding regulation.

9.5.5.3 The PVN Oxytocin-to-ARC POMC Pathway

Pharmacological and histological studies revealed that ARC POMC neurons are a direct target of oxytocin. To further determine whether PVN oxytocin neurons project to the ARC, a retrograde tracer was injected into the ARC of reporter rats expressing GFP in oxytocin neurons. A subset of PVN and SON oxytocin neurons was positive for the tracer (Maejima et al. 2014). PVN oxytocin neurons may also project to glutamatergic neurons in the ARC. Chemogenetic and optogenetic activation of oxytocin receptor-expressing glutamatergic neurons in the ARC that project to the PVN caused a reduction of food intake. These glutamatergic neurons did not express POMC (Fenselau et al. 2017). To determine whether or not ARC AgRP neurons receive monosynaptic inputs from PVN oxytocin neurons, cre-dependent AAV expressing ChR2-mCherry was injected into the PVN of oxytocin neuron-specific cre-expressing mice that also express GFP in AgRP neurons. Photostimulation of PVN oxytocin neurons failed to induce excitatory post-synaptic currents (EPSCs) in AgRP neurons (Krashes et al. 2014). These findings suggest that PVN oxytocin neurons provide monosynaptic inputs to POMC neurons but not AgRP neurons in the ARC. PVN oxytocin may regulate food intake by acting on both ARC POMC neurons and non-POMC glutamatergic neurons projecting to the PVN.

9.5.5.4 The PVN Oxytocin-to-VTA Dopamine Pathway

Pharmacological and electrophysiology studies suggested that oxytocin action in the midbrain VTA reduces the reward value of palatable food possibly by modulating the activity of VTA dopamine neurons. If oxytocin plays a role in reward-driven feeding, oxytocin neurons may project to midbrain dopamine neurons. To identify the synaptic input to VTA dopamine neurons, AAVs expressing cre-dependent TVA (the receptor for viruses containing the avian EnvA envelope glycoprotein) fused with mCherry (TC) and rabies glycoprotein (G) were injected into the VTA of knock-in mice that express cre recombinase in dopamine neurons. This was followed by the injection of an EnvA-pseudotyped, G-deleted, GFP-expressing rabies virus (RVdG) into the same VTA site. GFP-positive neurons were found across different brain regions including the PVN of the hypothalamus. A subset (6%) of PVN neurons that innervate VTA dopamine neurons express oxytocin mRNA, providing evidence for monosynaptic connections between PVN oxytocin neurons and VTA dopamine neurons (Beier et al. 2015). To further determine the input–output relationships of VTA dopamine neurons, TRIO (tracing the relationship between input and output) and cell-type-specific TRIO (cTRIO) techniques were used. TRIO relies on the axonal uptake of the canine adenovirus vector expressing cre recombinase (CAV-Cre) that efficiently transduces axon terminals. RVdG-mediated input tracing based on CAV-Cre injected at a projection site can reveal inputs to projection-defined VTA subpopulations. cTRIO further refines input tracing to VTA dopamine neurons that project to a specific output site by utilizing CAV that expresses a cre-dependent Flp recombinase in conjunction with AAVs expressing Flp-dependent TC and G in knock-in mice that express cre recombinase in dopamine neurons. cTRIO revealed that nucleus accumbens (NAc)-projecting VTA dopamine neurons receive monosynaptic input from diverse brain regions including the PVN (Beier et al. 2015).

In a separate study, retrobeads were injected into the VTA of mice expressing tdTomato under the control of the oxytocin promoter. Retrobead-labeled neurons were found in the PVN, but not in the SON. Approximately 20% of retrobead-positive neurons in the PVN were tdTomato-positive, providing evidence for a direct PVN oxytocinergic projection to the VTA. Cre-dependent AAV expressing ChR2 fused with either mCherry or eYFP was injected into the PVN of knock-in mice expressing cre recombinase in oxytocin neurons. Optogenetic activation of oxytocin somata in PVN or oxytocin terminals in VTA increased the firing rate of VTA dopamine neurons; this response was blocked by an oxytocin receptor antagonist (Xiao et al. 2017). Moreover, electrophysiology studies revealed that oxytocin or an oxytocin receptor agonist increased the firing rate in VTA dopamine neurons including those projecting to NAc (Hung et al. 2017, Xiao et al. 2017). Photostimulation of VTA dopamine cell bodies or dopamine terminals in NAc decreased reward-related feeding behavior as assessed by a two bottle choice paradigm (Mikhailova et al. 2016). Collectively, these findings suggest that PVN oxytocin neurons provide a stimulatory input directly to the NAc-projecting VTA dopamine neurons. It remains to be determined whether or not the PVN oxytocin-VTA dopamine-NAc neural pathway plays a role in the regulation of reward-driven feeding.

9.6 THE POSSIBILITY OF OXYTOCIN TREATMENT AS ANTI-OBESITY THERAPY

Impairments in hypothalamic oxytocin neurons contribute to the development of hyperphagia and obesity. A loss of function or deletion of Sim1, a transcription factor controlling the development of oxytocin neurons, results in hyperphagia and obesity (Kublaoui et al. 2008, Bonnefond et al. 2013). The number of PVN oxytocin neurons and the expression levels of oxytocin receptors is reduced in individuals with Prader–Willi syndrome (PWS) who are characterized by hyperphagic obesity (Swaab, Purba, and Hofman 1995, Martin et al. 1998, Bittel et al. 2007). In pre-clinical studies, sub-chronic oxytocin treatment has been proven to be effective in reducing food intake and body weight in high-fat diet-induced obese rodents, which is a rodent model of leptin-resistant obesity (Zhang and Cai 2011, Deblon et al. 2011, Morton et al. 2012, Blevins et al. 2016, Maejima, et al. 2017). Nasal administration of oxytocin decreases food intake and improves peripheral glucose metabolism in mice (Maejima et al. 2015). These findings have drawn much attention to oxytocin's therapeutic potential to treat hyperphagia and obesity. In clinical studies, intranasal administration of oxytocin reduced hunger-induced food intake in obese individuals (Zhang et al. 2013, Lawson et al. 2015, Thienel et al. 2016). Although intranasal oxytocin failed to reverse hyperphagia and obesity in PWS patients, it reduced food-related behavior, an indication of reduced interest in eating and food (Einfeld et al. 2014, Kuppens, Donze, and Hokken-Koelega 2016). Intranasal oxytocin reduced body weight in a patient with hypothalamic obesity who showed damages to the hypothalamus including the PVN and SON after surgical resection of a craniopharyngioma (Hsu et al. 2018). These findings support the possibility that intranasal delivery of oxytocin is a viable approach to the treatment of obesity that is characterized by leptin resistance (the majority of obese patients) and an impaired oxytocin system (i.e. PWS patients and survivors of craniopharyngioma).

9.7 PERSPECTIVES

Classical conventional pharmacological, histological, biochemical, and electrophysiological approaches initiated the elucidation of oxytocin's physiological function and the feasibility of oxytocin therapy in the treatment of obesity. This was followed by investigation of the detailed neural circuitry involving oxytocin neurons and its relationship to normal physiology and the pathophysiology of obesity using a combination of state-of-the-art genetic tools such as optogenetics and chemogenetics. These techniques have advanced our understanding of oxytocinergic neural circuitry (Figure 9.1) and its role in the regulation of energy balance. Nutrients, hormones, and neuromodulators affect the activity of oxytocin neurons in response to changes in the body's metabolic state. The increased activity of oxytocin neurons inhibits feeding and increases energy expenditure by altering the activity of specific neural circuits involving neurons in the hindbrain, hypothalamus, midbrain, and spinal cord that receive a projection of hypothalamic oxytocin neurons. Further investigation is necessary to fully understand the oxytocinergic neural circuitry and the role of each component of the neural circuitry in the regulation of the metabolism. Oxytocin treatment has been proven to be effective in reducing food intake and body weight in rodent models of leptin resistant obesity, a major form of human obesity. Thus, enhancing the activity of the specific oxytocinergic neural circuitry and its downstream mediators may serve as a beneficial therapeutic approach to the treatment of obesity.

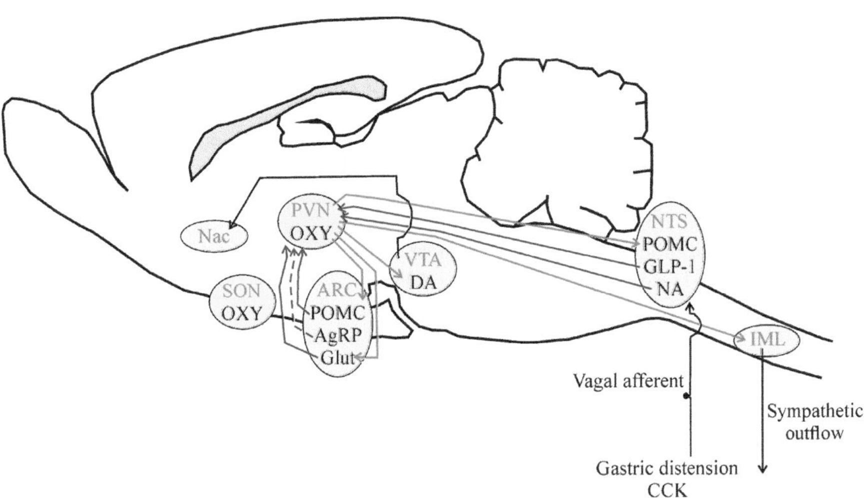

FIGURE 9.1 Schematic diagram of a sagittal view of the brain, illustrating the possible neural circuit involving PVN oxytocin (OXY) neurons that control energy balance. ARC: arcuate nucleus; DMV: dorsal motor nucleus of the vagus; IML: intermediolateral column of the spinal cord; Nac: nucleus accumbens; NTS: nucleus tractus solitarius; SON: supraoptic nucleus; PVN: paraventricular nucleus; VTA: ventral tegmental area; AgRP: agouti-related peptide; CCK: cholecystokinin; DA: dopamine; GLP-1: glucagon-like peptide-1; Glut: Glutamate; NA: noradrenaline; OXY: oxytocin; POMC: pro-opiomelanocortin. Red line: oxytocin neurons; blue line: input to PVN oxytocin neurons; black line: other neurons; dashed line: controversial data have been reported.

REFERENCES

Amico, J. A., R. R. Vollmer, H. M. Cai, J. A. Miedlar, and L. Rinaman. 2005. Enhanced initial and sustained intake of sucrose solution in mice with an oxytocin gene deletion. *Am J Physiol Regul Integr Comp Physiol* 289 (6):R1798–R1806. doi: 10.1152/ajpregu.00558.2005.

Arletti, R., A. Benelli, and A. Bertolini. 1989. Influence of oxytocin on feeding behavior in the rat. *Peptides* 10 (1):89–93.

Atasoy, D., J. N. Betley, H. H. Su, and S. M. Sternson. 2012. Deconstruction of a neural circuit for hunger. *Nature* 488 (7410):172–177.

Beier, K. T., E. E. Steinberg, K. E. DeLoach, S. Xie, K. Miyamichi, L. Schwarz, X. J. Gao, E. J. Kremer, R. C. Malenka, and L. Luo. 2015. Circuit Architecture of VTA Dopamine Neurons Revealed by Systematic Input-Output Mapping. *Cell* 162 (3):622–634. doi: 10.1016/j.cell.2015.07.015.

Bittel, D. C., N. Kibiryeva, S. M. Sell, T. V. Strong, and M. G. Butler. 2007. Whole genome microarray analysis of gene expression in Prader-Willi syndrome. *Am J Med Genet A* 143A (5):430–442. doi: 10.1002/ajmg.a.31606.

Blevins, J. E., T. J. Eakin, J. A. Murphy, M. W. Schwartz, and D. G. Baskin. 2003. Oxytocin innervation of caudal brainstem nuclei activated by cholecystokinin. *Brain Res* 993 (1–2):30–41.

Blevins, J. E., J. L. Graham, G. J. Morton, K. L. Bales, M. W. Schwartz, D. G. Baskin, and P. J. Havel. 2015. Chronic oxytocin administration inhibits food intake, increases energy expenditure, and produces weight loss in fructose-fed obese rhesus monkeys. *Am J Physiol Regul Integr Comp Physiol* 308 (5):R431–R438. doi: 10.1152/ajpregu.00441.2014.

Blevins, J. E., B. W. Thompson, V. T. Anekonda, J. M. Ho, J. L. Graham, Z. S. Roberts, B. H. Hwang, K. Ogimoto, T. Wolden-Hanson, J. Nelson, et al. 2016. Chronic CNS oxytocin signaling preferentially induces fat loss in high-fat diet-fed rats by enhancing satiety responses and increasing lipid utilization. *Am J Physiol Regul Integr Comp Physiol* 310 (7):R640–R658. doi: 10.1152/ajpregu.00220.2015.

Blouet, C., Y. H. Jo, X. Li, and G. J. Schwartz. 2009. Mediobasal hypothalamic leucine sensing regulates food intake through activation of a hypothalamus-brainstem circuit. *J Neurosci* 29 (26):8302–8311.

Bonnefond, A., A. Raimondo, F. Stutzmann, M. Ghoussaini, S. Ramachandrappa, D. C. Bersten, E. Durand, V. Vatin, B. Balkau, O. Lantieri, et al. 2013. Loss-of-function mutations in SIM1 contribute to obesity and Prader-Willi-like features. *J Clin Invest* 123 (7):3037–3041. doi: 10.1172/JCI68035.

Brownstein, M. J., J. T. Russell, and H. Gainer. 1980. Synthesis, transport, and release of posterior pituitary hormones. *Science* 207 (4429):373–378. doi: 10.1126/science.6153132.

Camerino, C. 2009. Low sympathetic tone and obese phenotype in oxytocin-deficient mice. *Obesity (Silver Spring)* 17 (5):980–984. doi: 10.1038/oby.2009.12.

Caquineau, C., G. Leng, X. M. Guan, M. Jiang, L. Van der Ploeg, and A. J. Douglas. 2006. Effects of alpha-melanocyte-stimulating hormone on magnocellular oxytocin neurones and their activation at intromission in male rats. *J Neuroendocrinol* 18 (9):685–691. doi: 10.1111/j.1365-2826.2006.01465.x.

Chini, B., and M. Manning. 2007. Agonist selectivity in the oxytocin/vasopressin receptor family: new insights and challenges. *Biochem Soc Trans* 35 (Pt 4):737–741. doi: 10.1042/BST0350737.

Cone, R. D. 2005. Anatomy and regulation of the central melanocortin system. *Nat Neurosci* 8 (5):571–578.

Csiffary, A., Z. Ruttner, Z. Toth, and M. Palkovits. 1992. Oxytocin nerve fibers innervate beta-endorphin neurons in the arcuate nucleus of the rat hypothalamus. *Neuroendocrinology* 56 (3):429–435. doi: 10.1159/000126259.

Dale, H. H. 1906. On some physiological actions of ergot. *J Physiol* 34 (3):163–206. doi: 10.1113/jphysiol.1906.sp001148.

Deblon, N., C. Veyrat-Durebex, L. Bourgoin, A. Caillon, A. L. Bussier, S. Petrosino, F. Piscitelli, J. J. Legros, V. Geenen, M. Foti, et al. 2011. Mechanisms of the anti-obesity effects of oxytocin in diet-induced obese rats. *PLoS One* 6 (9):e25565. doi: 10.1371/journal.pone.0025565.

Douglas, A. J., L. E. Johnstone, and G. Leng. 2007. Neuroendocrine mechanisms of change in food intake during pregnancy: a potential role for brain oxytocin. *Physiol Behav* 91 (4):352–365. doi: 10.1016/j.physbeh.2007.04.012.

Du Vigneaud, V., C. Ressler, and S. Trippett. 1953. The sequence of amino acids in oxytocin, with a proposal for the structure of oxytocin. *J Biol Chem* 205 (2):949–957.

Einfeld, S. L., E. Smith, I. S. McGregor, K. Steinbeck, J. Taffe, L. J. Rice, S. K. Horstead, N. Rogers, M. A. Hodge, and A. J. Guastella. 2014. A double-blind randomized controlled trial of oxytocin nasal spray in Prader Willi syndrome. *Am J Med Genet A* 164A (9):2232–2239. doi: 10.1002/ajmg.a.36653.

Fenselau, H., J. N. Campbell, A. M. Verstegen, J. C. Madara, J. Xu, B. P. Shah, J. M. Resch, Z. Yang, Y. Mandelblat-Cerf, Y. Livneh, et al. 2017. A rapidly acting glutamatergic ARC-->PVH satiety circuit postsynaptically regulated by alpha-MSH. *Nat Neurosci* 20 (1):42–51. doi: 10.1038/nn.4442.

Garfield, A. S., C. Li, J. C. Madara, B. P. Shah, E. Webber, J. S. Steger, J. N. Campbell, O. Gavrilova, C. E. Lee, D. P. Olson, et al. 2015. A neural basis for melanocortin-4 receptor-regulated appetite. *Nat Neurosci* 18 (6):863–871. doi: 10.1038/nn.4011.

Gimpl, G., and F. Fahrenholz. 2001. The oxytocin receptor system: structure, function, and regulation. *Physiol Rev* 81 (2):629–683. doi: 10.1152/physrev.2001.81.2.629.

Gould, B. R., and H. H. Zingg. 2003. Mapping oxytocin receptor gene expression in the mouse brain and mammary gland using an oxytocin receptor-LacZ reporter mouse. *Neuroscience* 122 (1):155–167. doi: 10.1016/s0306-4522(03)00283-5.

Herisson, F. M., J. R. Waas, R. Fredriksson, H. B. Schioth, A. S. Levine, and P. K. Olszewski. 2016. Oxytocin Acting in the Nucleus Accumbens Core Decreases Food Intake. *J Neuroendocrinol* 28 (4). doi: 10.1111/jne.12381.

Hsu, E. A., J. L. Miller, F. A. Perez, and C. L. Roth. 2018. Oxytocin and Naltrexone Successfully Treat Hypothalamic Obesity in a Boy Post-Craniopharyngioma Resection. *J Clin Endocrinol Metab* 103 (2):370–375. doi: 10.1210/jc.2017-02080.

Hung, L. W., S. Neuner, J. S. Polepalli, K. T. Beier, M. Wright, J. J. Walsh, E. M. Lewis, L. Luo, K. Deisseroth, G. Dolen, et al. 2017. Gating of social reward by oxytocin in the ventral tegmental area. *Science* 357 (6358):1406–1411. doi: 10.1126/science.aan4994.

Katoh, A., H. Fujihara, T. Ohbuchi, T. Onaka, T. Hashimoto, M. Kawata, H. Suzuki, and Y. Ueta. 2011. Highly visible expression of an oxytocin-monomeric red fluorescent protein 1 fusion gene in the hypothalamus and posterior pituitary of transgenic rats. *Endocrinology* 152 (7):2768–2774. doi: 10.1210/en.2011-0006.

Katoh, A., K. Shoguchi, H. Matsuoka, M. Yoshimura, J. I. Ohkubo, T. Matsuura, T. Maruyama, T. Ishikura, T. Aritomi, H. Fujihara, et al. 2014. Fluorescent visualisation of the hypothalamic oxytocin neurones activated by cholecystokinin-8 in rats expressing c-fos-enhanced green fluorescent protein and oxytocin-monomeric red fluorescent protein 1 fusion transgenes. *J Neuroendocrinol* 26 (5):341–347. doi: 10.1111/jne.12150.

Katsurada, K., Y. Maejima, M. Nakata, M. Kodaira, S. Suyama, Y. Iwasaki, K. Kario, and T. Yada. 2014. Endogenous GLP-1 acts on paraventricular nucleus to suppress feeding: projection from nucleus tractus solitarius and activation of corticotropin-releasing hormone, nesfatin-1 and oxytocin neurons. *Biochem Biophys Res Commun* 451 (2):276–281. doi: 10.1016/j.bbrc.2014.07.116.

Klockars, O. A., J. R. Waas, A. Klockars, A. S. Levine, and P. K. Olszewski. 2017. Neural Basis of Ventromedial Hypothalamic Oxytocin-Driven Decrease in Appetite. *Neuroscience* 366:54–61. doi: 10.1016/j.neuroscience.2017.10.008.

Knobloch, H. S., A. Charlet, L. C. Hoffmann, M. Eliava, S. Khrulev, A. H. Cetin, P. Osten, M. K. Schwarz, P. H. Seeburg, R. Stoop, et al. 2012. Evoked axonal oxytocin release in the central amygdala attenuates fear response. *Neuron* 73 (3):553–566. doi: 10.1016/j.neuron.2011.11.030.

Krashes, M. J., B. P. Shah, J. C. Madara, D. P. Olson, D. E. Strochlic, A. S. Garfield, L. Vong, H. Pei, M. Watabe-Uchida, N. Uchida, et al. 2014. An excitatory paraventricular nucleus to AgRP neuron circuit that drives hunger. *Nature* 507 (7491):238–242. doi: 10.1038/nature12956.

Ku, C. Y., A. Qian, Y. Wen, K. Anwer, and B. M. Sanborn. 1995. Oxytocin stimulates myometrial guanosine triphosphatase and phospholipase-C activities via coupling to G alpha q/11. *Endocrinology* 136 (4):1509–1515. doi: 10.1210/endo.136.4.7895660.

Kublaoui, B. M., T. Gemelli, K. P. Tolson, Y. Wang, and A. R. Zinn. 2008. Oxytocin deficiency mediates hyperphagic obesity of Sim1 haploinsufficient mice. *Mol Endocrinol* 22 (7):1723–1734. doi: 10.1210/me.2008-0067.

Kuppens, R. J., S. H. Donze, and A. C. Hokken-Koelega. 2016. Promising effects of oxytocin on social and food-related behaviour in young children with Prader-Willi syndrome: a randomized, double-blind, controlled crossover trial. *Clin Endocrinol (Oxf)* 85 (6):979–987. doi: 10.1111/cen.13169.

Lawson, E. A., D. A. Marengi, R. L. DeSanti, T. M. Holmes, D. A. Schoenfeld, and C. J. Tolley. 2015. Oxytocin reduces caloric intake in men. *Obesity (Silver Spring)* 23 (5):950–956. doi: 10.1002/oby.21069.

Liu, H., T. Kishi, A. G. Roseberry, X. Cai, C. E. Lee, J. M. Montez, J. M. Friedman, and J. K. Elmquist. 2003. Transgenic mice expressing green fluorescent protein under the control of the melanocortin-4 receptor promoter. *J Neurosci* 23 (18):7143–7154.

Llewellyn-Smith, I. J., D. O. Kellett, D. Jordan, K. N. Browning, and R. A. Travagli. 2012. Oxytocin-immunoreactive innervation of identified neurons in the rat dorsal vagal complex. *Neurogastroenterol Motil* 24 (3):e136–e146. doi: 10.1111/j.1365-2982.2011.01851.x.

Ludwig, M., and G. Leng. 2006. Dendritic peptide release and peptide-dependent behaviours. *Nat Rev Neurosci* 7 (2):126–136. doi: 10.1038/nrn1845.

Maejima, Y., M. Aoyama, K. Sakamoto, T. Jojima, Y. Aso, K. Takasu, S. Takenosihita, and K. Shimomura. 2017. Impact of sex, fat distribution and initial body weight on oxytocin's body weight regulation. *Sci Rep* 7 (1):8599. doi: 10.1038/s41598-017-09318-7.

Maejima, Y., Y. Iwasaki, Y. Yamahara, M. Kodaira, U. Sedbazar, and T. Yada. 2011. Peripheral oxytocin treatment ameliorates obesity by reducing food intake and visceral fat mass. *Aging (Albany NY)* 3 (12):1169–1177. doi: 10.18632/aging.100408.

Maejima, Y., R. S. Rita, P. Santoso, M. Aoyama, Y. Hiraoka, K. Nishimori, D. Gantulga, K. Shimomura, and T. Yada. 2015. Nasal oxytocin administration reduces food intake without affecting locomotor activity and glycemia with c-Fos induction in limited brain areas. *Neuroendocrinology* 101 (1):35–44. doi: 10.1159/000371636.

Maejima, Y., K. Sakuma, P. Santoso, D. Gantulga, K. Katsurada, Y. Ueta, Y. Hiraoka, K. Nishimori, S. Tanaka, K. Shimomura, et al. 2014. Oxytocinergic circuit from paraventricular and supraoptic nuclei to arcuate POMC neurons in hypothalamus. *FEBS Lett* 588 (23):4404–4412. doi: 10.1016/j.febslet.2014.10.010.

Maejima, Y., U. Sedbazar, S. Suyama, D. Kohno, T. Onaka, E. Takano, N. Yoshida, M. Koike, Y. Uchiyama, K. Fujiwara, et al. 2009. Nesfatin-1-regulated oxytocinergic signaling in the paraventricular nucleus causes anorexia through a leptin-independent melanocortin pathway. *Cell Metab* 10 (5):355–365. doi: 10.1016/j.cmet.2009.09.002.

Maejima, Y., S. Takahashi, K. Takasu, S. Takenoshita, Y. Ueta, and K. Shimomura. 2017. Orexin action on oxytocin neurons in the paraventricular nucleus of the hypothalamus. *Neuroreport* 28 (6):360–366. doi: 10.1097/WNR.0000000000000773.

Maejima, Y., S. Yokota, K. Nishimori, and K. Shimomura. 2018. The Anorexigenic Neural Pathways of Oxytocin and Their Clinical Implication. *Neuroendocrinology* 107 (1):91–104. doi: 10.1159/000489263.

Martin, A., M. State, G. M. Anderson, W. M. Kaye, J. M. Hanchett, C. W. McConaha, W. G. North, and J. F. Leckman. 1998. Cerebrospinal fluid levels of oxytocin in Prader-Willi syndrome: a preliminary report. *Biol Psychiatry* 44 (12):1349–1352.

McEwen, B. B. 2004. General introduction to vasopressin and oxytocin: structure/metabolism, evolutionary aspects, neural pathway/receptor distribution, and functional aspects relevant to memory processing. *Adv Pharmacol* 50:1–50, 655–708. doi: 10.1016/S1054-3589(04)50001-7.

Miedlar, J. A., L. Rinaman, R. R. Vollmer, and J. A. Amico. 2007. Oxytocin gene deletion mice overconsume palatable sucrose solution but not palatable lipid emulsions. *Am J Physiol Regul Integr Comp Physiol* 293 (3):R1063–R1068. doi: 10.1152/ajpregu.00228.2007.

Mikhailova, M. A., C. E. Bass, V. P. Grinevich, A. M. Chappell, A. L. Deal, K. D. Bonin, J. L. Weiner, R. R. Gainetdinov, and E. A. Budygin. 2016. Optogenetically-induced tonic dopamine release from VTA-nucleus accumbens projections inhibits reward consummatory behaviors. *Neuroscience* 333:54–64. doi: 10.1016/j.neuroscience.2016.07.006.

Monnikes, H., G. Lauer, C. Bauer, J. Tebbe, T. T. Zittel, and R. Arnold. 1997. Pathways of Fos expression in locus ceruleus, dorsal vagal complex, and PVN in response to intestinal lipid. *Am J Physiol* 273 (6):R2059–R2071. doi: 10.1152/ajpregu.1997.273.6.R2059.

Morton, G. J., B. S. Thatcher, R. D. Reidelberger, K. Ogimoto, T. Wolden-Hanson, D. G. Baskin, M. W. Schwartz, and J. E. Blevins. 2012. Peripheral oxytocin suppresses food intake and causes weight loss in diet-induced obese rats. *Am J Physiol Endocrinol Metab* 302 (1):E134–E144. doi: 10.1152/ajpendo.00296.2011.

Motojima, Y., M. Kawasaki, T. Matsuura, R. Saito, M. Yoshimura, H. Hashimoto, H. Ueno, T. Maruyama, H. Suzuki, H. Ohnishi et al. 2016. Effects of peripherally administered cholecystokinin-8 and secretin on feeding/drinking and oxytocin-mRFP1 fluorescence in transgenic rats. *Neurosci Res* 109:63–69. doi: 10.1016/j.neures.2016.02.005.

Mullis, K., K. Kay, and D. L. Williams. 2013. Oxytocin action in the ventral tegmental area affects sucrose intake. *Brain Res* 1513:85–91. doi: 10.1016/j.brainres.2013.03.026.

Noble, E. E., C. J. Billington, C. M. Kotz, and C. Wang. 2014. Oxytocin in the ventromedial hypothalamic nucleus reduces feeding and acutely increases energy expenditure. *Am J Physiol Regul Integr Comp Physiol* 307 (6):R737–R745. doi: 10.1152/ajpregu.00118.2014.

Olszewski, P. K., A. Klockars, A. M. Olszewska, R. Fredriksson, H. B. Schioth, and A. S. Levine. 2010. Molecular, immunohistochemical, and pharmacological evidence of oxytocin's role as inhibitor of carbohydrate but not fat intake. *Endocrinology* 151 (10):4736–4744. doi: 10.1210/en.2010-0151.

Olszewski, P. K., M. M. Wirth, T. J. Shaw, M. K. Grace, C. J. Billington, S. Q. Giraudo, and A. S. Levine. 2001. Role of alpha-MSH in the regulation of consummatory behavior: immunohistochemical evidence. *Am J Physiol Regul Integr Comp Physiol* 281 (2):R673–R680. doi: 10.1152/ajpregu.2001.281.2.R673.

Onaka, T., S. M. Luckman, I. Antonijevic, J. R. Palmer, and G. Leng. 1995. Involvement of the noradrenergic afferents from the nucleus tractus solitarii to the supraoptic nucleus in oxytocin release after peripheral cholecystokinin octapeptide in the rat. *Neuroscience* 66 (2):403–412. doi: 10.1016/0306-4522(94)00609-9.

Ong, Z. Y., A. L. Alhadeff, and H. J. Grill. 2015. Medial nucleus tractus solitarius oxytocin receptor signaling and food intake control: the role of gastrointestinal satiation signal processing. *Am J Physiol Regul Integr Comp Physiol* 308 (9):R800–R806. doi: 10.1152/ajpregu.00534.2014.

Ong, Z. Y., D. M. Bongiorno, M. A. Hernando, and H. J. Grill. 2017. Effects of Endogenous Oxytocin Receptor Signaling in Nucleus Tractus Solitarius on Satiation-Mediated Feeding and Thermogenic Control in Male Rats. *Endocrinology* 158 (9):2826–2836. doi: 10.1210/en.2017-00200.

Otero-Garcia, M., C. Agustin-Pavon, E. Lanuza, and F. Martinez-Garcia. 2016. Distribution of oxytocin and co-localization with arginine vasopressin in the brain of mice. *Brain Struct Funct* 221 (7):3445–3473. doi: 10.1007/s00429-015-1111-y.

Ott, V., G. Finlayson, H. Lehnert, B. Heitmann, M. Heinrichs, J. Born, and M. Hallschmid. 2013. Oxytocin reduces reward-driven food intake in humans. *Diabetes* 62 (10):3418–3425. doi: 10.2337/db13-0663.

Ott, I., and J. C. Scott. 1910. The action of infundibulin upon the mammary secretion. *Proc Soc Exp Biol Med* 8:48–49.

Peris, J., K. MacFadyen, J. A. Smith, A. D. de Kloet, L. Wang, and E. G. Krause. 2017. Oxytocin receptors are expressed on dopamine and glutamate neurons in the mouse ventral tegmental area that project to nucleus accumbens and other mesolimbic targets. *J Comp Neurol* 525 (5):1094–1108. doi: 10.1002/cne.24116.

Renaud, L. P., M. Tang, M. J. McCann, E. M. Stricker, and J. G. Verbalis. 1987. Cholecystokinin and gastric distension activate oxytocinergic cells in rat hypothalamus. *Am J Physiol* 253 (4 Pt 2):R661–R665. doi: 10.1152/ajpregu.1987.253.4.R661.

Rinaman, L. 1998. Oxytocinergic inputs to the nucleus of the solitary tract and dorsal motor nucleus of the vagus in neonatal rats. *J Comp Neurol* 399 (1):101–109.

Ross, H. E., C. D. Cole, Y. Smith, I. D. Neumann, R. Landgraf, A. Z. Murphy, and L. J. Young. 2009. Characterization of the oxytocin system regulating affiliative behavior in female prairie voles. *Neuroscience* 162 (4):892–903. doi: 10.1016/j.neuroscience.2009.05.055.

Russell, J. A., G. Leng, and A. J. Douglas. 2003. The magnocellular oxytocin system, the fount of maternity: adaptations in pregnancy. *Front Neuroendocrinol* 24 (1):27–61. doi: 10.1016/s0091-3022(02)00104-8.

Sawchenko, P. E., and L. W. Swanson. 1982. Immunohistochemical identification of neurons in the paraventricular nucleus of the hypothalamus that project to the medulla or to the spinal cord in the rat. *J Comp Neurol* 205 (3):260–272.

Sofroniew, M. V. 1980. Projections from vasopressin, oxytocin, and neurophysin neurons to neural targets in the rat and human. *J Histochem Cytochem* 28 (5):475–478. doi: 10.1177/28.5.7381192.

Sofroniew, M. V. 1983. Morphology of vasopressin and oxytocin neurones and their central and vascular projections. *Prog Brain Res* 60:101–114. doi: 10.1016/S0079-6123(08)64378-2.

Song, Z., and H. E. Albers. 2018. Cross-talk among oxytocin and arginine-vasopressin receptors: Relevance for basic and clinical studies of the brain and periphery. *Front Neuroendocrinol* 51:14–24. doi: 10.1016/j.yfrne.2017.10.004.

Sutton, A. K., H. Pei, K. H. Burnett, M. G. Myers, Jr., C. J. Rhodes, and D. P. Olson. 2014. Control of food intake and energy expenditure by Nos1 neurons of the paraventricular hypothalamus. *J Neurosci* 34(46):15306–15318. doi: 10.1523/JNEUROSCI.0226-14.2014.

Swaab, D. F., J. S. Purba, and M. A. Hofman. 1995. Alterations in the hypothalamic paraventricular nucleus and its oxytocin neurons (putative satiety cells) in Prader-Willi syndrome: a study of five cases. *J Clin Endocrinol Metab* 80 (2):573–579.

Swanson, L. W., and P. E. Sawchenko. 1983. Hypothalamic integration: organization of the paraventricular and supraoptic nuclei. *Annu Rev Neurosci* 6:269–324.

Takayanagi, Y., Y. Kasahara, T. Onaka, N. Takahashi, T. Kawada, and K. Nishimori. 2008. Oxytocin receptor-deficient mice developed late-onset obesity. *Neuroreport* 19 (9):951–955. doi: 10.1097/WNR.0b013e3283021ca9.

Tang, Y., Z. Chen, H. Tao, C. Li, X. Zhang, A. Tang, and Y. Liu. 2014. Oxytocin activation of neurons in ventral tegmental area and interfascicular nucleus of mouse midbrain. *Neuropharmacology* 77:277–284. doi: 10.1016/j.neuropharm.2013.10.004.

Thienel, M., A. Fritsche, M. Heinrichs, A. Peter, M. Ewers, H. Lehnert, J. Born, and M. Hallschmid. 2016. Oxytocin's inhibitory effect on food intake is stronger in obese than normal-weight men. *Int J Obes (Lond)* 40 (11):1707–1714. doi: 10.1038/ijo.2016.149.

Ueta, Y., H. Kannan, T. Higuchi, H. Negoro, and H. Yamashita. 1993. CCK-8 excites oxytocin-secreting neurons in the paraventricular nucleus in rats--possible involvement of noradrenergic pathway. *Brain Res Bull* 32 (5):453–459. doi: 10.1016/0361-9230(93)90290-r.

Verbalis, J. G., M. J. McCann, C. M. McHale, and E. M. Stricker. 1986. Oxytocin secretion in response to cholecystokinin and food: differentiation of nausea from satiety. *Science* 232 (4756):1417–1419. doi: 10.1126/science.3715453.

Wu, Z., Y. Xu, Y. Zhu, A. K. Sutton, R. Zhao, B. B. Lowell, D. P. Olson, and Q. Tong. 2012. An obligate role of oxytocin neurons in diet induced energy expenditure. *PLoS One* 7 (9):e45167. doi: 10.1371/journal.pone.0045167.

Xi, D., C. Long, M. Lai, A. Casella, L. O'Lear, B. Kublaoui, and J. D. Roizen. 2017. Ablation of Oxytocin Neurons Causes a Deficit in Cold Stress Response. *J Endocr Soc* 1 (8):1041–1055. doi: 10.1210/js.2017-00136.

Xiao, L., M. F. Priest, J. Nasenbeny, T. Lu, and Y. Kozorovitskiy. 2017. Biased Oxytocinergic Modulation of Midbrain Dopamine Systems. *Neuron* 95 (2):368–384 e5. doi: 10.1016/j.neuron.2017.06.003.

Yoshida, M., Y. Takayanagi, K. Inoue, T. Kimura, L. J. Young, T. Onaka, and K. Nishimori. 2009. Evidence that oxytocin exerts anxiolytic effects via oxytocin receptor expressed in serotonergic neurons in mice. *J Neurosci* 29 (7):2259–2271. doi: 10.1523/JNEUROSCI.5593-08.2009.

Young, W. S., 3rd, A. Iacangelo, X. Z. Luo, C. King, K. Duncan, and E. I. Ginns. 1999. Transgenic expression of green fluorescent protein in mouse oxytocin neurones. *J Neuroendocrinol* 11 (12):935–939. doi: 10.1046/j.1365-2826.1999.00410.x.

Zhang, G., H. Bai, H. Zhang, C. Dean, Q. Wu, J. Li, S. Guariglia, Q. Meng, and D. Cai. 2011. Neuropeptide exocytosis involving synaptotagmin-4 and oxytocin in hypothalamic programming of body weight and energy balance. *Neuron* 69 (3):523–535. doi: 10.1016/j.neuron.2010.12.036.

Zhang, G., and D. Cai. 2011. Circadian intervention of obesity development via resting-stage feeding manipulation or oxytocin treatment. *Am J Physiol Endocrinol Metab* 301 (5):E1004–E1012. doi: 10.1152/ajpendo.00196.2011.

Zhang, B. J., K. Kusano, P. Zerfas, A. Iacangelo, W. S. Young, 3rd, and H. Gainer. 2002. Targeting of green fluorescent protein to secretory granules in oxytocin magnocellular neurons and its secretion from neurohypophysial nerve terminals in transgenic mice. *Endocrinology* 143 (3):1036–1046. doi: 10.1210/endo.143.3.8700.

Zhang, H., C. Wu, Q. Chen, X. Chen, Z. Xu, J. Wu, and D. Cai. 2013. Treatment of obesity and diabetes using oxytocin or analogs in patients and mouse models. *PLoS One* 8 (5):e61477. doi: 10.1371/journal.pone.0061477.

10 Lessons Learned about Metabolism from Traditional and Novel Tools for Studying the Structure and Function of the Vagus Nerve

Guillaume de Lartigue, Arashdeep Singh, Alan de Araujo, Calyn B. Maske and Macarena Vergara
University of Florida, USA

CONTENTS

10.1 INTRODUCTION

Interoception refers to the process by which the nervous system senses and integrates signals originating from within the body [1]. The vagus nerve is a critical neural pathway for conveying information about the internal condition of the body to the brain. Bundled within the vagus nerve are afferent and efferent fibers that send information in opposite directions. The afferent fibers sense, encode, and communicate internal signals from most organs of the thoracic and abdominal cavities [2]. Thus, the sensory component of the vagus nerve is essential for interoception as is highlighted by its involvement in a broad range of physiological processes critical for survival [2,3]. The information acquired about the internal state helps guide decisions and behaviors by balancing internal needs with demands of the external world [4]. Disruption of vagal afferent signaling, and interoceptive awareness, has been implicated in a number of pathophysiological, emotional, and cognitive disease states [1,5–8].

Of all the organs supplied by the vagus nerve, the gastrointestinal tract is the most densely innervated [2]. In response to a meal, gustatory and post-ingestive information about the quantity and type of nutrients ingested is sensed by vagal afferent fibers in the gut and is communicated to the brain [9]. Thus, the vagus nerve serves as an interoceptive feedback mechanism to inhibit food intake [9]. Disruption of the gut–brain axis is a feature of obesity and the importance of this system in energy homeostasis is underscored by the effectiveness of bariatric surgery in treating obesity by targeting the gut and vagus nerve [10].

Our understanding of the vagus nerve has been constrained by the technical limitations associated with studying a complex nerve in which sensory and motor fibers are bundled together, with heterogeneous neuronal populations carrying a range of signals between the brain and a vast number of peripheral organs. Previous studies that combined traditional tools in ingenious ways has highlighted the need to study cellular components of the vagus nerve based on the stimuli they respond to, their innervation patterns, and their genetic composition. Over the past couple of decades, technological advances have made it possible to visualize, map, record, and manipulate select groups of CNS neurons *in vivo*. In the last five years, these tools have been utilized to study vagal neurons, resulting in a number of landmark findings [11–15] and a renewed interest in the gut–brain axis.

As the field transitions towards a molecular and genetic era, we review techniques that have laid the foundation for our current understanding of the vagal gut–brain axis and the role of the vagus nerve in metabolism. Subsequently we describe recent technologies that are revolutionizing our ability to study the structure and function of this system at the molecular and cellular level. For each technique, both old and new, we provide an overview, describe the protocol, highlight advantages and limitations, and conclude with what we have learned from studies using these approaches. The sections are organized both chronologically and based on the type of scientific questions that the techniques address with a focus on structure and function.

10.2 TRACERS

The concept that structural architecture can lead to insight about function is epitomized by the field of interoception. Much of what we now understand about the role of the vagus nerve in gut–brain signaling derives in large part from tracing studies mapping the circuitry between the brain and visceral organs. Two separate categories of tracers have been used that are characterized by their direction of travel. Retrograde tracers are transported from the periphery back to the cell body. Anterograde tracers are transported from the soma to their terminals in the periphery.

10.2.1 Retrograde Tracers

Retrograde transport is a useful tool to label cell bodies of axonal projections (Figure 10.1.A). The landmark discovery that horseradish peroxidase (HRP) could be taken up by axon terminals and transported a long distance to label a motor neuron revolutionized the field [16,17]. HRP was not extensively used due to its poor uptake at injection sites; however, this initiated the search for new retrograde tracers with more efficient uptake that could be visualized without amplification. A plethora of retrograde tracer options are now available [18,19]. The most widely used retrograde tracers to label the vagus nerve include wheat germ albumin (WGA), the non-toxic B subunit of cholera toxin B (CTB) that is conjugated to fluorescent reporters, or inorganic fluorescent tracers DiI, True Blue, and FluoroGold. WGA can travel transsynaptically which can confound interpretation. CTB is a highly sensitive retrograde tracer because it is taken up at axon terminals by a receptor-mediated mechanism, making it more sensitive than the original tracers. CTB is commercially available conjugated to a range of new-generation fluorescent probes that are water-soluble, exceptionally bright, and photostable.

10.2.1.1 Protocol

Retrograde tracers (e.g. CTB, 0.5% w/v in 0.1 M phosphate buffer, pH 6.0) can be pressure injected into the wall of peripheral organs via a pulled glass micropipette [20]. Useful suggestions for handling and preparing CTB have been previously described [21]. Intraperitoneal (IP) injection of fluorogold (20 μg/ml in saline) is useful to assess abdominal innervation patterns. It is necessary to wait five to seven days after injection before collecting the nodose ganglia to allow sufficient time for retrograde transport. For tissue

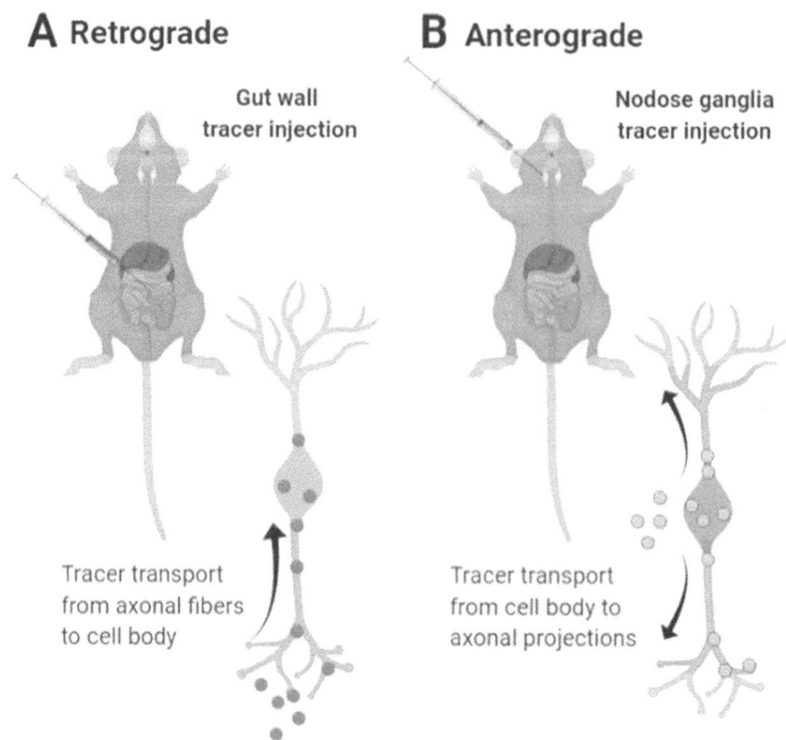

FIGURE 10.1 Retrograde and anterograde tracing of the vagus. (**A**) Retrograde tracer injection into peripheral organs will be picked up by vagal sensory fibers and trafficked back to the cell body, resulting in labeling of nodose ganglia cells that innervate the target region. (**B**) Anterograde tracer injection into the nodose ganglia will be transported from the cell body into the axonal processes, resulting in tracer labeling of fibers in peripheral organs and the brainstem.

collection, nodose ganglia can be extracted without perfusion and left in 4% w/v paraformaldehyde for up to 2 h before transfer to a cryoprotectant solution; from perfused animals, the nodose ganglia should be placed immediately into 25% w/v sucrose solution. Nodose ganglia are cryosectioned at 5–15 μm and examined for the presence of the tracer.

10.2.1.2 Advantages

By taking advantage of the wide spectrum of CTB conjugates it is possible to target multiple peripheral sites within the same animal. This can help assess the topographical organization of the ganglia – whether individual neurons innervate separate peripheral sites – and/or the plasticity of projections in response to experimental manipulations. Retrograde tracing is often combined with immunohistochemistry, *in situ* hybridization of nodose ganglia tissue, or electrophysiology of dissociated neurons allows phenotyping of neuronal subpopulations. Recently, single-cell sequencing was performed from manually selected retrograde-labeled vagal sensory neurons [12]. Fluorogold produces a very intense fluorescent labeling that fills the neurons. The endogenous fluorescence does not bleach easily and survives enzymatic breakdown in live animals for many months.

10.2.1.3 Limitations

Retrograde tracing often requires large injection volumes that can leak out of the target tissue and result in false-positive findings [22,23]. CTB is also taken up by fibers of passage, although this is not a significant concern when studying the vagal sensory neuron innervation of peripheral organs. CTB conjugated to fluorescent probes primarily label the soma; however, immunohistochemical staining of CTB with peroxidase and DAB-Ni will improve the labeling of cell bodies and their processes [24]. The intense white fluorescence of fluorogold (FG) results in a wide excitation spectrum, making it less ideal for experiments requiring a combination of multiple tracers or co-localization with antibodies.

10.2.2 Anterograde

Anterograde tracers hijack the transport mechanisms used by cells to traffic organelles and macromolecules (e.g. actin and myosin). The development of highly sensitive anterograde tracers that are reliably taken up and fill the entire cell has enabled detailed mapping of neuronal projections (Figure 10.1.B). Thus, anterograde tracing has served two critical functions in advancing our understanding of gut–brain signaling: (1) mapping the anatomical distribution of vagal sensory neurons within peripheral organs, and (2) identifying an array of specialized terminal endings with distinct morphologies and functions.

The 10kDa biotinylated dextran amine (BDA) is the most effective non-viral anterograde tracer. BDA is water-soluble and can be delivered into nodose ganglia by pressure injection. The mechanism of BDA uptake is unknown but is likely to be endocytic for intact neurons. BDA is preferentially transported in the anterograde direction [25], at a rate of 15–20 mm per week [26]. BDA remains stable for weeks post-injection and homogenously fills the entire neuron, allowing for detailed morphological analysis. Biotin can be readily visualized with fluorophore-conjugated avidin.

10.2.2.1 Protocol

BDA (10% w/v, 10-kDa BDA in 0.1 M PBS) can be pressure injected into the nodose ganglia (rat: 1 μl; mouse: 0.5 μl). Briefly, fasted animals (4–6 h mice, 12–18 h rats) treated with atropine are anesthetized and the nodose ganglia is exposed via a ventral midline neck incision. For each nodose ganglia, a glass capillary (rat: 20-μm tip, beveled 30° angle; mouse: 15-μm tip, beveled 45° angle) is inserted under the sheath [20,27].

Two to three weeks is a sufficient length of time to label central and peripheral terminals. To image the fibers, the tissue is fixed by transcardial perfusion or post-dissection. The target region of interest can be prepared as a whole mount or sectioned with a vibratome or cryostat. When using dextrans conjugated to fluorescent probes no additional staining is required. For biotinylated dextrans, the tissue should be incubated in Alexa Fluor-conjugated streptavidin or using an avidin-biotinylated peroxidase reaction for visualization.

10.2.2.2 Advantages

Broadly, anterograde tracing allows extremely precise mapping of fiber tracts, and the analysis of the compartmentation of large fascicles and association bundles. Thus, this approach is an affordable, simple, and reliable way to map fiber tracts and study terminal projection patterns and morphology of terminal endings. BDA has no specific genetic requirement and can therefore be used in any animal species. BDA can be labeled and visualized at least two months after injection, and therefore can be combined with experimental manipulation. However, it should be noted that we have observed poor labeling of fluorescently conjugated dextrans in tissue collected six weeks after initial nodose ganglia injection. Fluorescently conjugated and immunolabeled dextran retain the fluorescent intensity and detailed labeling patterns for greater than 12 months in fixed tissue with no noticeable increase in background fluorescence [28].

10.2.2.3 Limitations

There is evidence that BDA can be taken up by damaged axons and transported in both anterograde and retrograde directions [26,29–31]. We have noticed sparse labeling of vagal efferent neurons in the dorsal motor nucleus of the vagus (DMNV), presumably caused by damage to efferent fibers during the nodose ganglia injection. Although these are a fairly insignificant fraction of the total labeled fibers, this is a confound. Ensuring that nodose injections are performed parallel rather perpendicular to the vagus nerve reduces the extent of labeled neurons in the DMNV.

BDA is taken up by all cell bodies in the nodose ganglia. Therefore, its utility is restricted to mapping projections from the bulk of vagal sensory neurons. This approach does not allow the resolution of cell-type-specific mapping of innervation patterns. Viral strategies have largely resolved this issue and can also extend to mapping the downstream polysynaptic circuitry within the brain. Viral tracing is discussed in more detail in Section 10.4.2.

10.2.3 What We Have Learned from Tracing Approaches

The basic anatomy of the vagus nerve was originally described by Galen in the second century [32]. Since then, tracing experiments have been instrumental in delineating vagal afferent and efferent anatomy and providing insight into their separate functions. The cell bodies of vagal efferent fibers are located in the DMNV and send projections to peripheral organs. Conversely, vagal afferent cell bodies reside in two peripherally located nodose ganglia and send information to the brain. Afferent and efferent fibers are co-bundled within the vagus nerve and innervate most of the organs of the thoracic and abdominal cavities. Within the organs, the innervation patterns are distinct and, importantly, afferent fibers out-number efferent fibers by 8–9 to 1 [33].

Retrograde tracing experiments were initially used to determine the extent of vagal innervation of peripheral organs. This approach provided quantitative evidence that the gastrointestinal tract is heavily innervated by the vagal afferent and efferent neurons, along with the majority of organs in the abdominal and thoracic cavities

[34–38], by combining retrograde tracing with electrophysiological recordings from dissociated nodose ganglia (NG) neurons [39] and IHC to identify functional and molecular phenotypes of neurons with known innervation patterns [12,39,40]. Retrograde tracing also indicated that there is little viscerotopic organization in nodose ganglia, with heterogeneous neuronal populations innervating different organs comingling [34]. The interpretation of these data, however, has been confounded by reports that conventional retrograde tracers can leak outside the site of injection to contaminate neighboring organs [23,41]. These concerns may be more pronounced for organs like the pancreas with less defined borders but highlight the importance of including appropriate controls and bolstering retrograde studies with separate lines of evidence [14].

Anterograde tracing experiments confirmed that the vagus nerve innervates the entire length of the gastrointestinal tract [42,43], suggesting that it plays an important role in the control of feeding. In the gut, vagal efferent fibers terminate on enteric neurons, highlighting the importance of motor neurons in the control of motility of and secretion in the gastrointestinal (GI) tract. Vagal sensory neurons innervate both the muscular layer and the mucosa, including the villi of the small intestine [44,45], suggesting that these fibers are ideally positioned to sense mechanical and chemical stimuli. The exquisite resolution of vagal afferent endings in the gut achieved with anterograde tracers led to the identification of a number of morphologically distinct terminal structures. These findings reinforce the idea that these nerves could serve separate chemo- or mechanoreceptive functions [46]. Vagal sensory neurons send dense central projections that terminate solely in the nucleus tractus solitarius (NTS) and show some degree of a viscerotopic organization along the rostro-caudal axis [34].

Recent advances in genetically modified viral tracers that can be used to target defined cellular components of a neuronal circuit have significantly improved our ability to address unanswered questions about vagal circuits. The viral toolbox is discussed in detail in Section 10.4.2.

10.3 METHODS TO STUDY THE FUNCTION OF THE VAGUS NERVE

Although studies that define anatomy and structure can provide insight into function, ultimately these remain descriptive and/or correlative. To define the function of the vagus nerve it is therefore important to use different approaches that can empirically demonstrate a cause and effect relationship. Causality requires that a condition be both necessary (i.e. effect A does not occur without cause B) and sufficient (i.e. cause B will produce effect A). More specifically as it relates to studying the function of the vagus nerve, we need to demonstrate that stimulating the nerve will result in a physiological or behavioral outcome and that deletion of the vagus nerve prevents this same outcome. In this section we discuss the tools that have most extensively been used to define the function of the vagus nerve. We first discuss vagal nerve stimulation as the primary approach used to investigate sufficiency, and then discuss a number of surgical and pharmacological tools utilized to examine necessity.

10.3.1 Vagal Nerve Stimulation

Most of the available tools to study the vagus nerve rely on impairing vagal function to determine its necessity. Vagus nerve stimulation (VNS) has been the most extensively used method to empirically gauge the sufficiency of the vagus nerve and has been predominantly used in the literature to assess the therapeutic value of the vagus nerve for treating disease. VNS involves implanting electrodes on the vagus nerve and using electrical pulses that stimulate afferent and efferent firing (Figure 10.2.A). Clinically, VNS has proven effective for the treatment of epilepsy and refractory depression. VNS is well tolerated and safe [9], with only minor adverse effects

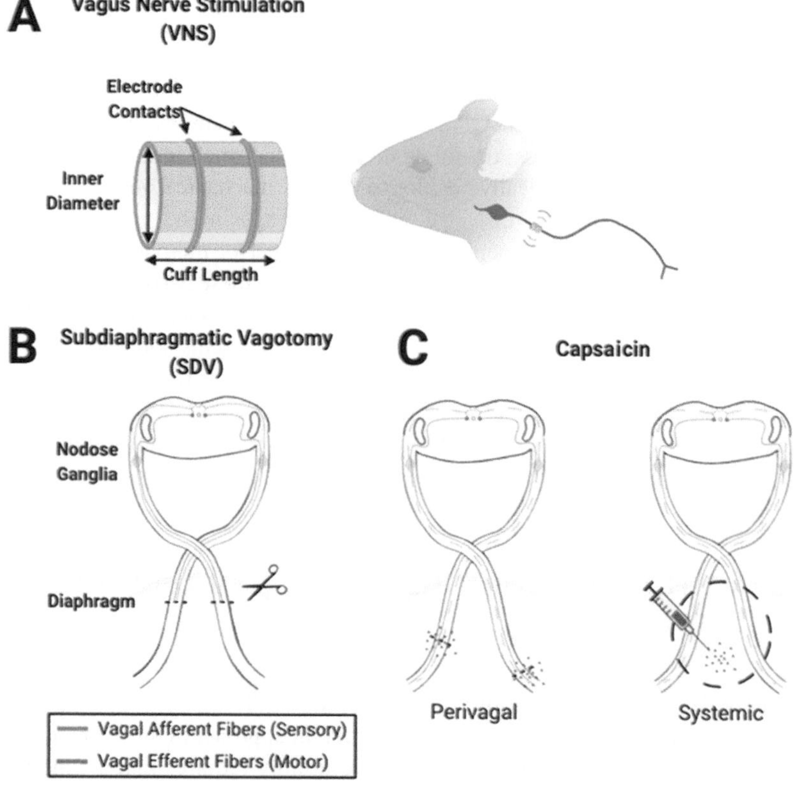

FIGURE 10.2 Techniques for examining vagus nerve function. (**A**) Vagus nerve stimulation in rodents involves implanting electrode cuff around the cervical vagus nerve and using electrical pulses to stimulate afferent and efferent firing. Illustration of a nerve cuff electrode with key design parameters and schematic of cuff placement. (**B**) Subdiaphragmatic vagotomy (SDV) involves resecting the dorsal and ventral vagal nerve trunks below the diaphragm. This method results in complete loss of vagal afferent and efferent signaling to abdominal organs. (**C**) Systemic or perivagal capsacin treatment targets TRPV1-expressing primary sensory neurons, resulting in excitotoxic cell death in ~70% of vagal afferents. This method often has off-target effects due to TRPV1 expression in sensory neurons of the dorsal root ganglia and trigeminal ganglia.

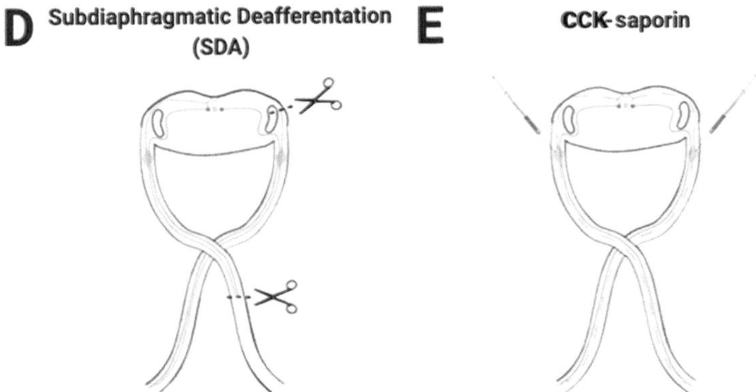

FIGURE 10.2 (Continued) (**D**) Subdiaphragmatic deafferentation (SDA) consists of transecting the subdiaphragmatic trunk of the dorsal vagus nerve, along with a unilateral intracranial vagal rhizotomy. This method completely eliminates vagal afferents while preserving ~50% of vagal efferent motor fibers. (**E**) Nodose ganglia injection of CCK-saporin causes cell death in CCK receptor-expressing vagal afferent neurons. This method results in ~80% elimination of gut-derived vagal afferent sensory signaling while preserving 100% of vagal efferent motor signaling.

reported since receiving Food and Drug Administration (FDA) approval in 1997. Recently, transcutaneous auricular VNS has been used as a non-invasive approach to study the role of the vagus nerve in human subjects.

10.3.1.1 Electrode Design

Although VNS in humans and animals is similar in principle, the considerations for designing and performing VNS studies differ greatly. In this section we focus on VNS in animal research. The first thing to consider in planning a VNS study is the electrodes (Figure 10.2.A). Electrodes in this case refers to an electrical conductor, typically made of metal, that allow the transfer of electrical energy to tissue. Thus, a key component for reliable peripheral nerve stimulation is a robust and stable physical connection between the electrode and the nerve. For acute studies, it is sufficient to suspend the dissociated intact nerve onto a hook-shaped wire electrode. For chronic studies, where repeated or continuous electrical stimulation is administered to the vagus nerve of awake and behaving animals, it is best to employ a cuff design. Cuff electrodes have contacts on the inside of a cylindrical non-conducting sheath that is wrapped around the nerve that ensures a robust physical connection while the sheath reduces current leakage to surrounding tissue [47–49].

Electrode fabrication can be done in-house, but customizable commercial options are also available (e.g. Cortec, Microprobes, World Precision Instruments, Micro-Leads Neuro). When designing electrodes for VNS there are four key factors that need to be considered: (1) conduction material; (2) contact configuration including the number of contacts, space between contacts, and distance between last contact and end of cuff; (3) inner diameter of the cuff; and (4) method of closing and securing the cuff. A detailed guide for electrode design can be found elsewhere [50–55];

TABLE 10.1
Example electrode design parameters

Electrode Component	Example Parameter
Conduction Material	0.2–0.25 mm platinum-iridium (9:1 ratio)
Contact Configuration	Bipolar hooks: 0.5 mm apart Tripolar hooks: 2.5 mm apart
Cuff Inner Diameter (ID)	Mice: 0.3 mm ID with 0.5-mm-spaced bipolar configuration Rat: 0.3–0.6 mm ID with 0.5-mm-spaced bipolar configuration
Distance Between Last Contact and End of Cuff	Mice: 1.5 mm Rat: 3x distance between electrodes
Cuff Closure and Anchoring	Suture or self-closing

however, Table 10.1 includes examples that have been used successfully in the literature. The angle of the cuff, type of cuff lead connectors, whether to encase wires in silicone, and how the cuff is closed are down to investigator preference and will not impact stimulation outcomes.

In unstimulated control animals, it is possible to implant either a functional cuff electrode or a silicon casing with no electrodes. The latter is more cost effective and partially replicates the mechanical stimulation that likely occurs, but is not as heavy as the casing with stimulation electrodes and does not reliably replicate the tethering that occurs in experimental animals. Additional commercially available equipment is required as a large one-off expense. Specifically, the externalized leads of the electrodes need to be connected to a pulse generator and current controlled stimulus isolator to apply electrical stimulation.

10.3.1.2 Protocol

Electrodes can be implanted anywhere along the length of the vagus nerve. For simplicity, they are often positioned unilaterally on the cervical vagus nerve. Left vagus nerve stimulation is typically favored; however, the rationale for this is largely based on (1) early canine studies reporting a few cases of higher bradycardia after right VNS [56,57], which was correlated with (2) asymmetrical innervation of the heart in human [58,59]. However, stimulation of the right cervical vagus nerve in humans [60], rodents [61], or monkeys [62] does not result in increased cardiac events, differences in blood pressure, or heart rate relative to left VNS [63]. There are rare examples in the literature of electrodes implanted on the subdiaphragmatic trunk(s) in rodents, while there are no reports of selective VNS of individual subdiaphragmatic branches. Irrespective of the site of electrode implantation, leads must first be exteriorized through the back of the neck and then electrodes positioned on the nerve.

For cervical electrode implantation, fasted animals (4–6 h mice, 12–18 h rats) treated with atropine are anesthetized and a small incision is made in the skin between the shoulder plates. The animals are then rotated to the supine position and an incision is made in the ventral midline of the neck. A subcutaneous tunnel is created toward the dorsum opening, and the leads of the electrode are fed through. The leads should be taped down to prevent them from pulling back out. The vagus nerve and carotid artery are exposed by retracting salivary glands and muscles. The nerve is then isolated from surrounding fascia and the carotid artery. The open cuff is positioned under the nerve, and once in place, the cuff is closed and fixed to subcutaneous tissue with a non-absorbable suture. For acute cervical VNS experiments, it is possible to cut the nerve below the electrode cuff to ascertain the role of efferent fibers. For this it is helpful to first tie the nerve caudal to the cuff with a 6–0 silk suture and then cut the nerve below the suture knot. The suture serves to prevent the cuff from detaching from the nerve.

For subdiaphragmatic implantation, the procedure is similar. A laparotomy is performed and an additional small hole is made into the abdominal muscle before subsequently tunneling the leads subcutaneously to the small incision in the dorsum as described above. The leads are attached with non-absorbable suture to abdominal muscle. With the animal in the supine position, the liver lobes are retracted and the hepatoduodenal ligament cut. The stomach is retracted to reveal the esophagus. The ventral trunk is more easily accessible as it lies on top of the esophagus; however, the dorsal trunk can be revealed by manipulating the position of the stomach and gently retracting the omentum. Upon isolating, the vagal trunk is carefully placed into the subdiaphragmatic cuff electrode. The electrode is tightly fixed to the surrounding tissue with non-absorbable tissue.

For VNS, a number of different parameters can be controlled. These including current intensity, pulse width, pulse frequency, and duration of the ON and OFF periods of stimulation. As can be seen from Table 10.2, a wide range of stimuli have been used in rodents, with no standardized parameters established.

10.3.1.3 Advantages

VNS is a useful method to assess the sufficiency of the vagus nerve for a given outcome. A major advantage of this technique is that it can be applied in awake, freely behaving animals performing complicated tasks to provide insight into the role of the vagus nerve in a myriad of complex behaviors. It has been predominantly exploited to assess whether targeting the vagus nerve can be a viable strategy for treating pathophysiology in animal models of disease [9,64]. VNS is safe and clinically approved for the treatment of epilepsy and depression [9], which makes VNS studies in animals highly translatable. There is considerable enthusiasm for the field of electroceuticals as a novel drug-free approach to treating diseases [64–68]. As a result,

TABLE 10.2
Example stimulation parameters

	Human	**Rodents**
Frequency (Hz)	20–30	0.05–34.00
Pulse width (msec)	0.13–0.50	0.1–0.5
Amplitude (mA)	1.5–2.5	0.25–5.00 (or 0.15–4.00 V)
Duty cycle	30 sec ON and 5 min OFF	Continuous, or as humans
Waveform	Asymmetric biphasic pulses	Monophasic rectangular pulses

this is a rapidly advancing field that has resulted in miniaturized, wireless devices with a view to being applied in closed-loop systems [69].

Transcutaneous auricular vagus nerve stimulation (taVNS) is a relatively new noninvasive stimulation approach. The electrodes are placed on the cochlea to provide stimulation of the auricular branch of the vagus nerve. The fact that it is low cost, non-invasive, temporary, and simple to use makes it an attractive alternative to conventional surgically implanted VNS. This tool is opening the door for the study of the vagus nerve in human subjects, allowing rapid translation of VNS research for treating central and peripheral diseases [70]. Recent studies defining the topographical organization of human vagal fascicular structures [71,72] may lead to more precise and targeted stimulation of fibers that innervate specific organs.

10.3.1.4 Limitations

A major limitation of VNS is that the mechanism by which it mediates its effects are poorly understood. Stimulating the vagus nerve has been demonstrated to activate both afferent and efferent pathways, thus this approach cannot distinguish if the outcomes are mediated by central or peripheral signals. In acute studies, this limitation can be partially offset by chemically or surgically abolishing the afferent component. Surgical ablation of efferent signaling causes confusion since it prevents both the direct effect of efferent stimulation and indirect vago-vagal signaling.

VNS is typically performed by implanting electrodes unilaterally on the left cervical vagus nerve. This approach results in two separate issues. First, as discussed above, the rationale for exclusively stimulating the left vagus nerve is not fully justified. Moreover, we have recently demonstrated in two separate studies that there is lateral asymmetry between the left and right vagus nerve. Specifically, the left and right vagus nerve respond differently to metabolic stimuli [73]; and the right, but not left, sensory neurons innervate the substantia nigra and cause dopamine release in the dorsal striatum, with reward behaviors only observed when stimulating the right sensory vagus nerve [14]. Thus, it is important to consider counterbalancing the VNS of each side or stimulate both left and right vagus nerves. Second, the vagus nerve innervates a large number of organs in the thoracic and abdominal cavity, and all the fibers innervating these organs run through the cervical vagus nerve. Thus, cervical VNS broadly stimulates all these organs to control their function, and causes mass activation of neurons in the dorsal vagal complex. For studies investigating the gut–brain axis, stimulation of the subdiaphragmatic trunk or selective subdiaphragmatic branches would be more informative. Targeting fascicles is a promising avenue in human VNS, but the rodent vagus nerve only has one fascicle.

From the technical side, there are five issues that limit the widespread use of VNS in rodent studies. First, the implants are relatively large which favors implantation on the cervical vagus nerve and makes it harder to perform bilateral stimulation in smaller animals. Second, the leads must be connected to a pulse generator, so the animals are usually tethered either before or during experiments, although newer wireless systems are now becoming available [74]. Third, the stimulation parameters are not standardized and greatly vary between experiments, making direct comparisons difficult. Fourth, VNS does not allow dynamic modulation on millisecond time scales. Finally, scarring around the cuff is typically visible within two months of implantation, resulting in a higher voltage requirement to have the same effect over time [75,76]. Of notable concern, a recent study presented compelling evidence that cuff electrodes implanted chronically for longer than two weeks may lead to impaired vagal efferent signaling in rats [77]. This was demonstrated by evidence of impaired retrograde labeling of vagal efferent neurons in the DMV and reduced motor function in rats with chronic compared to acute VNS [77]. Importantly, the classical verification approaches, including electrophysiological responses to VNS as well as visual and histological analysis of the nerves, showed no obvious signs of damage. It remains to be determined if this occurs universally, but it strongly supports using retrograde tracing for post hoc verification of the integrity of the efferent circuit with chronic cuff electrode implants.

Many of these limitations can now be addressed with new viral mediated tools. These molecular and genetic approaches to assess the sufficiency of defined neuronal populations are discussed in more detail in Section 10.4.2.2.

10.3.1.5 What We Have Learned from VNS

Findings from VNS studies are consistent with the idea that the vagus nerve is sufficient to convey negative feedback control of ingestion. VNS causes a reduction in food intake and weight loss in lean dogs, rabbits, minipigs, and rats [9]. Furthermore, VNS results in increased amplitude of gastric contractions, increased gastric emptying, and decreased acid output, suggesting that the vagus nerve also modulates GI motility, digestion, and absorption [9].

VNS in animal models of diet-induced obesity suggests that it can prevent excess weight gain, adiposity, and food intake compared to unstimulated controls [9,78,79]. There is largely consensus across a range of studies despite vastly different experimental designs, although it has been correctly pointed out by Pellot et al. that most of these preclinical VNS studies were performed by a few groups, and in many cases the experimental details are insufficiently described [79]. The mechanisms of VNS mediated weight loss and hypophagia remain poorly understood. VNS was found to alter the food preference of minipigs, and this was reinforced by the recent finding of a vagally mediated gut-reward circuit [78]. Furthermore, low grade inflammation is a hallmark of obesity, and VNS robustly reduces inflammation [80]. However, it remains unclear whether the metabolic effects of VNS are mediated by an afferent or efferent mechanism, since both have been reported. Furthermore, VNS studies examining meal pattern analysis, energy expenditure, or pair-feeding have yet to be performed.

In human studies the outcomes are more variable. Stimulation of the left cervical vagus caused weight loss in some [81–83], but not all, studies [84,85]. Important caveats to these experiments are that: they were predominantly retrospective uncontrolled studies in patients treated for epilepsy, stimulation parameters varied vastly between patients, and unilateral cervical stimulation is likely a suboptimal site of stimulation. Some of the reports indicate that body mass index may be a predictor for weight loss with VNS [81,84]. Thus, although the preclinical and human data show some promise, it remains premature to conclude that VNS can be an effective weight loss treatment. Notably none of the preclinical studies report weight loss, and large controlled clinical studies using subdiaphragmatic VNS in an obese population are still needed.

10.3.2 Tools to Inhibit Vagal Signaling

10.3.2.1 Vagotomy

Historically, vagotomy was the first approach used to assign a function to the vagus nerve. Vagotomy was famously used by Pavlov in his dog studies on the neural control of gastric secretion in 1889 to demonstrate that the vagus nerve was necessary for sham-feeding-induced gastric secretion. In these acute experiments, the cervical vagus nerve was cut on one side and after a couple of weeks recovery the other cervical trunk was cut. Subdiaphragmatic truncal vagotomy (SDV) was first reported in 1922 by Latarjet [86,87] and this approach was popularized by Dragstedt as a clinical treatment for peptic ulcers [88]. SDV was extensively used as a tool to study the gut–brain axis in animal studies starting in the 1970s and 1980s, after it was found to promote extensive weight loss in hypothalamic lesion-induced obesity [89] and abolished cholecystokinin (CCK)-induced satiation [90]. In obese human patients, vagotomy was reported to cause weight loss [91]. To date, SDV remains the most commonly used approach to study gut–brain signaling.

10.3.2.1.1 Protocol

SDV involves resection of the vagal nerve trucks below the diaphragm (Figure 10.2.B). Vagotomy is a relatively simple procedure involving a midline abdominal incision via which the liver lobes and stomach are retracted to expose the diaphragm. The dorsal and ventral vagal trunks are isolated from the esophagus and approximately 1 cm of each nerve is resected. It is recommended that a 3-0 suture is tied to the end of the nerve endings to reduce the amount of regrowth. Rats typically lose 10–30% body weight in the first 10–14 days before rebounding to levels near sham-operated controls. Providing liquid diet and wet mash for several days post-op reduces the amount of weight loss, time of recovery, and attrition.

10.3.2.1.2 Advantages

SDV is cheap, requiring only a surgical set-up, and relatively easy to learn and perform. It is particularly useful for determining whether the vagus nerve as a whole is involved in conveying visceral signals to the brain. Another advantage is that it can be performed in any mammalian model.

10.3.2.1.3 Limitations

SDV results in the complete loss of vagal afferent and efferent signaling to all abdominal organs, and therefore this method lacks specificity. It does not distinguish between (1) vagal afferent activation of central neurons, or (2) parasympathetic mediated motor control of end organs by either higher order control of DMV neurons or a vago-vagal reflex. Furthermore, the site of vagal afferent terminals responsible for mediating the effect cannot be determined. It is widely assumed that vagal afferent neurons respond to stimuli at their terminal endings; however, receptors are expressed on cell bodies in the nodose ganglia and on the plasma membrane along the axon [92]. Thus, circulating factors that activate receptors above the vagotomy may still be able to activate central circuits.

It is important to wait to perform any tests in vagotomized animals until food intake and body weight has returned to the pre-surgical baseline to reduce false positive rates caused by illness. In mice, survival has been reported at least two weeks post-surgery [93,94]. In case of high mortality rates, Heineke–Mikulicz pyloroplasty has been reported to ameliorate pyloric stenosis and increase mouse survival [95]. Notably, the vagus nerve is capable of regenerating. In rats, Powley et al. observed nerve fibers within the stomach as early as 18 weeks [96] post-op, although it remains disorganized and partial 45 weeks post-surgery [97]. Clinically, reinnervation is not sufficient to restore function even several decades after resection [98]. Thus, in rodent studies it is critical to histologically verify the completeness of the vagotomy at the end of the study. This can be achieved by intraperitoneal injection of a retrograde tracer (e.g. CTB) and quantifying labeling in the dorsal medial nucleus of the vagus as described by Powley et al. [99].

10.3.2.2 Selective Vagotomy

Selective vagotomy can be a useful approach to gain anatomical insight into the function of the vagus nerve. Five abdominal vagal branches innervate different sites along the GI tract [2]. The right cervical vagus becomes the dorsal vagus below the diaphragm due to rotation of the stomach during development and divides into (1) the posterior gastric and (2) the celiac branches. The posterior gastric branch innervates the dorsal side of the stomach and supplies the proximal duodenum. The celiac branch innervates the small and large intestines. The left cervical vagus becomes the ventral vagus below the diaphragm, then divides into (3) the anterior gastric, (4) the accessory celiac, and (5) the common hepatic branches. The anterior gastric branch supplies the ventral side of the stomach, pyloric sphincter, and proximal duodenum. The accessory celiac branch merges with the celiac branch to innervate the small and large intestines. The common hepatic branch splits into the hepatic branch and the gastroduodenal branch. The hepatic branch innervates the liver hilus, hepatic portal vein, and extrahepatic bilary duct. The gastroduodenal branch innervates the antrum, pylorus, proximal duodenum, and pancreas.

10.3.2.2.1 Protocol

In the rat, detailed anatomical description of subdiaphragmatic vagus branching was reported by Prechtl and Powley [100]. This serves as a useful reference guide to identify individual branches. Branching is generally similar in most other species, including the mouse and human [2]. The animals are prepared as for SDV.

- Hepatic: The anterior ligament and the membranous connection of the left lobe of the liver to the diaphragm are cut and the esophagus is moved to the left side of the abdomen. This reveals a neurovascular bundle that includes the hepatic branch of the vagus nerve. The common hepatic branch makes a distinct bifurcation from the anterior vagal trunk several millimeters proximal to the cardia. This branch is isolated, ligated with silk sutures, and cauterized.
- Celiac: Both the celiac and accessory celiac branches are transected by removing the posterior vagal trunk.

- Gastric: The ventral vagal trunk is located at the gastroesophageal border and divides into two, both of which should be isolated and cauterized. The dorsal gastric branch can be visualized by manipulating the position of the stomach and gently retracting the omentum to expose the dorsal gastroesophageal border and then cauterized [101].
- Sham: Sham surgery involves isolating the branches only.

10.3.2.2.2 Advantages

The advantages are similar to SDV but provide more detailed anatomical specificity. Selective vagotomy approaches have been primarily used as a way to gain insight into the role of individual organs in the control of physiological processes.

10.3.2.2.3 Limitations

As with SDV, selective vagotomy cannot distinguish between afferent and efferent signaling. While there is no question that cutting an abdominal vagal branch provides more specificity than SDV, none of the branches exclusively innervate a single organ and there is significant redundancy in organ innervation between the branches. Therefore, while impaired signaling or function in response to selective vagotomy is a significant advance, the role of an individual organ needs to be interpreted with caution. Conversely, the absence of an effect following selective vagotomy is difficult to interpret. Notably, common hepatic branch vagotomy is often mischaracterized as demonstrating a role for vagal signaling to and from the liver [102]. Anterograde tracing from the left nodose ganglia has revealed that some of the common hepatic branch fibers enter the liver hilus, but the majority innervate the antrum and pylorus of the stomach, proximal duodenum, and pancreas [103]. Furthermore, retrograde tracing studies demonstrated that significantly fewer nodose ganglia neurons were labeled in the left nodose ganglia after injection of horseradish peroxidase into the wall of the liver hilus and bile duct compared to when injected into the common hepatic branch [104]. Not only does the common hepatic branch innervate other organs, but retrograde tracing of the liver hilus also labels neurons in the right nodose ganglia [104] that travel along the dorsal celiac branch [103]. Thus, some vagal innervation remains following common hepatic branch vagotomy.

10.3.2.3 Capsaicin

Capsaicin, an active component in chili peppers, has been extensively used to inhibit sensory fiber signaling. Capsaicin's effects are mediated by the transient receptor potential cation channel subfamily V member 1 (TRPV1) [105], a nonselective cation channel with high calcium permeability. TRPV1 is highly expressed in small-diameter primary sensory neurons in dorsal root ganglia (DRG), trigeminal ganglia (TG) [106,107], and nodose ganglia [108], where it acts as an integrator of noxious thermal and chemical stimuli [109–111]. Activation of TRPV1 depolarizes the membrane and elicits repetitive firing of action potentials, triggering neuropeptide secretion from nerve endings [112–114]. Endogenously, TRPV1-expressing neurons broadly signal somatosensory information to the brain related to itch, temperature, and pain [115–120]. However, the specific role of TRPV1 on gut-innervating vagal sensory neurons remains unclear since these neurons are not thought to be involved in pain.

Capsaicin treatment as a mechanism for studying afferent neuron function was first described by Jancso et al. in 1977 [121]. Prolonged exposure to high concentrations of capsaicin hyperactivates TRPV1 channels and results in necrotic cell death [105]. Neurotoxic mechanisms are proposed to include long-lasting impairment of mitochondrial function from a large influx of calcium and/or osmotic lysis resulting from TRPV1-mediated sodium transport [122]. *In vivo*, capsaicin has been administered systemically or applied topically to the vagus nerve (Figure 10.2.C). Systemic administration of capsaicin results in nodose ganglia neuron cell death within 24 h, and this is accompanied by extensive degeneration of vagal afferent axons and terminals in the gut [123]. Neurogenesis of nodose ganglia neurons was reported a month after capsaicin treatment, and cell loss was restored to control levels by two months post-injection [124].

10.3.2.3.1 Protocol

Systemic capsaicin simply involves IP injection of capsaicin or a vehicle (8:1:1 in saline:tween-80:ethanol) in animals under anesthesia. In rats, three separate IP injections totaling 125 mg/kg capsaicin (25, 50, 50 mg/kg) are typically administered over a 24-h period (at 0, 6, and 24 h). In mice, one or two IP injections of 50 mg/kg capsaicin are administered 48 h apart; alternatively, increasing concentrations starting at 5 mg/kg and rising to 25 mg/kg are administered daily for 5–7 days. Notably some animals suffer respiratory distress and require assistance with positive pressure ventilation; pre-treatment of atropine (0.5 mg/kg) can help reduce acute actions of capsaicin on cardiovascular and respiratory systems. To assess the effectiveness of capsaicin treatment in abolishing sensory fibers, an eye-wipe-response test to mild corneal stimulation with 1% NH_4OH is used. In vehicle-treated animals, this test results in an immediate wipe of the stimulated eye, but not in capsaicin-treated animals.

Perivagal (topical) application of capsaicin allows more precise deafferentation of the vagus nerve and targeting select branches can provide some level of organ specificity. This approach involves isolating the vagal branch of interest and positioning the vagus over a sterilized parafilm to shield the surrounding area before a cotton pellet soaked in 1% CAP solution (8:1:1 saline/DMSO/ethanol) is applied to the nerve for 30 min, adding a further 1% capsaicin solution drop-wise to the cotton pellet at 5–10 min intervals. The cotton and parafilm are carefully removed and the surrounding area thoroughly lavaged and dried with a sterile swab. For the sham procedure, the vagus nerve is treated with a vehicle alone for 30 min.

10.3.2.3.2 Advantages

Capsaicin is a very useful pharmacological tool for studying the gut–brain axis because it provides insight into afferent signaling. By targeting TRPV1 neurons it mostly spares efferent neurons, enteric neurons, and central neurons, thereby improving on vagotomy. Systemic application of capsaicin is a convenient way to screen for the overall role of extrinsic afferent fibers in physiological and pathological conditions. The popularity of systemic capsaicin is undoubtedly related to the technical simplicity, with no expensive resources or extensive training required. Although perivagal capsaicin requires invasive surgery, it is also a relatively simple procedure, and the insight gained vastly improves on systemic capsaicin. When performed correctly, perivagal capsaicin reduces off-target effects and deletes afferent signaling from individual nerves (i.e. vagus nerve) and/or select nerve branches (i.e. hepatic, gastric, celiac).

10.3.2.3.3 Limitations

The results from any capsaicin experiment should be interpreted cautiously. This approach lacks specificity to the vagus nerve and more recent evidence suggests that the efferent pathway may not be completely spared [125]. Furthermore, TRPV1 nodose ganglia neurons account for a large but incomplete fraction and therefore a lack of effect does not rule out a role for sensory vagal neurons.

This is especially the case with systemic capsaicin, but also applies to perivagal capsaicin. TRPV1 is expressed in sensory neurons of the vagus nerve, dorsal root ganglia, and trigeminal ganglia. However, TRPV1 has also been identified in the vasculature and discrete brain neurons. Using a LacZ reporter in a TRPV1-cre mouse line, TRPV1-expressing neurons were identified in the intrafascicular nucleus, entorhinal cortex, periaqueductal gray, olfactory bulb, hippocampus, supramammillary nucleus, dorsomedial hypothalamus, posterior hypothalamus, and raphe nucleus [126]. TRPV1 is also expressed in microglia, and TRPV1 activation results in phagocytosis, cell migration, cytokine production, ROS generation, and cell death [127–132]. Several studies have also reported functional TRPV1 expression in arterial smooth muscle cells [126,133,134]. Thus, systemic capsaicin will ubiquitously activate all TRPV1 neurons expressed on most peripheral sensory neurons, central neurons, and arterial cells, and therefore can confound interpretation.

While perivagal capsaicin circumvents many of the possible off-target effects described above, it is important to note that high concentrations of capsaicin are used, raising the possibility that the observed effects are due at least in part to non-selective actions on ion channels or receptors, other than capsaicin-sensitive TRPV1 receptors. In fact, it has been shown that vagal efferent neurons are impaired following perivagal application of capsaicin marked by dendritic degeneration, altered neurochemical phenotype, decreased excitability, and accompanied by functional changes in GI motility [125]. These findings highlight that the selectivity of capsaicin for afferent neurons is not absolute, which is compounded with the fact that not all vagal afferents are capsaicin sensitive: capsaicin targets primarily unmyelinated c-fibers, and a small number of thinly myelinated Aδ fibers which together make-up approximately 70% of all vagal fibers. Given this information, it is worth carefully considering the utility of this approach for studying gut–brain signaling, especially in light of newly developed and validated approaches that provide far superior specificity.

10.3.2.4 Subdiaphragmatic Deafferentation

Subdiaphragmatic deafferentation (SDA) is often referred to as the gold standard for studying gut–brain signaling. This procedure involves rhizotomy of vagal afferent (or efferent for a defferentation) rootlets on one side combined with resection of the contralateral subdiaphragmatic vagal trunk (Figure 10.2.D). In this way, all of the vagal afferent signals below the diaphragm are abolished, while half of the efferent information is spared, thereby retaining at least partial extrinsic motor control of the gastrointestinal tract.

10.3.2.4.1 Procedure

Two separate approaches have been developed to reach the rootlets.

Ventral Access

This approach was first reported by Smith et al. in 1985 [135], before the procedure was more fully described by Norgren and Smith in 1994 [136]. An incision is made in the neck between the chin and shoulders. The salivary glands as well as the sternohyoid and omohyoid muscles are retracted to expose the carotid and cervical vagus nerve. The occipital bone is exposed and thinned with a dental drill until fracturing is observed without puncturing the dura. An incision is made through the dura, and the cerebrospinal fluid is absorbed, before widening the incision using blunt dissection. There are several efferent rootlets that are thinner in appearance and lie ventrally, making them easily accessible, while afferent rootlets enter the medulla dorsomedially in two to three bundles and are therefore located deeper under the efferent rootlets. A vein runs parallel to the afferent rootlets, thus it is recommended to pinch the rootlets before cutting. A flinch response occurs following resection of afferent, but not efferent, rootlets which provide some confirmation that the correct bundles are severed at the time of surgery. It is recommended that gel foam be inserted before closing the incision to limit cerebrospinal fluid drainage.

Dorsal Access

The advantage of the dorsal approach is that the afferent rootlets are more easily accessible [137]. In this approach the animal is mounted in a stereotaxic instrument with a 40-degree dorsoflex. The muscles are retracted and the rectus capitus dorsalis is scraped to expose the occipital bone. The surface of the bone is thinned using a dental drill to expose the dura mater. Blunt dissection is used to remove the dura and expose the vagal and glossopharyngeal afferent rootlets. It is recommended that the afferent rootlets are pinched distal to the cut to minimize bleeding. Gel foam should be packed to minimize cerebrospinal fluid drainage before closing the incision site.

Contralateral Subdiaphragmatic Vagotomy

After afferent rootlet resection, the contralateral vagal trunk should be cut below the diaphragm. It is important to stress that due to partial rotation of the stomach during development the left cervical vagus crosses over to form the right (or posterior) subdiaphragmatic vagus. Thus, care should be taken to resect the correct subdiaphragmatic trunk. Furthermore, this cut should occur above its bifurcation; for the left vagus nerve this should be above the posterior gastric and the celiac branches. It is recommended that proximal and distal stumps of the vagus are tied off with a 3-0 silk suture to prevent regrowth.

10.3.2.4.2 Advantages

SDA has been considered the gold standard for studying gut–brain signaling because at least some partial motor function of the GI tract is retained since efferent fibers are spared on one side. SDA results in far improved division of vagal afferent and efferent function compared to vagotomy, with fewer complications related to gastric dumping. Whereas capsaicin only abolishes TRPV1 expressing c-fibers that account for approximately 70% of vagal afferents and can have off-target effects, SDA completely abolishes 100% of all vagal afferents. Thus, SDA is a significant improvement on vagotomy and capsaicin to address the role of vagal afferent neurons in the control of physiological processes, including feeding behavior.

10.3.2.4.3 Limitations

As is evident from the description of the procedure above, SDA is a time consuming and highly technically challenging procedure. This presumably explains why this approach has not been more widely employed. Another technical limitation is that, unlike vagotomy or capsaicin, SDA cannot be performed in all model systems. It has been predominantly used in rats, with no published report to date of SDA in mice. More broadly, interpretation of the results from SDA are confounded in four different ways. First, in rats both vagal and glossopharyngeal axons are encapsulated within a common bundle in the foramen, thus 50% of glossopharyngeal afferents are cut during rhizotomy. Second, half of the subdiaphragmatic vagal efferent fibers are damaged. Retaining half of vagal efferent fibers appears to prevent gross disruption of GI function, but it is not possible to rule out subtle interference. Third, as discussed above with vagotomy, receptors expressed on vagal afferent cell bodies can theoretically signal information to the hindbrain, thereby leading to false negative results. Finally, and most importantly, SDA deafferentation lacks organ specificity. Signals from all subdiaphragmatic organs are abolished and half of the information from thoracic organs is lost. As a consequence, the site of action at which vagal afferent fibers sense signals cannot be identified. If multiple organs convey opposing information in response to the same stimulus, the lack of organ specificity could result in false negative results.

10.3.2.5 What We Have Learned from Approaches Inhibiting the Vagus Nerve

SDV and capsaicin have been extensively used to study the role of the vagus nerve in a wide range of physiological and pathological conditions [32,138–142]. A thorough review of this literature is beyond the scope of this chapter, but the consensus of these approaches is that the vagus nerve conveys negative-feedback signals that inhibit food intake. Chemical or physical lesioning identifies a role in sensing both the quantity and types of nutrients consumed. Specifically inhibiting the vagus nerve prevents activation of NTS neurons in response to a meal [143], and increases food intake following mechanical distension [144,145] or after a preload with lipids [146], carbohydrates [147], or protein [148]. From a mechanistic standpoint, it was shown that an intact vagus nerve was necessary to mediate the satiety effects of hormones, secreted in response to a meal from enteroendocrine cells along the length of the small intestine. The well characterized role of CCK on satiation are blunted when the vagus nerve is disrupted [90,149,150] by preventing activation of NTS neurons [151,152]. The requirement of an intact vagus nerve was also found to be necessary for the anorexigenic effects of serotonin [153], PYY [154], and GLP1 [155]. Importantly the vagus nerve was not required for the anorexigenic effects of GIP, suggesting that it is not universally required for satiation. Interestingly, the appetite stimulating effect of the gastric hormone ghrelin was abolished in rats with SDV or capsaicin [156,157], but not SDA [158], and vagotomy prevented ghrelin's ability to stimulate food intake in humans [159]. These data suggest that the vagus nerve can play a role in either termination or initiation of a meal.

The role of the vagus nerve in energy balance has been clouded by the fact that experiments have used diets ranging in caloric value. When these are separated, a clearer picture emerges. In response to low caloric diets, subdiaphragmatic vagotomy causes smaller, more frequent meals in both rats [160] and mice [149]. Similarly, i.p. capsaicin increases meal frequency in rats [161]. Thus, while hormonal data suggests a role for the vagus nerve in meal termination, data from freely behaving animals fed low caloric diets are more consistent with a role for the vagus nerve in control of the duration to the next meal. It should be noted that vagotomy also profoundly alters gastric secretion and motility [162]. This has led to the idea that the discordance between meal patterns in vagotomized animals in response to hormone or low-calorie diets is due to the nausea and discomfort caused by food being dumped into the small intestine which may be relieved by eating smaller more frequent meals [163]. Data from a more selective vagal deafferentation approach discussed in Section 10.4.1.1 suggests that, although the vagus nerve mediates the satiating effects of individual gut hormones, its primary summative role is in controlling the duration between meals. The mechanisms for this may be explained by recent studies using vagotomy and/or capsaicin, demonstrating that the vagus nerve is required for hippocampal-dependent episodic memory [11] and conditioned learning [164].

In animals fed palatable, high-calorie foods, both capsaicin and SDA lead to increased meal size in rats, although the hyperphagia is transient in capsaicin-treated animals [165–167], and there is a compensatory reduction in meal frequency in SDA treated rats [168]. These data suggest a potential role for promoting overeating in response to high calorie diets. In accordance with this idea, subdiaphragmatic vagotomy abolishes obesity associated with (1) bilateral destruction of the ventromedial hypothalamus [169–171], (2) a genetic mouse model of obesity in which the Mc4r gene is knocked out globally [95], and (3) a rodent model of diet induced obesity [172]. Capsaicin was found to have more modest weight loss effects in obese rats [172]. Clinically, vagotomy has been demonstrated to result in long-lasting weight loss accompanied with improved glucose homeostasis, increased satiation, and reduced hunger in obese patients [173–179]. Although vagotomy is not an optimal treatment for obesity because of the nausea and variable weight loss outcomes, it may explain some of the mechanisms of bariatric surgery [180].

Altogether, these approaches demonstrate that the vagus nerve is necessary to convey moment-to-moment feedback to the brain about the quantity and makeup of a meal and control food intake. Some of the conflicting results may be explained by the lack of standardized diets and/or the limitations of the approaches that have been used. The development of new molecular and genetic tools that allow more precise targeting of vagal afferent neuron subpopulations will provide greater insight into the role of gut–brain neural circuits in the control of food intake. These techniques are described in more detail in the next section.

10.4 NOVEL MOLECULAR AND GENETIC TOOLS

A consistent limitation of the approaches described in the previous sections is their lack of specificity. The ingenious combination of multiple approaches provided early evidence of separate neuronal subsets with distinct anatomy and functions. The development of numerous molecular and genetic tools have improved our ability to study these neuronal subsets in a cell-type-specific, spatially defined manner with increasing temporal control. Over the past decade the application of these molecular and genetic tools to study the vagus nerve have revolutionized the field. In this section we first describe various approaches that enable cell-type specificity, and then discuss molecular options that can be used to visualize, monitor, map, and manipulate defined neuronal populations.

10.4.1 Cell-Type Specificity

The nodose ganglia is composed of heterogeneous sensory neurons with different genetic expression [181,182], anatomical innervation patterns [13,15,183], sensory modalities [15,184–186], and neuronal structures [13,182,187–197]. The neurons are intermingled within the ganglia with no clear organization, making them neither readily distinguishable nor accessible for selective manipulation. A number of approaches have recently been developed that enable precise targeting of subsets of neurons based on their cell-type-specific characteristics, including receptor expression, transcriptional regulation, and innervation patterns.

10.4.1.1 CCK-saporin

Receptor-targeted pharmacological cell lesioning is a powerful approach to study cell-specific function without the requirement of a genetic mutant. Nodose ganglia injection of the neurotoxin saporin conjugated to the gastrointestinal hormone cholecystokinin (CCK) is a recently validated approach for gut-specific vagal deafferentation [20] (Figure 10.2.E). Since vagal afferent and efferent neurons are localized at different sites, injection of CCK-saporin into nodose ganglia targets afferent neurons while leaving efferent neurons intact. The ribosomal inhibitor saporin causes rapid cell death if it enters into a cell [198]. CCK-A receptor-expressing vagal sensory neurons extensively innervate the gut [199,200]. Therefore, conjugating saporin to the CCK provides both a way of targeting gut-innervating sensory neurons and a mechanism for transporting saporin into the cell, by taking advantage of the fact that G-protein coupled receptors are internalized in response to ligand binding [201]. Because there is no transport mechanism for unconjugated saporin into mammalian cells, it is inert in its native form [202], making it an ideal control. It is important to note that CCK-saporin causes cell death, and therefore causes vagal deafferentation rather than merely inhibiting CCK receptor signaling.

10.4.1.1.1 Procedure

Nodose ganglia injection (rat: 1.0–1.5 μl; mouse: <0.5 μl) is performed as described in Section 10.4.2.1 injecting either CCK-SAP (250–400 ng/μl) or SAP (250–400 ng/μl) per nodose ganglia. For optimal delivery it is recommended to inject across two sites, rostral and caudal to the laryngeal nerve branch. Providing liquid diet and wet food mash post-op has been reported to improve recovery.

A CCK satiation test allows functional verification of the loss of vagal afferent signaling. A counterbalanced within-subject design in which fasted animals receive IP injection of CCK (2.5–4.0 μg/kg) or saline at dark onset can be used to exclude animals that have >25% CCK induced reduction in food intake compared to saline. Pressure injection of a retrograde tracer (e.g. 0.5% cholera toxin B; 5 μl total volume) in the wall of the stomach and duodenum allows secondary post hoc histological validation of both vagal deafferentation and sparing of efferent neurons of the DMNV.

10.4.1.1.2 Advantages

Nodose ganglia injection of CCK-SAP is currently the most effective approach to induce selective vagal deafferentation of the gut. Retrograde tracing studies demonstrate that CCK-SAP selectively eliminates ~80% of GI-derived vagal sensory signaling below the diaphragm while preserving 100% of motor signaling. CCK-SAP injection deletes vagal sensory neurons that innervate the mucosal and muscular layers of the stomach and at least the upper part of the small intestine [20]. These data suggest that multiple different sensory modalities are abolished following CCK-saporin mediated ablation.

CCK-SAP injection in nodose ganglia shares many of the advantages of vatogotomy and capsaicin, with far fewer limitations. It is a relatively simple procedure that is quick to perform (<30 minutes). This approach has been validated in rats and mice, but can theoretically be employed in any vertebrate species. CCK-SAP causes cell death within hours, an important advantage over viral mediated deletion which takes approximately 2 weeks to take effect (discussed in Section 10.4.2). We have reported impaired CCK satiation lasting at least three months after surgery [203]. Thus this approach is no more invasive than vagotomy, subdiaphragmatic deafferentation, or perivagal capsaicin, but provides gut-specificity and superior separation between afferent and efferent signals. Unlike SDV and SDA that can continue to signal circulating factors that act at receptors above the resection, CCK-saporin injection ablates the perykaria and therefore is not sensitive to circulating factors.

10.4.1.1.3 Limitations

Nodose ganglia surgery has a learning curve and requires the use of some specialized equipment for pressure injection that may make this approach less accessible than vagotomy and systemic capsaicin. The approach does not abolish all gut-brain signaling; tracing studies suggest that signals from the lower GI tract and approximately 20% of afferent signals are retained. The fact that both chemosensory and mechanosensory vagal fibers are ablated is in most cases an advantage; however, in experiments seeking to delineate sensory modalities another approach is necessary.

10.4.1.1.4 What We Have Learned from This Approach

Since first being described a few years ago, CCK-SAP induced vagal deafferentation has been used to identify novel roles for vagal sensory gut-brain signaling in (1) reward [183], (2) hippocampal-dependent spatial working memory and contextual episodic memory [11], (3) satiety (rather than satiation) [203], and (4) protecting against diet-induced weight gain and hyperphagia [203].

10.4.1.2 Cre/Lox System

Cre-Lox recombination is a powerful and versatile tool for cell-specific genetic manipulation [204]. Cre recombinase is an enzyme produced by bacteriophages that can be inserted into a targeted mammalian cell population under the control of a cell-specific promoter. Cre catalyzes DNA recombination at LoxP target sites. Depending on the number and the orientation of the LoxP sites (Figure 10.3.A), Cre-mediated recombination is used to insert, delete, or invert select genes. A key component of this system relies on the cell specificity of Cre-recombinase expression. Two primary strategies have been employed to achieve cell specificity in vagal sensory neurons: transcriptional regulation and retrograde transport of viral constructs.

10.4.1.2.1 Promoters

A promoter is a sequence of DNA that regulates gene expression within a cell. The expression of genes at a developmentally appropriate or in tissue or cell-specific manner is regulated by a combination of gene regulatory elements, promoters, and their interaction with transcription factors. Thus, by inserting a cell-specific promoter in front of the Cre-recombinase gene it is possible to create conditional knockout or knockin mutants (Figure 10.3.B).

No single promoter has been identified to exclusively target sensory vagal neurons; however, two Cre lines have been preferentially used: a paired-like homeobox 2b (Phox2b)-Cre and a voltage gated sodium channel 1.8 (Nav1.8)-Cre. Phox2b-Cre is a transcription factor that is critically involved in the early differentiation of autonomic and viscerosensory pathways [205]. The neural precursors of many gut–brain axis neurons express Phox2b during development, including vagal afferent and efferent neurons, enteric and sympathetic ganglia neurons, along with some neurons of the dorsal vagal complex [206]. Nav1.8 is a tetrodotoxin-resistant, voltage-gated sodium channel implicated in nociception [207]. β-Galactosidase activity in these neurons is visible from embryonic day E15, and no positive staining was observed in the brain, spinal cord, or peripheral tissues [208]. Thus, the Nav1.8-Cre mouse is favored because it largely restricts Cre-expression in peripheral sensory neurons and allows separation between sensory and motor components of the vagus nerve.

10.4.1.2.1.1 Advantages The Cre/lox system is very efficient, ensuring that the majority of Cre-expressing cells will undergo recombination. Both Nav1.8 and Phox2b Cre lines have been successfully used to generate conditional knockout mice in which a single gene flanked by two loxP sites was deleted selectively from sensory neurons, or crossed to a diphtheria toxin A subunit-floxed mouse line to ablate Cre-expressing cells during development (see Table 10.3). These conditional knockout mice utilize an effective and simple breeding strategy and improved on previous studies by selectively targeting afferent neurons. Both Cre mouse lines are commercially available. The Nav1.8-Cre mice are available from Dr. Wood [208] and/or cryopreserved at the International Mouse Strain Resource. Phox2b-Cre mice are available from Jackson laboratories. A number of Phox2b-Cre mice exist. One

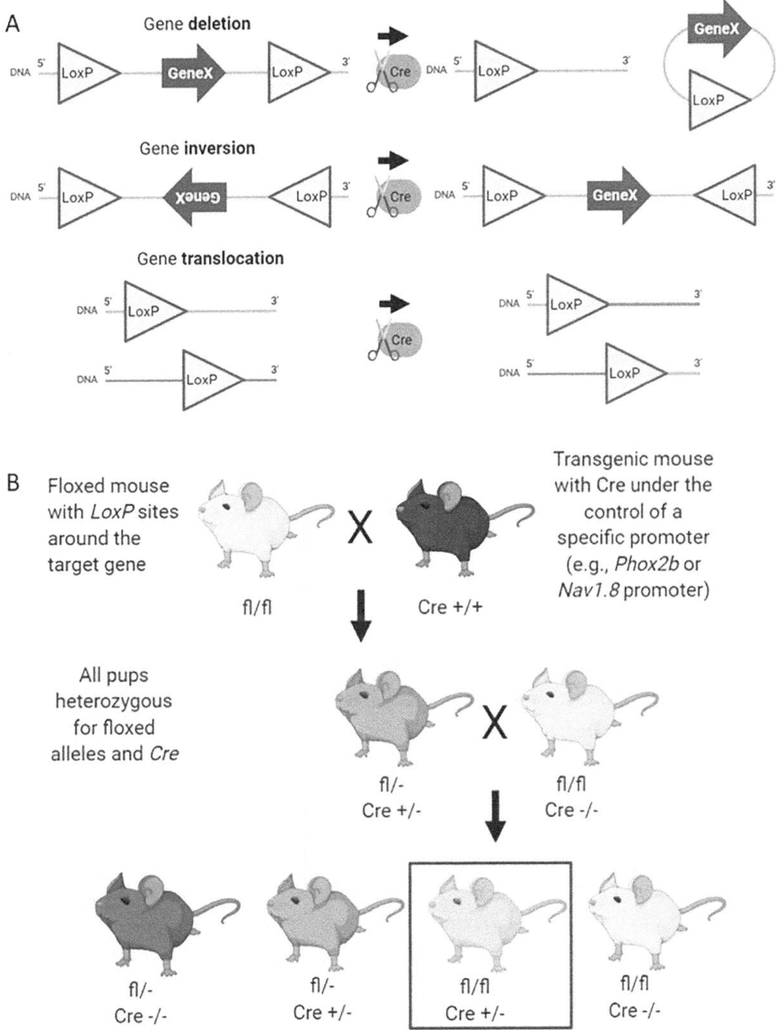

FIGURE 10.3 Cre-lox recombination. (**A**) The Cre-lox recombination uses a site-specific recombinase technology to manipulate specific regions in the DNA of cells. The Cre recombinase enzyme acts on the ***LoxP*** sites to create genetic modifications, such as gene deletion, inversion, and translocation. The type of gene editing will depend on the orientation and location of the ***LoxP*** sites. (**B**) Conditional genetic manipulation uses a combination of gene targeting approach and promoter-specific ***Cre*** expression to introduce DNA modifications to specific cell types. A homozygous mouse with ***LoxP***-flanked alleles around a specific gene is bread to a homozygous mouse for the ***Cre*** gene under the control of a specific promoter (e.g., ***Phox2b*** or ***Nav1.8*** promoter) to generate offspring heterozygous for both ***LoxP*** and ***Cre*** sequences. Mating these back to the homozygous ***LoxP***-flanked alleles will generate a combination of homozygous ***LoxP*** and heterozygous ***Cre*** alleles in approximately 25% of the progeny.

TABLE 10.3
Genetic models using Nav1.8-Cre and Phox2b-Cre transgenic mouse lines

Mouse Line	Gene	Protein	References
	Knockout		
Nav1.8-Cre	*LepR*	Leptin receptor	[210,211]
Phox2b-Cre	*Pparg*	PPARγ	[212]
Phox2b-Cre	*Cnr1*	CB1R	[213]
Phox2b-Cre	*Glp1r*	GLP-1 receptor	[214]
Phox2b-Cre	*Ppara*	PPARα	[215]
Phox2b-Cre	*Piezo1 and Piezo2*	PIEZO1 and PIEZO2	[216]
Mouse line	**Gene**	**Protein**	**References**
	Knockin		
Nav1.8-Cre	ChR2	Channelrhodopsin2	[217]
Nav1.8-Cre	Diphtheria Toxin A	DTA	[218]
Nav1.8-Cre	LacZ	β-galactosidase	[219]
Nav1.8-Cre	tdTomato	tdTomato	[220,221]
Phox2b-Cre	yfp	YFP	[222]
Phox2b-Cre	LacZ	β-galactosidase	[210]
Phox2b-Cre	tdTomato	tdTomato	[223]

Phox2b-Cre mouse line (Jackson Laboratories # 016223) was found to have no expression in sympathetic or enteric cells [209], making this the most useful Phox2b-Cre line for studying the vagus nerve.

10.4.1.2.1.2 Limitations There are limitations related to a germline Cre/lox strategy. This type of work is largely restricted to mice studies because of the large number of existing mutant mice. Cre rat lines are now becoming available, but rats with floxed transgene mutations are rare. Breeding mice is simple, but it is not quick or cheap and can represent certain challenges, including ectopic Cre expression patterns, variable recombination efficiency, and/or Cre toxicity [224]. Furthermore, when transgene expression is controlled by removal of a Cre-inducible stop codon, it is important to ensure that there is no transcriptional leakage when the stop codon fails to completely prevent transcription of the transgene. This concern can be mitigated by using a double-floxed inverse open reading frame strategy, since the inverted transgene cannot be transcribed in the absence of Cre recombination. When animals have germline mutations that result in deletion of a single gene or ablation of a cell type there is the possibility that compensatory mechanisms occur during development that may mask the phenotypic consequence of the deletion [225]. This can be overcome by using Cre-inducible mouse lines [226], but with inducible models it is important to test the expression of the transgene before and after tamoxifen-induced Cre expression. Notably, tamoxifen is a selective estrogen receptor antagonist, therefore exogenous control of the endogenous receptors will have an impact on the physiology of the animal. Injection of tamoxifen in control animals that lack inducible Cre expression are crucial controls, and allowing weeks between the final tamoxifen injection and the experiment can help to minimize the confounding effects of tamoxifen.

10.4.1.2.1.3 New Developments Ultimately, both Nav1.8 and Phox2b lack specificity to vagal sensory neurons. Thus, it is not possible to assign the phenotypical consequence of a knockdown or ablation to the sensory vagal neurons without confirming that gene expression is unaltered in other cells known to express these genes. Recently, single cell RNA sequencing of the nodose ganglia neurons retrograde labeled from the gastrointestinal tract identified individual genes that could serve as unique markers of functionally distinct vagal sensory neuron populations [12]. These genetic markers are not unique to the vagus nerve, but when combined with viral injection into the nodose ganglia can serve as a powerful tool to investigate the role of the diverse neuronal populations in the vagus nerve in controlling physiological processes of the gut–brain axis (Table 10.4).

The identification and generation of these novel mouse lines to genetically manipulate subpopulations of vagal sensory neurons is exciting, and a summary of available mouse lines along with their site of innervation is summarized in Table 10.4. However, it is important to note that additional validation is still warranted. Vagal afferent neurons innervate the majority of peripheral organs. It would be important to know the extent to which these genetic markers allow selective innervation of the gut, and what physiological consequence there might be of stimulating or inhibiting a subpopulation that innervates another organ such as the heart or lungs. It was

TABLE 10.4
New Cre mouse lines available to study gut–brain signaling

Cre Lines	Availability	Organ	Sensory Modality	Overlap with Other Genes	Thoracic Innervation (%)
Vglut2	Jax: 016963	Length of GI tract	All	All	30
Scn10a	MGI: 3053096	Length of GI tract	All	All	10
Oxtr	Jax 031303	Intestine	Mechanosensitive (IGLE)	Vip, Npy2r, P2ry1	15
Sst	Jax:018973	Antrum	Mucosal ending	Gpr65, Npy2r	20
Calca	MGI 5460801	Corpus and antrum	Mucosal ending	Npy2r	35
Vip	Jax: 010908	Intestine	Chemosensitive (mucosal)	Uts2bm, OxtR, Npy2r	20
Gpr65	Jax: 029282	Length of GI tract	Chemosensitive (mucosal)	P2ry1	20
Glp1r	JAX 029283	Primarily gastric, but also intestine	Gastric mechanosensitive (IGLE); intestine possibly chemosensitive (mucosal)	Vip, OxtR	30

Source: Summarized from [12].

demonstrated for example that the majority of these genetic markers innervate the thoracic cavity and that colocalization with Npy and P1Y2R suggests innervation of the lungs. Deconstructing the nodose ganglia into cellular subsets based on their genetic composition will unquestionably advance our understanding of sensory vagus nerve biology, but it is also important to note that in response to a meal a heterogeneous combination of neurons are likely activated. Therefore, defining and targeting functional ensembles will be a valuable next stepp.

10.4.1.2.2 Retrograde Viral Mediated Cre Expression

As discussed in more detail in the next section, viral vectors constitute an important class of tools for introducing transgenes into cells. Two viral vectors have been widely used in research animals to transport genetic material along axons to the soma of projection neurons: canine adnovirus-2 (CAV-2) and recombinant adenoassociated virus 2 retro (AAVrg). Importantly, both of these viral tools do not transport material across synapses, and therefore viral load is restricted to the projection neurons. We recently pioneered a new method for expressing transgenes selectively in vagal sensory neurons based on their site of innervation [183] (Figure 10.4). Retrograde virus expressing Cre recombinase is injected into the wall of various organs and a separate Cre-dependent viral construct injected in the nodose ganglia. CAV-2 has been extensively used to deliver Cre-recombinase to projection neurons [227–234]. However, in

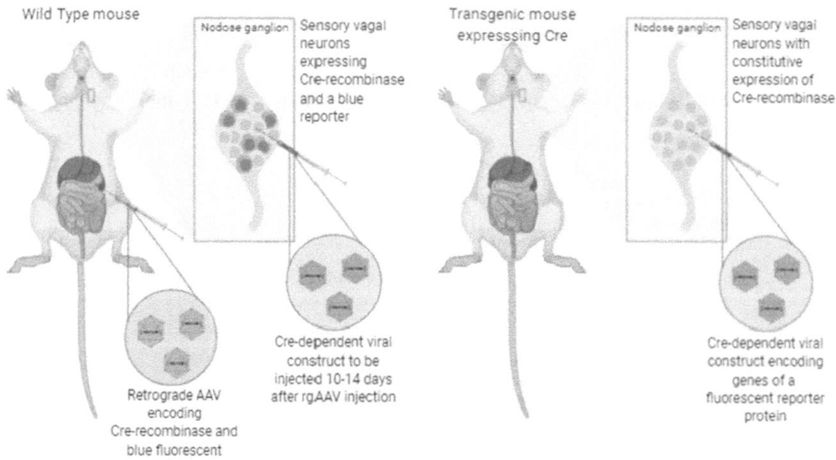

FIGURE 10.4 Genetic manipulation of sensory vagal neurons. (**A**) Using a combinatorial viral approach allows vagal sensory targeting based on their innervation patterns. First, a retrogradely transported, adeno associated virus carrying Cre recombinase is injected into the organ of choice. The virus will be bilaterally transported to the nodose ganglia. The second step consists in injecting a cre-inducible viral construct into nodose ganglia at least ten days after the organ-specific transfection. The transgenes introduced will only be expressed in the subpopulation of neurons that innervate the site of the first injection. (**B**) Transgenic mice that express Cre recombinase only require one injection of a cre-inducible viral construct into the nodose ganglia.

unpublished pilot studies we found that AAVrg had superior retrograde efficiency in nodose ganglia neurons when injected in the wall of the gut compared to CAV-2.

We have had mixed success with expressing other transgenes in AAVrg, possibly as a consequence of low copy numbers, whereas even low concentration of the Cre enzyme is sufficient to turn on the expression of Cre-dependent genes [235]. Importantly, we demonstrated that targeting nodose ganglia which innervate different organs resulted in different terminal fields in the NTS. Furthermore, stimulating nodose ganglia neurons that selectively innervate the upper gut resulted in reduction in food intake, but had no effect on respiratory or cardiovascular tone in contrast to lung or heart innervating vagal sensory neurons [13]. Thus, this dual viral mediated approach, utilizing AAVrg to deliver Cre-recombinase into vagal neurons, based on their site of innervation, is an important addition to the genetic toolkit for studying vagal circuits.

10.4.1.2.2.1 Protocol

The injection protocol is similar to that described in Section 10.2.1. A retrograde virus expressing Cre recombinase with a fluorescent reporter (AAVrg-hSyn-reporter-Cre; Addgene; 1013 PFU/ml; 3 μl) is delivered into the upper gut by micropressure pulses into the wall of the organ. Ten to fourteen days after AAVrg injection, a second virus can be injected into the nodose ganglia that expresses a Cre-inducible viral construct expressing a transgene of choice, as discussed in more detail in Section 10.4.2. It is important to verify co-localization of both viral constructs in vagal afferent neurons, and ideally confirm that the retrograde labeled neurons have restricted innervation patterns to the site of injection.

10.4.1.2.2.2 Advantages This approach allows targeted expression of a subpopulation of vagal sensory neurons based on their site of innervation, allowing for better organ specificity than other approaches. It also has the advantage of not requiring a genetically modified organism, potentially increasing general applicability to a variety of mammalian models. AAVrg studies can be done quickly, in 4–6 weeks, and at little cost.

10.4.1.2.2.3 Limitations As discussed above, AAVrg transport of other transgenes has resulted in low or no yield, thus this approach works best as a dual viral based approach. Variability in retrogradely targeted neurons is difficult to control between animals, which can be reduced by standardizing injection sites. Post hoc phenotyping and quantification of target neurons can empirically determine the extent of variability. It is also important to rule out leakage of retrograde virus from the target site in each animal. The injection sites into the gut may not be precise enough to distinguish between mechanosensitive and chemosensitive vagal afferent neurons that innervate the same organ.

10.4.1.2.2.4 What We Have Learned Using This Approach

To date there has only been one published report using this method. Using a combination of circuit mapping, stimulation, or ablation of neurons innervating the stomach and duodenum, the existence of a gut-reward circuit was identified. These neurons connect polysynaptically to dopamine producing neurons of the substantia nigra, cause dopamine release in the dorsal striatum, and cause hallmark behaviors of reward including conditioned preference and self-stimulation. Interestingly, there is lateral asymmetry of the left and right vagal sensory neurons that innervate the upper GI tract, with only the right nodose ganglia neurons innervated limbic regions or caused reward. It was also demonstrated that parasympathetic vagal motor neurons could be targeted and modulated. Stimulation of vagal motor neurons that innervate the upper gut caused significant increase in smooth muscle contraction and gut motility.

10.4.2 Viral Mediated Approaches to Study Vagal Afferent Neurons

Viruses have become an essential component of the research toolkit because of their ability to deliver genetic material in a cell-specific manner. The primary advantage of this approach over germline transmission is the tight spatial and temporal control of gene expression manipulation. Specifically, viral constructs can be injected at any point during the lifespan of the animal and can therefore be tailored to the experimental design. By injecting Cre-dependent genetic material into adult animals it bypasses ectopic expression of floxed alleles in transgenic mice that arise due to unanticipated Cre activity during development. Furthermore, injection of a virus into a discrete tissue (e.g. nodose ganglia) provides increased spatial resolution which, when combined with the viral promoter, tropism, Cre-recombinase technology offers far superior targeting of tissue and cell specificity.

The past decade has produced an explosion in the number and variety of genetic tools available, resulting in an unprecedented ability to precisely image and manipulate subsets of cells [236]. These tools are now being applied to the peripheral nervous system and have allowed significant advances in understanding how discrete populations of vagal afferent neurons respond to metabolic stimuli and the function of these neurons in controlling physiological functions in freely behaving animals. Recombinant adeno-associated viruses (rAAV) have been the preferred method for delivering genes to nodose ganglia neurons as a result of the nontoxic transduction of both replicating and non-replicating cells, coupled with long-term stable transgene expression [236]. Another advantage is the vast number of commercially available AAV with prepackaged constructs available from common vector cores, including the University of North Carolina, Stanford University, the Salk Institute for Biological Studies, and Addgene.

It is important to consider the serotype, promoter, and the genetic material to be inserted. A number of AAV serotypes exist, with different capsid protein sequences that determine the tropism (Figure 10.5). The three serotypes with the highest proneness for vagal sensory neurons are AAV5, AAV9, and AAVPhP.S. The majority of promoter options (CMV, CBA, EF1α) allow high constitutive expression in all nodose ganglia cells, while the truncated human *synapsin-1* (hSyn) promoter is effective for neuron-selective gene expression [237,238]. The genetic material should be selected according to the experimental question and can be broadly categorized to address circuit mapping, necessity, sufficiency, and activity.

10.4.2.1 Circuit Mapping

Circuit mapping aims to identify and characterize innervation patterns as well as the synaptic connections between neurons. The advantage of viral based approaches

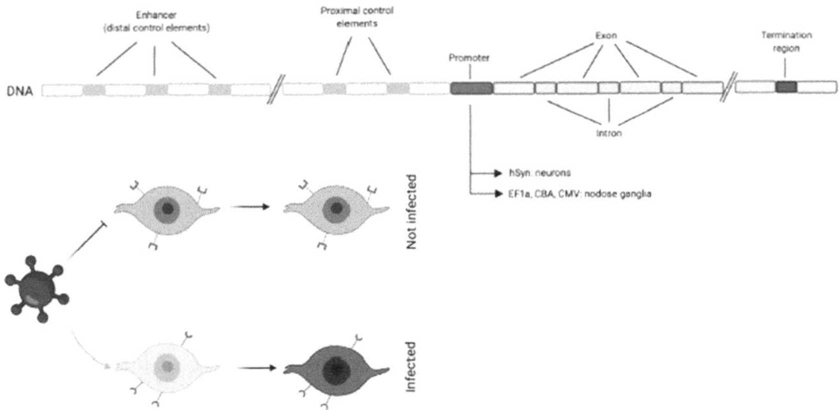

FIGURE 10.5 Viral specificity for targeting nodose ganglia. (**A**) The promoter of the viral construct will provide cell type specificity. The hSyn promoter will ensure only neurons express the viral construct. Ubiquitous promoters like EF1a, CBA, and CMV will allow expression in all cell types. (**B**) The AAV serotype will determine the tropism. The most effective serotypes for infecting nodose ganglia neurons are AAV5, AAV9, and AAVPhP.S. AAV retro is also effective at infecting nodoseganglia neurons when injected into the wall of peripheral organs.

over conventional tracing is the ability to express genetic payloads into a defined neuronal subtype. As discussed in Section 10.4.1.2.2, retrograde transport of Cre-recombinase provides a method for targeting neurons based on their innervation patterns. Viral based anterograde tracing allows detailed description of neuronal projections in a genetically defined population by driving the constitutive expressing of a fluorescent reporter to achieve high levels of fluorescent labeling.

The protocol for anterograde mapping of projection patterns involves injection of a viral vector that is not capable of transsynaptic spread, and remains there within the neuron, continuously amplifying the signal. Typically a Cre-dependent AAV vector expressing a fluorescent reporter under the control of a strong ubiquitous promoter is used (e.g. AAVPhP.S-hSyn-DIO-tdTomato, 1013 PFU/ml) and injected into the nodose ganglia as previously described in Section 10.2.1. Chang et al. were the first to use this approach, demonstrating that two genetically distinct populations of lung innervating vagal afferent neurons had different central projections patterns [13]. We also found that nodose ganglia neurons innervating different organs could also be distinguished based on the pattern of their terminal fields in the NTS [183]. Genetic markers of vagal afferent subtypes with distinct terminal morphologies and gut innervation patterns have been identified using this type of genetic guided mapping [15,181]. The absence of overlap between the projection fields of GLP1R expressing vagal sensory neurons with central GLP1 neurons provides anatomical evidence that the central and peripheral GLP1 system are independent [239]. Thus, this is a powerful approach that has led to significant advances in our understanding of the neurobiology of vagal sensory neurons. A Cre-dependent viral vector expressing Synaptophysin [240–242] or synaptobrevin [243] fused to fluorescent reporters have been utilized for cell-type-specific labeling of presynaptic boutons. This approach has been used to demonstrate the site of presynaptic terminals in the NTS [183].

10.4.2.1.1 Transsynaptic Circuit Tracing

Standard anterograde and retrograde neuronal tracers can reveal the locations of neurons and their projections, but fall short of defining neural circuits. The propensity of neurotropic viruses to spread among synaptically linked neurons in a single direction, and proliferate after spreading, allows clear labeling of transsynaptically connected cells making these vectors ideal tools for mapping neural circuits [18,244,245].

10.4.2.1.2 Polysynaptic Retrograde Tracing

Polysynaptic retrograde tracing provides insight into the source of information that is received by a neuron at the circuit level. Common neurotropic viruses that travel in the retrograde direction include the human simplex virus (HSV) [18], pseudorabies virus (PRV) [246], and rabies virus (RV) [247]. Because of its speed of spread and retrograde specificity PRV is often the polysynaptic retrograde virus of choice [18]. This approach has not been widely used to study vagal circuits, in part because sensory neurons are a primary sensor and therefore do not receive extensive polysynaptic inputs. Thus, polysynaptic retrograde tracing from nodose ganglia neurons would be limited to confirming the existence of synaptically connected cells in the periphery [248]. Nevertheless, this approach can be useful to demonstrate that specific brain nuclei receive vagal inputs. For example we recently performed bilateral injection of a PRV that expresses GFP (BarthaPRV-152) [249] into the midbrain and demonstrated that the dorsal striatum receives inputs from the right, but not left, nodose ganglia [183]. Neurotrophic viruses are cytotoxic, resulting in animal death within 4–6 days. Extra-synaptic transsynapting infection can occur when viral particles are released as a consequence of cell death [250], although this is mitigated by using the attenuated PRV strain (Bartha PRV) with highly selective retrograde transsynaptic spread [251,252]. A Cre-dependent PRV Bartha virus that expresses GFP has been developed and was used to define the feeding circuits of leptin receptor expressing or NPY expressing neurons of the arcuate nucleus [253].

10.4.2.1.3 Monosynaptic Retrograde Tracing

To understand the organization of neural circuits it is important to determine how the cells are connected. Although polysynaptic viral tracers determine all the neurons within the circuit, these viruses cross synapses at different rates which makes it difficult to interpret if two neurons are connected via a direct synaptic connection. To identify presynaptic partners a monosynaptic viral tracer that can be targeted to a genetically defined neuronal population is required. At its core, this approach utilizes a GFP expressing rabies virus (SAD19), known to exclusively spread transsynaptically in the retrograde direction. By deleting the gene responsible for transsynaptic spread, the mutated virus (SADΔG) is trapped in the infected cells [254]. The missing gene can be introduced selectively in a defined population of neurons to define monosynaptically connected neurons. SADΔG infects and labels all cells at the site of injection, thus an envelope protein (EnvA) has been added to restrict SADΔG infection to neurons that express the EnvA receptor

(TVA) [255]. This approach requires two separate viral injections. First an AAV with Cre-dependent expression of TVA, the deleted glycoprotein, and a red fluorescent reporter is injected into a defined region in a Cre animal. Second, after two weeks to allow sufficient expression, the EnvA coated SADΔG is injected within the same region.

Despite some variability in transsynaptic spread, and neurotoxicity that develops after several weeks, this approach is the gold standard for mapping monosynaptic partners. A number of recent publications have demonstrated the utility of this approach for the study of gut–brain neural circuits. A novel monosynaptic connection between enteroendocrine cells of the gut and vagal sensory neurons has been revealed [248]. Furthermore, a number of genetically defined NTS neuronal populations were demonstrated to receive vagal inputs [239,256]. Specifically, GLP1 producing neurons of the NTS were found to receive direct inputs from nodose ganglia neurons expressing oxytocin, but not GLP1, receptors [239].

10.4.2.1.4 Anterograde Polysynaptic Tracing

Anterograde polysynaptic tracing allows mapping of output circuits across multiple synapses. Unlike the wealth of viral strains that spread in the retrograde direction, the H129 strain of HSV1 is the only viral tool used to map polysynaptic anterograde circuits [257]. A number of H129 mutants have been developed that include expression of different fluorescent reporters [258]. Notably a cell-type-specific mutant was generated that places a red fluorescent reporter (tdTomato) and the replication gene (TK) under the control of Cre-recombinase to label Cre-expressing neurons along with their postsynaptic partners [259]. More recently a replication incompetent H129 mutant was developed that can be combined with a Cre-dependent helper virus expressing the missing TK gene for monosynaptic anterograde tracing [260].

H129 replicates and spreads rapidly and the reporter is visible in the starter cells after 24 hours when administered in its native form, or after 48 hours for the Cre-dependent variant. We have found that the virus crosses synapses approximately every 24 h. The cytotoxicity of the virus results in rapid deterioration of the animal's health within 4–7 days [183,259,261,262] and therefore limits the extent of transsynaptic spread and the ability to combine tracing with other physiological or behavioral experiments. Other notable limitations include variable infectivity of the virus that results in a high level of failure rates; delayed retrograde transmission has been reported, starting at 3–4 days post injection [263,264].

For nearly 30 years, H129 has been used to map motor circuits [257,265,266] and sensory circuits of the visual [267–269], oral [270], gastrointestinal [36], adipose [271,272], and respiratory [273] systems. Notably, Rinaman and Schwartz mapped the viscerosensory inputs from the ventral stomach and found labeling in the left nodose ganglia along with extensive brain-wide labeling in discrete nuclei associated with energy balance, which is consistent with the idea of the vagus nerve conveying feedback to the brain about the quantity of food consumed [36]. In addition, Cre-dependent H129 has recently identified a circuit connecting the duodenum with dopamine producing cells of the substantia nigra, and revealed an asymmetrical ascending CNS circuits of vagal sensory neurons from the left and right nodose ganglia [183].

10.4.2.1.5 Monosynaptic Anterograde Tracing

A couple of recent advances have made monosynaptic anterograde tracing possible. The most promising option is the H129 mutant that can only spread in the presence of a Cre-dependent helper virus [260], although this comes with the same toxicity caveat as other H129 variants. It has also been reported that highly concentrated AAV1 are capable of transsynaptic spread [274,275]. The lack of toxicity and the ability to transport genetic material to postsynaptic neurons makes AAV1 an attractive option. However, the efficiency of spread is low, with little to no transport across serotonergic, cholinergic, or noradrenergic projections, and the bidirectional transport of AAV1 may limit the utility. AAV1 has been demonstrated to be transported from nodose ganglia neurons into NTS neurons [256], although the efficiency of transport to label all synaptic partners requires further validation.

10.4.2.1.6 Functional Mapping

Transsynaptic labeling provides evidence for a structural synapse. A powerful new tool combining electrophysiological recordings with cell-specific optogenetic stimulation can demonstrate that the circuit is functional. Genetically defined cells and their axons expressing the light-activated ion channel, channelrhodopsin-2 (ChR2), can be activated with millisecond precision [276,277]. In a brain slice containing a mixed population of axons from various cell types, it is possible to selectively activate the axons from the defined neuronal population while simultaneously recording the evoked response from a putative postsynaptic neuron. This approach known as ChR2-assisted circuit mapping (CRACM) [278,279] is being used to map monosynaptic excitatory connectivity from genetically defined presynaptic vagal afferent neurons to putative postsynaptic NTS neurons.

10.4.2.2 Activation Strategies

Modulating the activity of precise neurons in live animals allows an understanding of the role of the neurons in behavior or disease. Here we describe three techniques that are allowed targeted control over neuronal control (Table 10.5). These tools can be divided based on the duration of their stimulatory effect.

TABLE 10.5
Viral constructs to stimulate vagal signaling of targeted cell populations

Activation Type	Constructs	Mechanism	References
Acute	Optogenetics (Channelrhodpsin)	Acute activation of neural activity with light	[280]
	Chemogenetics (hM3Dq, hM3Ds)	Acute activation of neural activity with chemokine	[281]
Chronic	NachBac	Chronic current leakage that increases excitability	[282]

10.4.2.2.1 Short-Term Transient Neural Activation

Optogenetics and chemogenetics technologies have revolutionized neuroscience. They both allow acute and reversible modulation of the neural activity of targeted populations. In both cases, Cre-dependent viral constructs (10^{13} PFU/ml) are injected into the NG as previously described in Section 10.2.1. In order to decide on the optimal activation strategy it is important to understand the advantages and limitations of these two approaches.

10.4.2.2.1.1 Optogenetics

Optogenetics is the introduction of algae-derived ion channels that allow temporal depolarization or the hyperpolarization of neurons in response to light pulses [280]. For neuronal activation, the non-selective cation channel, channelrhodopsin-2 (ChR2), is activated by blue light (470 nm) to depolarize targeted neurons with high temporal resolution [280]. ChR2 traffics to the membrane well at low levels but forms intracellular aggregates at high levels [283]. The most widely used variant is ChR2/H134R, which has increased sensitivity to light, rebounds quicker after light activation, and remains open longer than ChR2 [284]. A couple of far-red-shifted ChR2 (e.g. ChrimsonR, C1V1, ChETA) are also available, which allows combination of optogenetics with calcium imaging.

A light source needs to be targeted to shine on the perykaria or terminal endings. We have implanted optic posts at the base of the skull, targeted to the mid-NTS where vagal afferent neurons terminate (NTS: AP: –7.5 mm, ML: ±0.3 mm, DV: –5.0 mm) [183], although targeting nodose ganglia and peripheral organs with LED lights has also proven successful [285,286]. ChR2 stimulation is usually achieved using a blue light source (473 nm wavelength), which requires a stimulus generator to control the light pulses. Light pulse parameters typical range between 1 and 50 Hz frequency, and 1 and 10 mW light intensity, depending on neuronal subtypes and whether targeting the perykaria or terminal fields. We have previously found that 2–3 weeks after nodose ganglia injection of a virus, blue laser stimulation (1 Hz, 5 mW) of the central terminals of vagal afferent neurons reduces food intake [183].

The primary advantage of optogenetics is that it allows high temporal and spatial resolution of a genetically defined population of cells in an awake and behaving animal. The spatial resolution and cell specificity is a significant advance over VNS. ChR2 distributes throughout the neuron, which makes fluorescently tagged ChR2 a useful anterograde tracer, and the added spatial resolution can overcome some of the limitations inherent in Cre/Lox breeding strategies. Moderate intensity light does not interfere with neuronal function, is reversible, and allows millisecond time scale resolution which can be used to generate physiological patterns of neuronal activity [287]. However, this approach requires significant financial investment to administer and control light pulses [288]. Furthermore, fiber optic posts have to be implanted into the brain which adds an extra surgical step, requires correct placement, and will cause tissue damage. In optogenetic studies, the animals are often tethered to the light source, which restricts movement and can make some behavioral studies more challenging. Although light is not toxic to cells, light has been reported to alter the properties of NMDA receptors [289] and gene expression [290–293]. Heat caused by repeated high-intensity light stimulation can cause physical damage to the tissue. Many of these confounds can be minimized with appropriate controls, including implanting optic fibers and optogenetically stimulating negative controls.

10.4.2.2.1.2 Chemogenetics

Chemogenetics makes use of designer receptor exclusively activated by designer drugs (DREADDs), which are muscarinic G protein-coupled receptors that have been modified to have low affinity for endogenous ligands. Importantly, neither Gq- [294] nor Gs- [295] coupled receptors cause measurable electrophysiological, behavioral, or morphological consequences to cells under baseline conditions. In response to an exogenous "designer" ligand, that is physiologically inert, DREADD receptors can be transiently activated to modulate cell activity. In response to the designer drug, Gq-coupled hM3Dq receptors cause neuronal firing [281], while the Gs-coupled hM3Ds variant stimulates cyclic AMP signaling, resulting in increased excitability [296].

DREADDs can be activated by one of three "designer" drugs: clozapine-N-oxide (CNO), clozapine, and compound 21 (C21). Although these drugs are considered physiologically inert, it is important to include control animals without DREADDs to assess the potential off-target effects of these drugs. The original designer drug, CNO, can be diluted in normal saline made fresh every day, and administered IP or intracranially by microinjections at concentrations of 0.1–5.0 mg/kg. In mice, the effects of intraperitoneally injected CNO are observed in 10–15 min, a peak at 45–50 min, and a slow return to baseline over approximately 9 h [294]. Clozapine was identified as the active by-product of CNO, with superior blood–brain barrier permeability [297]. At doses of above 0.1 mg/kg, clozapine exhibits off-target antipsychotic effects on locomotor activity [298] and anxiety [299]. The pharmacokinetic properties of clozapine appear to be similar to CNO. C21 was identified in a screen for high affinity actuators of hM3Dq.

C21 is administered at 0.5–1.0 mg/kg [300]. Based on experiments in multiple different animal species, C21 has high brain penetrance but at higher doses (>1 mg/kg) may act on endogenous receptors [301]. In vagus nerve studies, we found that chemogenetic activation of hM3Dq in GLP-1R-expressing nodose ganglia neurons with CNO (IP, 2 mg/kg) reduced food intake over 12 hours in the dark phase, an effect that was maintained without compensation for 24 hours [239].

DREADDs provide a non-invasive way to manipulate the activity of genetically defined cells in a freely behaving animal. This approach requires no specialized instrumentation and can therefore be performed at low cost. DREADDs have low affinity for endogenous ligands and so have little constitutive activity. The drugs are widely accessible and can be administered through injection or in the drinking water, allowing animals to perform complex tasks or socialize unobstructedly. Repeated dosing of the ligand can cause desensitization as a result of well-characterized GPCR internalization and downregulation following ligand binding [302]. Compared with optogenetics, which allows high temporal control over neuronal modulation, chemogenetics is preferred in experiments where the activity of the neurons needs to be manipulated over a longer timeframe (hours to days). Thus, when deciding over chemogenetics or optogenetics, it is important to consider the cost, the length of time that the neuronal activity needs to be activated, and the temporal resolution required.

10.4.2.2.2 Chronic Stimulation

The bacterial sodium channel, NaChBac, is a useful molecular tool for upregulation of neuronal excitability. Neurons expressing NaChBac (AAV-Flex-eGFP-p2a-mNaChBac) increase spontaneous frequencies, action potential half-widths, and action potential voltage thresholds [303]. This approach therefore provides an alternative for long-term chronic activation of neurons at the expense of temporal resolution. This approach requires no specialized equipment. The plasmid is available from Addgene (#60658), but the viral preparation is not commercially available and needs to be packaged at cost.

10.4.2.3 Inhibition Strategies

There is a wide selection of viral tools available for inhibiting neurons (Table 10.6). To date only ablation and RNA interference have been tried and tested in nodose ganglia neurons, but there is no reason to suspect that silencing or crispr tools would not work. In selecting the most appropriate inhibition strategy, it is important to decide whether to inhibit a cell population or a specific protein within the cell. Both silencing and ablation tools are useful to determine if a subset of cells is a necessary component of a circuit, while knockdown tools can provide cellular mechanisms within the target cells.

Next it is important to determine the length of time over which the inhibition should last. Optogenetic and chemogenetic inhibition are transient and reversible, with optogenetics offering better temporal resolution and chemogenetics leading to longer inhibition caused by a more physiological mechanism involving ligand receptor binding. Although it is theoretically possible to chronically inhibit neural activity with optogenetics or chemogenetics, neither approach is optimal for

TABLE 10.6
Viral constructs to inhibit vagal signaling of targeted cell populations

Inhibition Type	Constructs	Mechanism	References
Silence	Optogenetics (e.g. Jaws, Arch, SwiChR, eNpHR)	Acute inhibition of neural activity with light	[304]
	Chemogenetics (e.g. hM4Di, KORD)	Acute inhibition of neural activity with chemokine	[281]
	non-inwardly rectifying variant of Kir2.1	Chronic current leakage that educes excitability	[305]
	Tetrodotoxin light chain (TelC)	Chronic inhibition of transmitter release	[306]
Ablate	Catalytic diptheria toxin fragment A (DTA)	Cytotoxic inhibition of protein synthesis	[307]
	Caspase	Commits cell to apoptosis	[308]
Gene targeting	RNA interference (shRNA, siRNA)	Degradation of specific mRNA to inhibit protein synthesis	[309]
	Crispr	Targeted gene deletion	[310]

long-term inhibition. Chronic light can cause local tissue damage as a result of heat that may confound the results, although new channelrhodopsin variants that remain open longer between light bursts (e.g. SwiChR) may partially address this issue. Chemogenetics work by administration of an inert chemokine to activate a modified G protein coupled receptor, therefore this approach is susceptible to desensitization over repeated administration. Thus, for chronic inhibition, two options are available that permanently cause hyperpolarization (Kir2.1) or blockade of transmitter release (TelC). The advantage of these silencing tools over other long-lasting ablation tools is that the cells remain viable and circuit structures are not disrupted. The limitation is that they only cause ~50% reduction in signaling [311–313]. For more complete chronic inhibition, cell ablation is highly effective. No direct comparisons have been performed between the AAV-FLEX-CASP3-TVeP and AAV-DIO-DTA viruses, but caspase mediated ablation consistently ablates >95% of the target population [183,308,312,313], while DTA results in incomplete ablation [314–316]. Furthermore, use of caspase allows targeted physiological cell death without inflammation, which reduces the impact on adjacent untargeted cells [317].

Gene targeting strategies can be used to impair the function of a gene, although a priori knowledge of the target gene is required. RNA interference uses a naturally occurring biological process in which a specific sequence of mRNA is degraded, resulting in targeted reduction in gene function. *In vivo*, short hairpin RNA (shRNA) is preferred over small interfering RNA (siRNA) because of its high potency and sustainable gene knockdown. There are multiple examples of successful viral mediated shRNA induced knockdown of individual genes in the sensory vagal neurons of rats [27,73,318] and mice [319]. It is critical to verify the efficiency of the knockdown (typically 50–80%) and use a control shRNA to demonstrate specificity. Clustered Regularly Interspaced Short Palindromic Repeats (CRISPR) is a gene editing tool that enables complete elimination of a precise gene using "molecular scissors." This approach has a lot of potential, although it is important to rule out the off-target deletion of genes with similar sequences. Viral-mediated gene editing of target cells *in vivo* has been achieved [320]; however, this approach has not yet been performed to edit genes in the vagus nerve.

10.4.2.4 Imaging

Developments in optical microscopy along with activity-dependent fluorescent sensor proteins have made it possible to monitor the activity of a select subset of neurons *in vivo*. Genetically encoded calcium indicators (GECI) provide an optical proxy for activity-dependent calcium transients. GECI have several advantages over traditional electrophysiological measurements [321]; they can target specific neuronal populations, allow recording from multiple neurons simultaneously, and are stably expressed for months without any apparent adverse effects, enabling repeated recordings over time [322]. The most recent GECI variants produce very high signal to noise ratio and are reported to detect calcium changes evoked by a single action potential [323].

Calcium imaging of culture vagal sensory neurons has been extensively performed [39,40,324,325]. However the *in vivo* calcium imaging approach for recording the natural activation profile of specific subsets of nodose ganglia neurons in response to intraluminal signals in live animals has only recently been developed [15]. Nodose ganglia neurons of an anesthetized animal, expressing a Cre-dependent GECI, were positioned on a coverslip under a confocal microscope by cutting central projections. It was demonstrated that subsets of intermingled vagal sensory neurons responding to distinct peripheral stimuli could be dissociated based on their genetic makeup, suggesting that the vagus nerve communicates to the brain via labeled lines [15]. A separate report using an intact nodose ganglia preparation confirmed that vagal sensory neurons are activated in response to post-ingestive sugar but not non-nutritive sweeteners [326].

Imaging the real time activity patterns of nodose ganglia neurons is unquestionably a very powerful approach that will be essential in defining the stimuli and temporal response patterns of sensory neuron subsets. The technically challenging preparation and prohibitively expensive microscopy equipment necessary for imaging will likely reduce the widespread use of this approach. Currently the use of single photon microscopy restricts imaging to the superficial neurons of the nodose ganglia. Furthermore, it should be noted that optical imaging results in very large datasets that can be complicated to analyze.

10.5 CONCLUSIONS

Our understanding of the importance of the gut–brain axis in the control of food intake, body weight, and glucose homeostasis has been profoundly influenced by studies using tracing, whole nerve recordings, and surgical or chemical lesioning of the vagus nerve. While individually these techniques do not fully delineate between sensory and motor components of the vagus nerve, nor the end-organs involved, in combination the limitations were minimized. Certainly, the use of new more precise tools has for the most part corroborated previous work. The use of traditional approaches therefore still have a role to play, especially in combination with molecular and genetic tools.

New, highly selective approaches that target neuronal subsets based on their innervation patterns, genetic composition, or functional activity are now being used to study the vagus nerve. These technological advances make it possible to trace projections, map circuits, profile cells, record real time activity, and modulate cell-type-specific vagal sensory neurons with greater precision and less invasively. As discussed above significant conceptual advancements have already resulted from the application of these tools, including the identification of a gut-reward circuit [14], the concept of labeled lines [15], the importance of mechanosensitive vagal fibers in meal termination [12], and the defensive role of the vagus nerve against diet-induced obesity [203]. In addition to the increased spatial and temporal resolution of these tools, they can be multiplexed to create nearly endless number of combinations that will enable significant advances over the next decade as they become more widely employed and improved viral constructs continue to be developed. It would be of particular interest to address basic questions about (1) the organization of the nodose ganglia, (2) the heterogeneity of projections and sensing of genetically defined neuronal subsets, (3) the range of stimuli sensed by individual neurons, (4) cellular signaling mechanisms, (5) the extent of neural plasticity, (6) the characteristics of neuronal ensembles within the vagus nerve that respond to complex meals, (7) how information is communicated to the brain, and (8) the central circuits that are recruited. These data will lay the foundation for developing more mechanistic hypotheses to understand the role of the vagus nerve in interoception, more complex motivated behaviors, and disease states.

Although the focus has been primarily on how these tools can be applied to better understand metabolic interoception along the gut–brain axis, it is important to note that these tools can be applied to address the structure and function of any neuronal subset in the vagus nerve innervating any organ. The tools for the study of the vagus nerve are primarily for use in rodents, and it will be important to determine the extent to which these model organisms translate to human physiology and pathology. New non-invasive tools to address the mechanistic underpinning of vagal signaling in humans are now available and early work suggests that there is promising convergence between species. The use of artificial intelligence and machine learning, coupled with recent technological advances, will hopefully result in the development of more clinically effective closed-loop therapeutic strategies based on a solid mechanistic framework.

REFERENCES

1. Khalsa, S.S., et al., *Interoception and mental health: A roadmap. Biol Psyc: Cogn Neurosci Neuroimag*, 2018. 3(6): pp. 501–513.
2. Berthoud, H.-R. and W.L. Neuhuber, *Functional and chemical anatomy of the afferent vagal system. Auton Neurosci*, 2000. 85(1): pp. 1–17.
3. de Lartigue, G., *Putative roles of neuropeptides in vagal afferent signaling. Physiol Behav*, 2014. 136: pp. 155–169.
4. Maniscalco, J.W. and L. Rinaman, *Vagal interoceptive modulation of motivated behavior. Physiology*, 2018. 33(2): pp. 151–167.
5. Martin, E., et al., *Interoception and disordered eating: A systematic review. Neurosci Biobehav Rev*, 2019. 107: pp. 166–191.
6. Breit, S., et al., *Vagus nerve as modulator of the brain–gut axis in psychiatric and inflammatory disorders. Frontiers in Psychiatry*, 2018. 9(44). doi: 10.3389/fpsyt.2018.00044
7. Bonaz, B., V. Sinniger, and S. Pellissier, *The vagus nerve in the neuro-immune axis: Implications in the pathology of the gastrointestinal tract. Front Immunol*, 2017. 8(1452).
8. Pavlov, V.A. and K.J. Tracey, *The vagus nerve and the inflammatory reflex--linking immunity and metabolism. Nat Rev Endocrinol*, 2012. 8(12): pp. 743–754.
9. de Lartigue, G., *Role of the vagus nerve in the development and treatment of diet-induced obesity. J Physiol*, 2016. 594(20): pp. 5791–5815.
10. Berthoud, H.R., A.C. Shin, and H. Zheng, *Obesity surgery and gut-brain communication. Physiol Behav*, 2011. 105(1): pp. 106–119.
11. Suarez, A.N., et al., *Gut vagal sensory signaling regulates hippocampus function through multi-order pathways. Nat Commun*, 2018. 9(1): pp. 2181.
12. Bai, L., et al., *Genetic Identification of Vagal Sensory Neurons That Control Feeding. Cell*, 2019. 179(5): pp. 1129–1143.
13. Chang, R.B., et al., *Vagal sensory neuron subtypes that differentially control breathing. Cell*, 2015. 161(3): pp. 622–633.
14. Han, W., et al., *A neural circuit for gut-induced reward. Cell*, 2018. 175(3): pp. 887–888.

15. Williams, E.K., et al., *Sensory neurons that detect stretch and nutrients in the digestive system. Cell*, 2016. 166(1): pp. 209–221.
16. Kristensson, K. and Y. Olsson, *Retrograde axonal transport of protein. Brain Res*, 1971. 29(2): pp. 363–365.
17. Kristensson, K., *Uptake and retrograde axonal transport of peroxidase in hypoglossal neurons. Electron microscopical localization in the neuronal perikaryon. Acta Neuropathol*, 1971. 19(1): pp. 1–9.
18. Saleeba, C., et al., A *student's guide to neural circuit tracing. Front Neurosci*, 2019. 13: pp. 897.
19. Kumar, P., *Retrograde tracing. Mat Meth*, 2020. 9: pp. 2713.
20. Diepenbroek, C., et al., *Validation and characterization of a novel method for selective vagal deafferentation of the gut. Am J Physiol Gastrointest Liver Physiol*, 2017. 313(4): pp. G342–g352.
21. Conte, W.L., H. Kamishina, and R.L. Reep, *Multiple neuroanatomical tract-tracing using fluorescent Alexa Fluor conjugates of cholera toxin subunit B in rats. Nat Protoc*, 2009. 4(8): pp. 1157–1166.
22. Fox, E.A. and T.L. Powley, *False-positive artifacts of tracer strategies distort autonomic connectivity maps. Brain Res Brain Res Rev*, 1989. 14(1): pp. 53–77.
23. Fox, E.A., *Tracer diffusion has exaggerated CNS maps of direct preganglionic innervation of pancreas. J Auton Nerv Syst*, 1986. 15(1): pp. 55–69.
24. Dederen, P.J.W.C., A.A.M. Gribnau, and M.H.J.M. Curfs, *Retrograde neuronal tracing with cholera toxin B subunit: comparison of three different visualization methods. Histochem J*, 1994. 26(11): pp. 856–862.
25. Olsson, Y., et al., *Fluorescein labelled dextrans as tracers for vascular permeability studies in the nervous system. Acta Neuropathol*, 1975. 33(1): pp. 45–50.
26. Veenman, C.L., A. Reiner, and M.G. Honig, *Biotinylated dextran amine as an anterograde tracer for single- and double-labeling studies. J Neurosci Methods*, 1992. 41(3): pp. 239–254.
27. Krieger, J.P., et al., *Knockdown of GLP-1 Receptors in Vagal Afferents Affects Normal Food Intake and Glycemia. Diabetes*, 2016. 65(1): pp. 34–43.
28. Walter, G.C., et al., *Versatile, high-resolution anterograde labeling of vagal efferent projections with dextran amines. J Neurosci Methods*, 2009. 178(1): pp. 1–9.
29. Glover, J.C., G. Petursdottir, and J.K.S. Jansen, *Fluorescent dextran-amines used as axonal tracers in the nervous system of the chicken embryo. J Neurosci Methods*, 1986. 18(3): pp. 243–254.
30. Todorova, N. and G.S. Rodziewicz, *Biotin-dextran: fast retrograde tracing of sciatic nerve motoneurons. J Neurosci Methods*, 1995. 61(1): pp. 145–150.
31. Reiner, A., et al., *Differential morphology of pyramidal tract-type and intratelencephalically projecting-type corticostriatal neurons and their intrastriatal terminals in rats. J Comp Neurol*, 2003. 457(4): pp. 420–440.
32. Woodward, E.R., *The history of vagotomy. Am J Surg*, 1987. 153(1): pp. 9–17.
33. Agostoni, E., et al., *Functional and histological studies of the vagus nerve and its branches to the heart, lungs and abdominal viscera in the cat. J Physiol*, 1957. 135(1): pp. 182–205.
34. Altschuler, S.M., et al., *Viscerotopic representation of the upper alimentary tract in the rat: Sensory ganglia and nuclei of the solitary and spinal trigeminal tracts. J Comp Neurol*, 1989. 283(2): pp. 248–268.
35. Rinaman, L., M.R. Roesch, and J.P. Card, *Retrograde transynaptic pseudorabies virus infection of central autonomic circuits in neonatal rats. Brain Res Dev Brain Res*, 1999. 114(2): pp. 207–216.

36. Rinaman, L. and G. Schwartz, *Anterograde transneuronal viral tracing of central viscerosensory pathways in rats. J Neurosci*, 2004. 24(11): pp. 2782–2786.
37. Sharkey, K.A., R.G. Williams, and G.J. Dockray, *Sensory substance P innervation of the stomach and pancreas. Demonstration of capsaicin-sensitive sensory neurons in the rat by combined immunohistochemistry and retrograde tracing. Gastroenterology*, 1984. 87(4): pp. 914–921.
38. Sterner, M.R., E.A. Fox, and T.L. Powley, *A retrograde tracer strategy using True Blue to label the preganglionic parasympathetic innervation of the abdominal viscera. J Neurosci Methods*, 1985. 14(4): pp. 273–280.
39. Daly, D.M., et al., *Impaired intestinal afferent nerve satiety signalling and vagal afferent excitability in diet induced obesity in the mouse. J Physiol*, 2011. 589(Pt 11): pp. 2857–2870.
40. Iwasaki, Y., et al., *Insulin activates vagal afferent neurons including those innervating pancreas via insulin cascade and Ca(2+) influx: its dysfunction In Irs2-Ko mice with hyperphagic obesity. PLoS One*, 2013. 8(6): pp. e67198.
41. Berthoud, H.-R., E.A. Fox, and W.L. Neuhuber, *Vagaries of adipose tissue innervation. Am J Phys Regul Integr Comp Phys*, 2006. 291(5): pp. R1240–R1242.
42. Berthoud, H.R., N.R. Carlson, and T.L. Powley, *Topography of efferent vagal innervation of the rat gastrointestinal tract. Am J Phys*, 1991. 260(1 Pt 2): pp. R200–R207.
43. Berthoud, H.R. and W.L. Neuhuber, *Functional and chemical anatomy of the afferent vagal system. Auton Neurosci*, 2000. 85(1–3): pp. 1–17.
44. Neuhuber, W.L., *Sensory vagal innervation of the rat esophagus and cardia: a light and electron microscopic anterograde tracing study. J Auton Nerv Syst*, 1987. 20(3): pp. 243–255.
45. Berthoud, H.R. and T.L. Powley, *Vagal afferent innervation of the rat fundic stomach: morphological characterization of the gastric tension receptor. J Comp Neurol*, 1992. 319(2): pp. 261–276.
46. Brookes, S.J.H., et al., *Extrinsic primary afferent signalling in the gut. Nat Rev Gastroenterol Hepatol*, 2013. 10(5): pp. 286–296.
47. Stein, R.B., et al., *Stable long-term recordings from cat peripheral nerves. Brain Res*, 1977. 128(1): pp. 21–38.
48. Barone, F.C., et al., *A bipolar electrode for peripheral nerve stimulation. Brain Res Bull*, 1979. 4(3): pp. 421–422.
49. Sauter, J.F., H.R. Berthoud, and B. Jeanrenaud, *A simple electrode for intact nerve stimulation and/or recording in semi-chronic rats. Pflugers Arch*, 1983. 397(1): pp. 68–69.
50. Loeb, G.E. and R.A. Peck, *Cuff electrodes for chronic stimulation and recording of peripheral nerve activity. J Neurosci Methods*, 1996. 64(1): pp. 95–103.
51. Merrill, D.R., M. Bikson, and J.G. Jefferys, *Electrical stimulation of excitable tissue: design of efficacious and safe protocols. J Neurosci Methods*, 2005. 141(2): pp. 171–198.
52. Foldes, E.L., et al., *Design, fabrication and evaluation of a conforming circumpolar peripheral nerve cuff electrode for acute experimental use. J Neurosci Methods*, 2011. 196(1): pp. 31–37.
53. Dweiri, Y.M., et al., *Fabrication of high contact-density, flat-interface nerve electrodes for recording and stimulation applications. J Vis Exp*, 2016(116) e54388, doi:10.3791/54388.
54. Caravaca, A.S., et al., *A novel flexible cuff-like microelectrode for dual purpose, acute and chronic electrical interfacing with the mouse cervical vagus nerve. J Neural Eng*, 2017. 14(6): pp. 066005.
55. Navarro, X., et al. *Neurobiological evaluation of thin-film longitudinal intrafascicular electrodes as a peripheral nerve interface. in 2007 IEEE 10th International Conference on Rehabilitation Robotics*. 2007.
56. Ardell, J.L. and W.C. Randall, *Selective vagal innervation of sinoatrial and atrioventricular nodes in canine heart. Am J Phys*, 1986. 251(4 Pt 2): pp. H764–H773.

57. Randall, W.C., et al., *Selective vagal innervation of the heart. Ann Clin Lab Sci*, 1986. 16(3): pp. 198–208.
58. Vagus nerve stimulation study group *A randomized controlled trial of chronic vagus nerve stimulation for treatment of medically intractable seizures. The vagus nerve stimulation study group. Neurology*, 1995. 45(2): pp. 224–230.
59. Rutecki, P., *Anatomical, physiological, and theoretical basis for the antiepileptic effect of vagus nerve stimulation. Epilepsia*, 1990. 31 Suppl 2: pp. S1–S6.
60. McGregor, A., et al., *Right-sided vagus nerve stimulation as a treatment for refractory epilepsy in humans. Epilepsia*, 2005. 46(1): pp. 91–96.
61. Krahl, S.E., S.S. Senanayake, and A. Handforth, *Right-sided vagus nerve stimulation reduces generalized seizure severity in rats as effectively as left-sided. Epilepsy Res*, 2003. 56(1): pp. 1–4.
62. Lockard, J.S., W.C. Congdon, and L.L. DuCharme, *Feasibility and safety of vagal stimulation in monkey model. Epilepsia*, 1990. 31 Suppl 2: pp. S20–S26.
63. Hotta, H., et al., *Vagus nerve stimulation-induced bradyarrhythmias in rats. Auton Neurosci*, 2009. 151(2): pp. 98–105.
64. Broncel, A., et al., *Vagal nerve stimulation as a promising tool in the improvement of cognitive disorders. Brain Res Bull*, 2020. 155: pp. 37–47.
65. Capilupi, M.J., S.M. Kerath, and L.B. Becker, *Vagus nerve stimulation and the cardiovascular system. Cold Spring Harb Perspect Med*, 2020. 10(2).
66. Ntiloudi, D., et al., *Pulmonary arterial hypertension: the case for a bioelectronic treatment. Bioelectron Med*, 2019. 5: pp. 20.
67. Ma, J., et al., *Vagus nerve stimulation as a promising adjunctive treatment for ischemic stroke. Neurochem Int*, 2019. 131: pp. 104539.
68. Bonaz, B., *Is-there a place for vagus nerve stimulation in inflammatory bowel diseases? Bioelectron Med*, 2018. 4: pp. 4.
69. Reddy, S., L. He, and S. Ramakrishana, *Miniaturized-electroneurostimulators and self-powered/rechargeable implanted devices for electrical-stimulation therapy. Biomed Sig Proc Con*, 2018. 41: pp. 255–263.
70. Neuser, M.P., et al., *Vagus nerve stimulation boosts the drive to work for rewards. Nat Commun*, 2020. 11(1): pp. 3555.
71. Ravagli, E., et al., *Optimization of the electrode drive pattern for imaging fascicular compound action potentials in peripheral nerve with fast neural electrical impedance tomography. Physiol Meas*, 2019. 40(11): pp. 115007.
72. Thompson, N., S. Mastitskaya, and D. Holder, *Avoiding off-target effects in electrical stimulation of the cervical vagus nerve: Neuroanatomical tracing techniques to study fascicular anatomy of the vagus nerve. J Neurosci Methods*, 2019. 325: pp. 108325.
73. Lee, S.J., et al., *Blunted vagal cocaine- and amphetamine-regulated transcript promotes hyperphagia and weight gain. Cell Rep*, 2020. 30(6): pp. 2028–2039.
74. Yao, G., et al., *Effective weight control via an implanted self-powered vagus nerve stimulation device. Nat Commun*, 2018. 9(1): pp. 5349.
75. Helmers, S.L., et al., *Application of a computational model of vagus nerve stimulation. Acta Neurol Scand*, 2012. 126(5): pp. 336–343.
76. Agnew, W.F. and D.B. McCreery, *Considerations for safety with chronically implanted nerve electrodes. Epilepsia*, 1990. 31 Suppl 2: pp. S27–S32.
77. Somann, J.P., et al., *Chronic cuffing of cervical vagus nerve inhibits efferent fiber integrity in rat model. J Neural Eng*, 2018. 15(3): pp. 036018.
78. Val-Laillet, D., et al., *Chronic vagus nerve stimulation decreased weight gain, food consumption and sweet craving in adult obese minipigs. Appetite*, 2010. 55(2): pp. 245–252.

79. Pelot, N.A. and W.M. Grill, *Effects of vagal neuromodulation on feeding behavior. Brain Res*, 2018. 1693(Pt B): pp. 180–187.
80. Chang, E.H., S.S. Chavan, and V.A. Pavlov, *Cholinergic control of inflammation, metabolic dysfunction, and cognitive impairment in obesity-associated disorders: mechanisms and novel therapeutic opportunities. Front Neurosci*, 2019. 13(263) doi: 10.3389/fnins.2019.00263.
81. Pardo, J.V., et al., *Weight loss during chronic, cervical vagus nerve stimulation in depressed patients with obesity: an observation. Int J Obes*, 2007. 31(11): pp. 1756–1759.
82. Abubakr, A. and I. Wambacq, *Long-term outcome of vagus nerve stimulation therapy in patients with refractory epilepsy. J Clin Neurosci*, 2008. 15(2): pp. 127–129.
83. Burneo, J.G., et al., *Weight loss associated with vagus nerve stimulation. Neurology*, 2002. 59(3): pp. 463.
84. Kansagra, S., et al., *The effect of vagus nerve stimulation therapy on body mass index in children. Epilepsy Behav*, 2010. 19(1): pp. 50–51.
85. Koren, M.S. and M.D. Holmes, *Vagus nerve stimulation does not lead to significant changes in body weight in patients with epilepsy. Epilepsy Behav*, 2006. 8(1): pp. 246–249.
86. Latarjet, A., *Resection des nerfs de l'estomac Technique operatoire. Resultats cliniques Bull Acad Med (Paris)* 1922. 67: pp. 661–691.
87. Latarjet A, W.P., *Quelques resultats de l'innervation gastrique. Presse Med* 1923. 2: pp. 993–995.
88. Dragstedt, L.R. and F.M. Owens, *Supra-diaphragmatic section of the vagus nerves in treatment of duodenal ulcer. Proc Soc Exp Biol Med*, 1943. 53(2): pp. 152–154.
89. Powley, T.L., and Opsahl, C.A. , *Ventromedial hypothalamic obesity abolished by subdiaphragmatic vagotomy. Am J Physiol*, 1974. 226(1): pp. 25–33.
90. Smith, G.P., et al., *Abdominal vagotomy blocks the satiety effect of cholecystokinin in the rat. Science*, 1981. 213(4511): pp. 1036.
91. Kral, J., *Vagotomy for treatment of severe obesity. Lancet*, 1978. 311(8059): pp. 307–308.
92. Moran, T.H., et al., *Transport of cholecystokinin (CCK) binding sites in subdiaphragmatic vagal branches. Brain Res*, 1987. 415(1): pp. 149–152.
93. Iwasaki, Y., et al., *Peripheral oxytocin activates vagal afferent neurons to suppress feeding in normal and leptin-resistant mice: a route for ameliorating hyperphagia and obesity. Am J Phys Regul Integr Comp Phys*, 2015. 308(5): pp. R360–R369.
94. Yoshii, Y., et al., *Complexity of stomach-brain interaction induced by molecular hydrogen in parkinson's disease model mice. Neurochem Res*, 2017. 42(9): pp. 2658–2665.
95. Dezfuli, G., et al., *Subdiaphragmatic vagotomy with pyloroplasty ameliorates the obesity caused by genetic deletion of the melanocortin 4 receptor in the mouse. Front Neurosci*, 2018. 12(104) doi: 10.3389/fnins.2018.00104.
96. Phillips, R.J., E.A. Baronowsky, and T.L. Powley, *Regenerating vagal afferents reinnervate gastrointestinal tract smooth muscle of the rat. J Comp Neurol*, 2000. 421(3): pp. 325–346.
97. Phillips, R.J., *Long-term regeneration of abdominal vagus: efferents fail while afferents succeed. J Comp Neurol*, 2003. 455(2): pp. 222-237.
98. Gruenberg, J.C., Conrad R., *Early vagotomies at henry ford hospital: an historical vignette and a follow-up. Henry Ford Hosp Med J*, 1977. 25(1): pp. 37–44.
99. Powley, T.L., E.A. Fox, and H.R. Berthoud, *Retrograde tracer technique for assessment of selective and total subdiaphragmatic vagotomies. Am J Phys*, 1987. 253(2 Pt 2): pp. R361–R370.
100. Prechtl, J.C. and T.L. Powley, *Organization and distribution of the rat subdiaphragmatic vagus and associated paraganglia. J Comp Neurol*, 1985. 235(2): pp. 182–195.

101. Horn, C.C. and J.C. Mitchell, *Does selective vagotomy affect conditioned flavor-nutrient preferences in rats? Physiol Behav*, 1996. 59(1): pp. 33–38.
102. Berthoud, H.R. and W.L. Neuhuber, *Vagal mechanisms as neuromodulatory targets for the treatment of metabolic disease. Ann N Y Acad Sci*, 2019. 1454(1): pp. 42–55.
103. Berthoud, H.R., M. Kressel, and W.L. Neuhuber, *An anterograde tracing study of the vagal innervation of rat liver, portal vein and biliary system. Anat Embryol (Berl)*, 1992. 186(5): pp. 431–442.
104. Magni, F. and C. Carobi, *The afferent and preganglionic parasympathetic innervation of the rat liver, demonstrated by the retrograde transport of horseradish peroxidase. J Auton Nerv Syst*, 1983. 8(3): pp. 237–260.
105. Holzer, P., II. *The elusive action of capsaicin on the vagus nerve. Am J Physiol-Gastr Liv Physiol*, 1998. 275(1): pp. G8–G13.
106. Caterina, M.J., et al., *The capsaicin receptor: a heat-activated ion channel in the pain pathway. Nature*, 1997. 389(6653): pp. 816–824.
107. Tominaga, M., *[Activation and regulation of nociceptive transient receptor potential (TRP) channels, TRPV1 and TRPA1]. Yakugaku Zasshi*, 2010. 130(3): pp. 289–294.
108. Tominaga, M., et al., *The cloned capsaicin receptor integrates multiple pain-producing stimuli. Neuron*, 1998. 21(3): pp. 531–543.
109. Szallasi, A. and P.M. Blumberg, *Vanilloid (Capsaicin) receptors and mechanisms. Pharmacol Rev*, 1999. 51(2): pp. 159–212.
110. van der Stelt, M. and V. Di Marzo, *Endovanilloids Eur J Biochem*, 2004. 271(10): pp. 1827–1834.
111. Zygmunt, P.M., et al., *Monoacylglycerols activate TRPV1 – A Link between Phospholipase C and TRPV1. PLoS ONE*, 2013. 8(12): pp. e81618.
112. Amann, R., *Desensitization of capsaicin-evoked neuropeptide release — Influence of Ca2+ and temperature. Naunyn Schmiedeberg's Arch Pharmacol*, 1990. 342(6): pp. 671–676.
113. Gamse, R., A. Molnar, and F. Lembeck, *Substance P release from spinal cord slices by capsaicin. Life Sci*, 1979. 25(7): pp. 629–636.
114. Maggi, C.A., et al., *Release of VIP- but not CGRP-like immunoreactivity by capsaicin from the human isolated small intestine. Neurosci Lett*, 1989. 98(3): pp. 317–320.
115. Asai, H., et al., *Heat and mechanical hyperalgesia in mice model of cancer pain. Pain*, 2005. 117(1–2): pp. 19–29.
116. Amaya, F., et al., *Local inflammation increases vanilloid receptor 1 expression within distinct subgroups of DRG neurons. Brain Res*, 2003. 963(1-2): pp. 190–196.
117. Shinoda, M., et al., *Involvement of TRPV1 in nociceptive behavior in a rat model of cancer pain. J Pain*, 2008. 9(8): pp. 687–699.
118. Hudson, L.J., et al., *VR1 protein expression increases in undamaged DRG neurons after partial nerve injury. Eur J Neurosci*, 2001. 13(11): pp. 2105–2114.
119. Rashid, M.H., et al., *Novel expression of vanilloid receptor 1 on capsaicin-insensitive fibers accounts for the analgesic effect of capsaicin cream in neuropathic pain. J Pharmacol Exp Ther*, 2003. 304(3): pp. 940–948.
120. Fukuoka, T., et al., *VR1, but not P2X(3), increases in the spared L4 DRG in rats with L5 spinal nerve ligation. Pain*, 2002. 99(1–2): pp. 111–120.
121. Jancsó, G., E. Kiraly, and A. Jancsó-Gábor, *Pharmacologically induced selective degeneration of chemosensitive primary sensory neurones. Nature*, 1977. 270(5639): pp. 741–743.
122. Holzer, P., *Capsaicin: cellular targets, mechanisms of action, and selectivity for thin sensory neurons. Pharmacol Rev*, 1991. 43(2): pp. 143–201.

123. Ritter, S. and T.T. Dinh, *Capsaicin-induced neuronal degeneration: silver impregnation of cell bodies, axons, and terminals in the central nervous system of the adult rat. J Comp Neurol*, 1988. 271(1): pp. 79–90.
124. Czaja, K., G.A. Burns, and R.C. Ritter, *Capsaicin-induced neuronal death and proliferation of the primary sensory neurons located in the nodose ganglia of adult rats. Neuroscience*, 2008. 154(2): pp. 621–630.
125. Browning, K.N., et al., *A critical re-evaluation of the specificity of action of perivagal capsaicin. J Physiol*, 2013. 591(6): pp. 1563–1580.
126. Cavanaugh, D.J., et al., *Trpv1 reporter mice reveal highly restricted brain distribution and functional expression in arteriolar smooth muscle cells. J Neurosci*, 2011. 31(13): pp. 5067–5077.
127. Kim, S.R., et al., *Transient receptor potential vanilloid subtype 1 mediates microglial cell death in vivo and in vitro via Ca²⁺-mediated mitochondrial damage and cytochrome <em>c</em> release. J Immunol*, 2006. 177(7): pp. 4322.
128. Sappington, R.M. and D.J. Calkins, *Contribution of TRPV1 to microglia-derived IL-6 and NFκB translocation with elevated hydrostatic pressure. Invest Ophthalmol Vis Sci*, 2008. 49(7): pp. 3004–3017.
129. Schilling, T. and C. Eder, *Importance of the non-selective cation channel TRPV1 for microglial reactive oxygen species generation. J Neuroimmunol*, 2009. 216(1): pp. 118–121.
130. Hassan, S., et al., *Cannabidiol enhances microglial phagocytosis via transient receptor potential (TRP) channel activation. Br J Pharmacol*, 2014. 171(9): pp. 2426–2439.
131. Miyake, T., et al., *Activation of mitochondrial transient receptor potential vanilloid 1 channel contributes to microglial migration. Glia*, 2015. 63(10): pp. 1870–1882.
132. Park, E.S., S.R. Kim, and B.K. Jin, *Transient receptor potential vanilloid subtype 1 contributes to mesencephalic dopaminergic neuronal survival by inhibiting microglia-originated oxidative stress. Brain Res Bull*, 2012. 89(3): pp. 92–96.
133. Kark, T., et al., *Tissue-specific regulation of microvascular diameter: opposite functional roles of neuronal and smooth muscle located vanilloid receptor-1. Mol Pharmacol*, 2008. 73(5): pp. 1405–1412.
134. Phan, T.X., et al., *Sex-dependent expression of TRPV1 in bladder arterioles. Am J Phys Renal Phys*, 2016. 311(5): pp. F1063–f1073.
135. Smith, G.P., C. Jerome, and R. Norgren, *Afferent axons in abdominal vagus mediate satiety effect of cholecystokinin in rats. Am J Phys Regul Integr Comp Phys*, 1985. 249(5): pp. R638–R641.
136. Norgren, R. and G.P. Smith, *A method for selective section of vagal afferent or efferent axons in the rat. Am J Phys*, 1994. 267(4 Pt 2): pp. R1136–R1141.
137. Walls, E.K., et al., *Selective vagal rhizotomies: a new dorsal surgical approach used for intestinal deafferentations. Am J Phys*, 1995. 269(5 Pt 2): pp. R1279–R1288.
138. Liu, B., et al., *Vagotomy and parkinson disease: A Swedish register-based matched-cohort study. Neurology*, 2017. 88(21): pp. 1996–2002.
139. Breen, D.P., G.M. Halliday, and A.E. Lang, *Gut-brain axis and the spread of α-synuclein pathology: Vagal highway or dead end? Mov Disord*, 2019. 34(3): pp. 307–316.
140. Kim, S., et al., *Transneuronal propagation of pathologic α-synuclein from the gut to the brain models parkinson's disease. Neuron*, 2019. 103(4): pp. 627–641.
141. De Couck, M., et al., *The role of the vagus nerve in cancer prognosis: a systematic and a comprehensive review. J Oncol*, 2018. 2018 pp. 1236787.
142. Fagerberg, S., et al., *Vagotomy and gallbladder function. Gut*, 1970. 11(9): pp. 789.

143. Timofeeva, E., E.D. Baraboi, and D. Richard, *Contribution of the vagus nerve and lamina terminalis to brain activation induced by refeeding. Eur J Neurosci*, 2005. 22(6): pp. 1489-1501.
144. Gonzalez, M.F. and J.A. Deutsch, *Vagotomy abolishes cues of satiety produced by gastric distension. Science*, 1981. 212(4500): pp. 1283.
145. Traub, R.J., J.N. Sengupta, and G.F. Gebhart, *Differential c-fos expression in the nucleus of the solitary tract and spinal cord following noxious gastric distention in the rat. Neuroscience*, 1996. 74(3): pp. 873–884.
146. Mönnikes, H., et al., *Pathways of Fos expression in locus ceruleus, dorsal vagal complex, and PVN in response to intestinal lipid. Am J Phys*, 1997. 273(6): pp. R2059–R2071.
147. Yamamoto, T. and K. Sawa, *c-Fos-like immunoreactivity in the brainstem following gastric loads of various chemical solutions in rats. Brain Res*, 2000. 866(1-2): pp. 135–143.
148. Yox, D.P., H. Stokesberry, and R.C. Ritter, *Vagotomy attenuates suppression of sham feeding induced by intestinal nutrients. Am J Phys*, 1991. 260(3 Pt 2): pp. R503–R508.
149. Powley, T.L., et al., *Gastrointestinal tract innervation of the mouse: afferent regeneration and meal patterning after vagotomy. Am J Phys Regul Integr Comp Phys*, 2005. 289(2): pp. R563–r574.
150. Joyner, K., G.P. Smith, and J. Gibbs, *Abdominal vagotomy decreases the satiating potency of CCK-8 in sham and real feeding. Am J Phys*, 1993. 264(5 Pt 2): pp. R912–R916.
151. Sayegh, A.I. and R.C. Ritter, *Vagus nerve participates in CCK-induced Fos expression in hindbrain but not myenteric plexus. Brain Res*, 2000. 878(1-2): pp. 155–162.
152. Baptista, V., K.N. Browning, and R.A. Travagli, *Effects of cholecystokinin-8s in the nucleus tractus solitarius of vagally deafferented rats. Am J Phys Regul Integr Comp Phys*, 2007. 292(3): pp. R1092–R1100.
153. Wu, X.Y., et al., *Neurochemical phenotype of vagal afferent neurons activated to express C-FOS in response to luminal stimulation in the rat. Neuroscience*, 2005. 130(3): pp. 757–767.
154. Koda, S., et al., *The role of the vagal nerve in peripheral PYY3-36-induced feeding reduction in rats. Endocrinology*, 2005. 146(5): pp. 2369–2375.
155. Abbott, C.R., et al., *The inhibitory effects of peripheral administration of peptide YY3–36 and glucagon-like peptide-1 on food intake are attenuated by ablation of the vagal–brainstem–hypothalamic pathway. Brain Res*, 2005. 1044(1): pp. 127–131.
156. Date, Y., et al., *The role of the gastric afferent vagal nerve in ghrelin-induced feeding and growth hormone secretion in rats. Gastroenterology*, 2002. 123(4): pp. 1120–1128.
157. Davis, E.A., et al., *Ghrelin signaling regulates feeding behavior, metabolism, and memory through the vagus nerve.* bioRxiv, 2020: pp. 2020.06.16.155762.
158. Arnold, M., et al., *Gut vagal afferents are not necessary for the eating–stimulatory effect of intraperitoneally injected ghrelin in the rat. J Neurosci*, 2006. 26(43): pp. 11052–11060.
159. le Roux, C.W., et al., *Ghrelin does not stimulate food intake in patients with surgical procedures involving vagotomy. J Clin Endocrinol Metab*, 2005. 90(8): pp. 4521–4524.
160. Snowdon, C.T. and A.N. Epstein, *Oral and intragastric feeding in vagotomized rats. J Comp Physiol Psychol*, 1970. 71(1): pp. 59–67.
161. Reidelberger, R., et al., *Role of capsaicin-sensitive peripheral sensory neurons in anorexic responses to intravenous infusions of cholecystokinin, peptide YY-(3-36), and glucagon-like peptide-1 in rats. Am J Physiol Endocrinol Metab*, 2014. 307(8): pp. E619–E629.

162. Skak-Nielsen, T., J.J. Holst, and O.V. Nielsen, *Role of gastrin-releasing peptide in the neural control of pepsinogen secretion from the pig stomach. Gastroenterology*, 1988. 95(5): pp. 1216–1220.
163. Snowdon, C.T., *Gastrointestinal sensory and motor control of food intake. J Comp Physiol Psychol*, 1970. 71(1): pp. 68–76.
164. Tellez, L.A., et al., *A gut lipid messenger links excess dietary fat to dopamine deficiency. Science*, 2013. 341(6147): pp. 800–802.
165. Chavez, M., et al., *Chemical lesion of visceral afferents causes transient overconsumption of unfamiliar high-fat diets in rats. Am J Phys*, 1997. 272(5 Pt 2): pp. R1657–R1663.
166. Kelly, L., et al., *Capsaicin-treated rats permanently overingest low- but not high-concentration sucrose solutions. Am J Phys Regul Integr Comp Phys*, 2000. 279(5): pp. R1805–R1812.
167. Kelly, L.A., M. Chavez, and H.R. Berthoud, *Transient overconsumption of novel foods by deafferentated rats: effects of novel diet composition. Physiol Behav*, 1999. 65(4–5): pp. 793–800.
168. Schwartz, G.J., et al., *Gut vagal afferent lesions increase meal size but do not block gastric preload-induced feeding suppression. Am J Phys*, 1999. 276(6): pp. R1623–R1629.
169. Inoue, S. and G.A. Bray, *The effects of subdiaphragmatic vagotomy in rats with ventromedial hypothalamic obesity. Endocrinology*, 1977. 100(1): pp. 108–114.
170. Cox, J.E. and T.L. Powley, *Prior vagotomy blocks VMH obesity in pair-fed rats. Am J Phys*, 1981. 240(5): pp. E573–E583.
171. Sclafani, A., P.F. Aravich, and M. Landman, *Vagotomy blocks hypothalamic hyperphagia in rats on a chow diet and sucrose solution, but not on a palatable mixed diet. J Comp Physiol Psychol*, 1981. 95(5): pp. 720–734.
172. Stearns, A.T., et al., *Relative contributions of afferent vagal fibers to resistance to diet-induced obesity. Dig Dis Sci*, 2012. 57(5): pp. 1281–1290.
173. Gortz, L., et al., *Truncal vagotomy reduces food and liquid intake in man. Physiol Behav*, 1990. 48(6): pp. 779–781.
174. Kral, J.G., *Vagotomy for treatment of severe obesity. Lancet*, 1978. 1(8059): pp. 307–308.
175. Kral, J.G., *Vagotomy as a treatment for morbid obesity. Surg Clin North Am*, 1979. 59(6): pp. 1131–1138.
176. Kral, J.G., *Effects of truncal vagotomy on body weight and hyperinsulinemia in morbid obesity. Am J Clin Nutr*, 1980. 33(2 Suppl): pp. 416–419.
177. Kral, J.G., *Surgical treatment of obesity. Med Clin North Am*, 1989. 73(1): pp. 251–264.
178. Kral, J.G. and L. Görtz, *Truncal vagotomy in morbid obesity. Int J Obes*, 1981. 5(4): pp. 431–435.
179. Takahashi, T. and C. Owyang, *Characterization of vagal pathways mediating gastric accommodation reflex in rats. J Physiol*, 1997. 504 (Pt 2): pp. 479–488.
180. Hankir, M.K., et al., *Gastric bypass surgery recruits a gut PPAR-α-Striatal D1R pathway to reduce fat appetite in obese rats. Cell Metab*, 2017. 25(2): pp. 335–344.
181. Bai, L., et al., *Genetic identification of vagal sensory neurons that control feeding. Cell*, 2019. 179(5): pp. 1129–1143.
182. Kupari, J., et al., *An atlas of vagal sensory neurons and their molecular specialization. Cell Rep*, 2019. 27(8): pp. 2508–2523 .
183. Han, W., et al., *A neural circuit for gut-induced reward. Cell*, 2018. 175(3): pp. 665–678 .

184. Kentish, S.J., et al., *Gastric vagal afferent modulation by leptin is influenced by food intake status. J Physiol*, 2013. 591(7): pp. 1921–1934.
185. Blackshaw, L.A., D. Grundy, and T. Scratcherd, *Involvement of gastrointestinal mechano- and intestinal chemoreceptors in vagal reflexes: an electrophysiological study. J Auton Nerv Syst*, 1987. 18(3): pp. 225–234.
186. Schwartz, G.J. and T.H. Moran, *Duodenal nutrient exposure elicits nutrient-specific gut motility and vagal afferent signals in rat. Am J Phys*, 1998. 274(5): pp. R1236–R1242.
187. Thoren, P., E. Noresson, and S.E. Ricksten, *Resetting of cardiac C-fiber endings in the spontaneously hypertensive rat. Acta Physiol Scand*, 1979. 107(1): pp. 13–18.
188. Ricco, M.M., et al., *Interganglionic segregation of distinct vagal afferent fibre phenotypes in guinea-pig airways. J Physiol*, 1996. 496 (Pt 2): pp. 521–530.
189. Zhuo, H., H. Ichikawa, and C.J. Helke, *Neurochemistry of the nodose ganglion. Prog Neurobiol*, 1997. 52(2): pp. 79–107.
190. Mazzone, S.B. and B.J. Canning, *Synergistic interactions between airway afferent nerve subtypes mediating reflex bronchospasm in guinea pigs. Am J Phys Regul Integr Comp Phys*, 2002. 283(1): pp. R86–R98.
191. Carr, M.J. and B.J. Undem, *Pharmacology of vagal afferent nerve activity in guinea pig airways. Pulm Pharmacol Ther*, 2003. 16(1): pp. 45–52.
192. Mazzone, S.B., N. Mori, and B.J. Canning, *Synergistic interactions between airway afferent nerve subtypes regulating the cough reflex in guinea-pigs. J Physiol*, 2005. 569(Pt 2): pp. 559–573.
193. Yu, S., B.J. Undem, and M. Kollarik, *Vagal afferent nerves with nociceptive properties in guinea-pig oesophagus. J Physiol*, 2005. 563(Pt 3): pp. 831–842.
194. Nassenstein, C., et al., *Phenotypic distinctions between neural crest and placodal derived vagal C-fibres in mouse lungs. J Physiol*, 2010. 588(Pt 23): pp. 4769–4783.
195. Usoskin, D., et al., *Unbiased classification of sensory neuron types by large-scale single-cell RNA sequencing. Nat Neurosci*, 2015. 18(1): pp. 145–153.
196. Wang, J., et al., *Distinct and common expression of receptors for inflammatory mediators in vagal nodose versus jugular capsaicin-sensitive/TRPV1-positive neurons detected by low input RNA sequencing. PLoS One*, 2017. 12(10): pp. e0185985.
197. Chou, Y.L., N. Mori, and B.J. Canning, *Opposing effects of bronchopulmonary C-fiber subtypes on cough in guinea pigs. Am J Phys Regul Integr Comp Phys*, 2018. 314(3): pp. R489–R498.
198. Eiklid, K., S. Olsnes, and A. Pihl, *Entry of lethal doses of abrin, ricin and modeccin into the cytosol of HeLa cells. Exp Cell Res*, 1980. 126(2): pp. 321–326.
199. Berthoud, H.R., *The vagus nerve, food intake and obesity. Regul Pept*, 2008. 149(1-3): pp. 15–25.
200. Burdyga, G., et al., *Expression of cannabinoid CB1 receptors by vagal afferent neurons is inhibited by cholecystokinin. J Neurosci*, 2004. 24(11): pp. 2708–2715.
201. Belouzard, S., D. Delcroix, and Y. Rouille, *Low levels of expression of leptin receptor at the cell surface result from constitutive endocytosis and intracellular retention in the biosynthetic pathway. J Biol Chem*, 2004. 279(27): pp. 28499–28508.
202. Wiley, R.G. and D.A. Lappi, *Targeted toxins in pain. Adv Drug Deliv Rev*, 2003. 55(8): pp. 1043–1054.
203. McDougle, M., et al., *Intact vagal gut-brain signalling prevents hyperphagia and excessive weight gain in response to high-fat high-sugar diet. Acta Physiol (Oxford)*, 2020. 2020: pp. e13530.
204. Tsien, J.Z., *Cre-Lox Neurogenetics: 20 Years of Versatile Applications in Brain Research and Counting. Front Genet*, 2016. 7: pp. 19.

205. Brunet, J.F. and A. Pattyn, *Phox2 genes - from patterning to connectivity. Curr Opin Genet Dev*, 2002. 12(4): pp. 435–440.
206. Tiveron, M.C., M.R. Hirsch, and J.F. Brunet, *The expression pattern of the transcription factor Phox2 delineates synaptic pathways of the autonomic nervous system. J Neurosci*, 1996. 16(23): pp. 7649–7660.
207. Dib-Hajj, S.D., et al., *Sodium channels in normal and pathological pain. Annu Rev Neurosci*, 2010. 33: pp. 325–347.
208. Stirling, L.C., et al., *Nociceptor-specific gene deletion using heterozygous NaV1.8-Cre recombinase mice. Pain*, 2005. 113(1–2): pp. 27–36.
209. Rossi, J., et al., *Melanocortin-4 receptors expressed by cholinergic neurons regulate energy balance and glucose homeostasis. Cell Metab*, 2011. 13(2): pp. 195–204.
210. Scott, M.M., et al., *Leptin receptor expression in hindbrain Glp-1 neurons regulates food intake and energy balance in mice. J Clin Invest*, 2011. 121(6): pp. 2413–2421.
211. de Lartigue, G., C.C. Ronveaux, and H.E. Raybould, *Deletion of leptin signaling in vagal afferent neurons results in hyperphagia and obesity. Mol Metab*, 2014. 3(6): pp. 595–607.
212. Liu, C., et al., *PPARγ in vagal neurons regulates high-fat diet induced thermogenesis. Cell Metab*, 2014. 19(4): pp. 722–730.
213. Vianna, C.R., et al., *Cannabinoid receptor 1 in the vagus nerve is dispensable for body weight homeostasis but required for normal gastrointestinal motility. J Neurosci*, 2012. 32(30): pp. 10331–10337.
214. Varin, E.M., et al., *distinct neural sites of GLP-1R expression mediate physiological versus pharmacological control of incretin action. Cell Rep*, 2019. 27(11): pp. 3371–3384.e3.
215. Caillon, A., et al., *The OEA effect on food intake is independent from the presence of PPARα in the intestine and the nodose ganglion, while the impact of OEA on energy expenditure requires the presence of PPARα in mice. Metabolism*, 2018. 87: pp. 13–17.
216. Zeng, W.Z., et al., *PIEZOs mediate neuronal sensing of blood pressure and the baroreceptor reflex. Science*, 2018. 362(6413): pp. 464–467.
217. Egerod, K.L., et al., *Profiling of G protein-coupled receptors in vagal afferents reveals novel gut-to-brain sensing mechanisms. Mol Metab*, 2018. 12: pp. 62–75.
218. Udit, S., et al., *Na(v)1.8 neurons are involved in limiting acute phase responses to dietary fat. Mol Metab*, 2017. 6(10): pp. 1081–1091.
219. Stirling, L.C., et al., *Nociceptor-specific gene deletion using heterozygous NaV1.8-Cre recombinase mice. Pain*, 2005. 113(1-2): pp. 27–36.
220. Gautron, L., et al., *Genetic tracing of Nav1.8-expressing vagal afferents in the mouse. J Comp Neurol*, 2011. 519(15): pp. 3085–3101.
221. Serlin, H.K. and E.A. Fox, *Abdominal vagotomy reveals majority of small intestinal mucosal afferents labeled in na(v) 1.8cre-rosa26tdTomato mice are vagal in origin. J Comp Neurol*, 2020. 528(5): pp. 816–839.
222. D'Autréaux, F., et al., *Homeoprotein Phox2b commands a somatic-to-visceral switch in cranial sensory pathways. Proc Natl Acad Sci U S A*, 2011. 108(50): pp. 20018–20023.
223. Gautron, L., J.F. Zechner, and V. Aguirre, *Vagal innervation patterns following Roux-en-Y gastric bypass in the mouse. Int J Obes*, 2013. 37(12): pp. 1603–1607.
224. Schmidt-Supprian, M. and K. Rajewsky, *Vagaries of conditional gene targeting. Nat Immunol*, 2007. 8(7): pp. 665–668.
225. El-Brolosy, M.A. and D.Y.R. Stainier, *Genetic compensation: A phenomenon in search of mechanisms. PLoS Genet*, 2017. 13(7): pp. e1006780.
226. Feil, S., N. Valtcheva, and R. Feil, *Inducible cre mice. Methods Mol Biol*, 2009. 530: pp. 343-363.

227. Beyeler, A., et al., *Divergent routing of positive and negative information from the amygdala during memory retrieval. Neuron*, 2016. 90(2): pp. 348–361.
228. Carter, M.E., et al., *Genetic identification of a neural circuit that suppresses appetite. Nature*, 2013. 503(7474): pp. 111–114.
229. Darvas, M. and R.D. Palmiter, *Restriction of dopamine signaling to the dorsolateral striatum is sufficient for many cognitive behaviors. Proc Natl Acad Sci U S A*, 2009. 106(34): pp. 14664–14669.
230. Hnasko, T.S., et al., *Cre recombinase-mediated restoration of nigrostriatal dopamine in dopamine-deficient mice reverses hypophagia and bradykinesia. Proc Natl Acad Sci U S A*, 2006. 103(23): pp. 8858–8863.
231. Kim, E.J., et al., *Three types of cortical layer 5 neurons that differ in brain-wide connectivity and function. Neuron*, 2015. 88(6): pp. 1253–1267.
232. Ruder, L., A. Takeoka, and S. Arber, *Long-distance descending spinal neurons ensure quadrupedal locomotor stability. Neuron*, 2016. 92(5): pp. 1063–1078.
233. Senn, V., et al., *Long-range connectivity defines behavioral specificity of amygdala neurons. Neuron*, 2014. 81(2): pp. 428–437.
234. Wu, Q., M.S. Clark, and R.D. Palmiter, *Deciphering a neuronal circuit that mediates appetite. Nature*, 2012. 483(7391): pp. 594–597.
235. Nagy, A., *Cre recombinase: the universal reagent for genome tailoring. Genesis*, 2000. 26(2): pp. 99–109.
236. Betley, J.N. and S.M. Sternson, *Adeno-associated viral vectors for mapping, monitoring, and manipulating neural circuits. Hum Gene Ther*, 2011. 22(6): pp. 669–677.
237. Glover, C.P., et al., *Adenoviral-mediated, high-level, cell-specific transgene expression: a SYN1-WPRE cassette mediates increased transgene expression with no loss of neuron specificity. Mol Ther*, 2002. 5(5 Pt 1): pp. 509–516.
238. Kugler, S., E. Kilic, and M. Bahr, *Human synapsin 1 gene promoter confers highly neuron–specific long–term transgene expression from an adenoviral vector in the adult rat brain depending on the transduced area. Gene Ther*, 2003. 10(4): pp. 337–347.
239. Brierley DI, Holt MK, Singh A, de Araujo A, McDougle M, Vergara M, Afaghani MH, Lee SJ, Scott K, Maske C, Langhans W, Krause E, de Kloet A, Gribble FM, Reimann F, Rinaman L, de Lartigue G, Trapp S. *Central and peripheral GLP-1 systems independently suppress eating. Nat Metab*. 2021 Feb;3(2):258–273.
240. Li, L., et al., *Visualizing the distribution of synapses from individual neurons in the mouse brain. PLoS One*, 2010. 5(7): pp. e11503.
241. Oh, S.W., et al., *A mesoscale connectome of the mouse brain. Nature*, 2014. 508(7495): pp. 207–214.
242. Lerner, T.N., et al., *Intact-brain analyses reveal distinct information carried by snc dopamine subcircuits. Cell*, 2015. 162(3): pp. 635–647.
243. Land, B.B., et al., *Medial prefrontal D1 dopamine neurons control food intake. Nat Neurosci*, 2014. 17(2): pp. 248–253.
244. Li, J., et al., *Trans-synaptic neural circuit-tracing with neurotropic viruses. Neurosci Bull*, 2019. 35(5): pp. 909–920.
245. Kumar, P., *Retrograde Tracing. Mat Meth*, 2019. 2019: 9.
246. Li, B., et al., *Studies on neuronal tracing with pseudorabies virus. Bing Du Xue Bao*, 2014. 30(3): pp. 333–337.
247. Kelly, R.M. and P.L. Strick, *Rabies as a transneuronal tracer of circuits in the central nervous system. J Neurosci Methods*, 2000. 103(1): pp. 63–71.

248. Kaelberer, M.M., et al., *A gut-brain neural circuit for nutrient sensory transduction. Science*, 2018. 361(6408).
249. Smith, B.N., et al., *Pseudorabies virus expressing enhanced green fluorescent protein: A tool for in vitro electrophysiological analysis of transsynaptically labeled neurons in identified central nervous system circuits. Proc Natl Acad Sci U S A*, 2000. 97(16): pp. 9264–9269.
250. Ugolini, G., H.G. Kuypers, and A. Simmons, *Retrograde transneuronal transfer of herpes simplex virus type 1 (HSV 1) from motoneurones. Brain Res*, 1987. 422(2): pp. 242–256.
251. Loewy, A.D., *Viruses as transneuronal tracers for defining neural circuits. Neurosci Biobehav Rev*, 1998. 22(6): pp. 679–684.
252. Enquist, L.W., *Exploiting circuit-specific spread of pseudorabies virus in the central nervous system: insights to pathogenesis and circuit tracers. J Infect Dis*, 2002. 186 Suppl 2: pp. S209–S214.
253. DeFalco, J., et al., *Virus-assisted mapping of neural inputs to a feeding center in the hypothalamus. Science*, 2001. 291(5513): pp. 2608–2613.
254. Wickersham, I.R., et al., *Retrograde neuronal tracing with a deletion-mutant rabies virus. Nat Methods*, 2007. 4(1): pp. 47–49.
255. Wickersham, I.R., et al., *Monosynaptic restriction of transsynaptic tracing from single, genetically targeted neurons. Neuron*, 2007. 53(5): pp. 639–647.
256. Chen, J., et al., *A vagal-nts neural pathway that stimulates feeding. Curr Biol*, 2020. 30(20): pp. 3986–98.e5.
257. Zemanick, M.C., P.L. Strick, and R.D. Dix, *Direction of transneuronal transport of herpes simplex virus 1 in the primate motor system is strain-dependent. Proc Natl Acad Sci U S A*, 1991. 88(18): pp. 8048–8051.
258. Li, D., et al., *Anterograde neuronal circuit tracers derived from herpes simplex virus 1: development, application, and perspectives. Int J Mol Sci*, 2020. 21(16): 5937 doi:10.3390/ijms21165937.
259. Lo, L. and D.J. Anderson, *A Cre-dependent, anterograde transsynaptic viral tracer for mapping output pathways of genetically marked neurons. Neuron*, 2011. 72(6): pp. 938–950.
260. Zeng, W.B., et al., *Anterograde monosynaptic transneuronal tracers derived from herpes simplex virus 1 strain H129. Mol Neurodegener*, 2017. 12(1): pp. 38.
261. Bolovan, C.A., N.M. Sawtell, and R.L. Thompson, *ICP34.5 mutants of herpes simplex virus type 1 strain 17syn+ are attenuated for neurovirulence in mice and for replication in confluent primary mouse embryo cell cultures. J Virol*, 1994. 68(1): pp. 48–55.
262. Sedarati, F. and J.G. Stevens, *Biological basis for virulence of three strains of herpes simplex virus type 1. J Gen Virol*, 1987. 68 (Pt 9): pp. 2389–2395.
263. Su, P., et al., *Evaluation of retrograde labeling profiles of HSV1 H129 anterograde tracer. J Chem Neuroanat*, 2019. 100: pp. 101662.
264. Wojaczynski, G.J., et al., *The neuroinvasive profiles of H129 (herpes simplex virus type 1) recombinants with putative anterograde-only transneuronal spread properties. Brain Struct Funct*, 2015. 220(3): pp. 1395–1420.
265. Kelly, R.M. and P.L. Strick, *Cerebellar loops with motor cortex and prefrontal cortex of a nonhuman primate. J Neurosci*, 2003. 23(23): pp. 8432–8444.
266. Dum, R.P., D.J. Levinthal, and P.L. Strick, *The spinothalamic system targets motor and sensory areas in the cerebral cortex of monkeys. J Neurosci*, 2009. 29(45): pp. 14223–14235.

267. Labetoulle, M., et al., *Neuronal pathways for the propagation of herpes simplex virus type 1 from one retina to the other in a murine model. J Gen Virol*, 2000. 81(Pt 5): pp. 1201–1210.
268. Sun, N., M.D. Cassell, and S. Perlman, *Anterograde, transneuronal transport of herpes simplex virus type 1 strain H129 in the murine visual system. J Virol*, 1996. 70(8): pp. 5405–5413.
269. Garner, J.A. and J.H. LaVail, *Differential anterograde transport of HSV type 1 viral strains in the murine optic pathway. J Neurovirol*, 1999. 5(2): pp. 140–150.
270. Barnett, E.M., et al., *Anterograde tracing of trigeminal afferent pathways from the murine tooth pulp to cortex using herpes simplex virus type 1. J Neurosci*, 1995. 15(4): pp. 2972–2984.
271. Vaughan, C.H. and T.J. Bartness, *Anterograde transneuronal viral tract tracing reveals central sensory circuits from brown fat and sensory denervation alters its thermogenic responses. Am J Phys Regul Integr Comp Phys*, 2012. 302(9): pp. R1049–R1058.
272. Song, C.K., G.J. Schwartz, and T.J. Bartness, *Anterograde transneuronal viral tract tracing reveals central sensory circuits from white adipose tissue. Am J Phys Regul Integr Comp Phys*, 2009. 296(3): pp. R501–R511.
273. McGovern, A.E., et al., *Transneuronal tracing of airways-related sensory circuitry using herpes simplex virus 1, strain H129. Neuroscience*, 2012. 207: pp. 148–166.
274. Zingg, B., et al., *AAV-mediated anterograde transsynaptic tagging: mapping corticocollicular input-defined neural pathways for defense behaviors. Neuron*, 2017. 93(1): pp. 33–47.
275. Zingg, B., et al., *Synaptic specificity and application of anterograde transsynaptic aav for probing neural circuitry. J Neurosci*, 2020. 40(16): pp. 3250–3267.
276. Boyden, E.S., et al., *Millisecond-timescale, genetically targeted optical control of neural activity. Nat Neurosci*, 2005. 8(9): pp. 1263–1268.
277. Li, X., et al., *Fast noninvasive activation and inhibition of neural and network activity by vertebrate rhodopsin and green algae channelrhodopsin. Proc Natl Acad Sci U S A*, 2005. 102(49): pp. 17816–17821.
278. Petreanu, L., et al., *Channelrhodopsin-2-assisted circuit mapping of long-range callosal projections. Nat Neurosci*, 2007. 10(5): pp. 663–668.
279. Wang, H., et al., *High-speed mapping of synaptic connectivity using photostimulation in Channelrhodopsin-2 transgenic mice. Proc Natl Acad Sci U S A*, 2007. 104(19): pp. 8143–8148.
280. Diester, I., et al., *An optogenetic toolbox designed for primates. Nat Neurosci*, 2011. 14(3): pp. 387–397.
281. Armbruster, B.N., et al., *Evolving the lock to fit the key to create a family of G protein-coupled receptors potently activated by an inert ligand. Proc Natl Acad Sci U S A*, 2007. 104(12): pp. 5163–5168.
282. Rothwell, P.E., et al., *Autism-associated neuroligin-3 mutations commonly impair striatal circuits to boost repetitive behaviors. Cell*, 2014. 158(1): pp. 198–212.
283. Lin, J.Y., et al., *Characterization of engineered channelrhodopsin variants with improved properties and kinetics. Biophys J*, 2009. 96(5): pp. 1803–1814.
284. Lin, J.Y., *A user's guide to channelrhodopsin variants: features, limitations and future developments. Exp Physiol*, 2011. 96(1): pp. 19–25.
285. Nussinovitch, U. and L. Gepstein, *Optogenetics for in vivo cardiac pacing and resynchronization therapies. Nat Biotechnol*, 2015. 33(7): pp. 750–754.
286. Kim, W.S., Hong, S., Gamero, M. et al. *Organ-specific, multimodal, wireless optoelectronics for high-throughput phenotyping of peripheral neural pathways. Nat Commun* 12, 157 (2021). https://doi.org/10.1038/s41467-020-20421-8

287. Kim, H., et al., *Prefrontal parvalbumin neurons in control of attention. Cell*, 2016. 164(1–2): pp. 208–218.
288. Zhang, F., et al., *Optogenetic interrogation of neural circuits: technology for probing mammalian brain structures. Nat Protoc*, 2010. 5(3): pp. 439–456.
289. Leszkiewicz, D.N., K. Kandler, and E. Aizenman, *Enhancement of NMDA receptor-mediated currents by light in rat neurones in vitro. J Physiol*, 2000. 524 Pt 2: pp. 365–374.
290. Cheng, K.P., et al., B*lue light modulates murine microglial gene expression in the absence of optogenetic protein expression. Sci Rep*, 2016. 6: pp. 21172.
291. Volkov, O., et al., *Structural insights into ion conduction by channelrhodopsin 2. Science*, 2017. 358(6366).
292. Tyssowski, K.M. and J.M. Gray, *Blue light increases neuronal activity-regulated gene expression in the absence of optogenetic proteins. eNeuro*, 2019. 6(5).
293. Duke, C.G., et al., *Blue light-induced gene expression alterations in cultured neurons are the result of phototoxic interactions with neuronal culture media. eNeuro*, 2020. 7(1).
294. Alexander, G.M., et al., *Remote control of neuronal activity in transgenic mice expressing evolved G protein-coupled receptors. Neuron*, 2009. 63(1): pp. 27–39.
295. Farrell, M.S., et al., *A Galphas DREADD mouse for selective modulation of cAMP production in striatopallidal neurons. Neuropsychopharmacology*, 2013. 38(5): pp. 854–862.
296. Wang, Q. and F.M. Zhou, *cAMP-producing chemogenetic and adenosine A2a receptor activation inhibits the inwardly rectifying potassium current in striatal projection neurons. Neuropharmacology*, 2019. 148: pp. 229–243.
297. Gomez, J.L., et al., *Chemogenetics revealed: DREADD occupancy and activation via converted clozapine. Science*, 2017. 357(6350): pp. 503–507.
298. Cho, J., et al., *Optimizing clozapine for chemogenetic neuromodulation of somatosensory cortex. Sci Rep*, 2020. 10(1): pp. 6001.
299. Manzaneque, J.M., P.F. Brain, and J.F. Navarro, *Effect of low doses of clozapine on behaviour of isolated and group-housed male mice in the elevated plus-maze test. Prog Neuro-Psychopharmacol Biol Psychiatry*, 2002. 26(2): pp. 349–355.
300. Jendryka, M., et al., *Pharmacokinetic and pharmacodynamic actions of clozapine-N-oxide, clozapine, and compound 21 in DREADD-based chemogenetics in mice. Sci Rep*, 2019. 9(1): pp. 4522.
301. Bonaventura, J., et al., *Chemogenetic ligands for translational neurotheranostics. bioRxiv*, 2018.
302. DeWire, S.M., et al., *Beta-arrestins and cell signaling. Annu Rev Physiol*, 2007. 69: pp. 483–510.
303. Patel, J.M., et al., *Sensory perception drives food avoidance through excitatory basal forebrain circuits. elife*, 2019. 8.
304. Zhang, F., et al., *Multimodal fast optical interrogation of neural circuitry. Nature*, 2007. 446(7136): pp. 633–639.
305. Lin, C.W., et al., *Genetically increased cell-intrinsic excitability enhances neuronal integration into adult brain circuits. Neuron*, 2010. 65(1): pp. 32–39.
306. Yu, K., et al., *The central amygdala controls learning in the lateral amygdala. Nat Neurosci*, 2017. 20(12): pp. 1680–1685.
307. Soumier, A. and E. Sibille, *Opposing effects of acute versus chronic blockade of frontal cortex somatostatin-positive inhibitory neurons on behavioral emotionality in mice. Neuropsychopharmacology*, 2014. 39(9): pp. 2252–2262.
308. Yang, C.F., et al., *Sexually dimorphic neurons in the ventromedial hypothalamus govern mating in both sexes and aggression in males. Cell*, 2013. 153(4): pp. 896–909.

309. Brummelkamp, T.R., R. Bernards, and R. Agami, *A system for stable expression of short interfering RNAs in mammalian cells. Science*, 2002. 296(5567): pp. 550–553.
310. Wu, X., et al., *Genome-wide binding of the CRISPR endonuclease Cas9 in mammalian cells. Nat Biotechnol*, 2014. 32(7): pp. 670–676.
311. Yang, J., Y.N. Jan, and L.Y. Jan, *Control of rectification and permeation by residues in two distinct domains in an inward rectifier K+ channel. Neuron*, 1995. 14(5): pp. 1047–1054.
312. Schiavo, G., M. Matteoli, and C. Montecucco, *Neurotoxins affecting neuroexocytosis. Physiol Rev*, 2000. 80(2): pp. 717–766.
313. Mochida, S., et al., *Light chain of tetanus toxin intracellularly inhibits acetylcholine release at neuro-neuronal synapses, and its internalization is mediated by heavy chain. FEBS Lett*, 1989. 253(1–2): pp. 47–51.
314. Inutsuka, A., et al., *Concurrent and robust regulation of feeding behaviors and metabolism by orexin neurons. Neuropharmacology*, 2014. 85: pp. 451–460.
315. Foster, E., et al., *Targeted ablation, silencing, and activation establish glycinergic dorsal horn neurons as key components of a spinal gate for pain and itch. Neuron*, 2015. 85(6): pp. 1289–1304.
316. Wu, Z., et al., *Galanin neurons in the medial preoptic area govern parental behaviour. Nature*, 2014. 509(7500): pp. 325–330.
317. Fujikawa, D.G., et al., *Caspase-3 is not activated in seizure-induced neuronal necrosis with internucleosomal DNA cleavage. J Neurochem*, 2002. 83(1): pp. 229–240.
318. Davis, E.A., et al., *Ghrelin signaling regulates feeding behavior, metabolism, and memory through the vagus nerve.* bioRxiv, 2020.
319. Iwasaki, Y., et al., *GLP-1 release and vagal afferent activation mediate the beneficial metabolic and chronotherapeutic effects of D-allulose. Nat Commun*, 2018. 9(1): pp. 113.
320. Xu, J., et al., *Genetic identification of leptin neural circuits in energy and glucose homeostases. Nature*, 2018. 556(7702): pp. 505–509.
321. Richard Sun, X., et al., *SnapShot: Optical control and imaging of brain activity. Cell*, 2012. 149(7): pp. 1650–1650.
322. Zariwala, H.A., et al., *A Cre-dependent GCaMP3 reporter mouse for neuronal imaging in vivo. J Neurosci*, 2012. 32(9): pp. 3131–3141.
323. Akerboom, J., et al., *Optimization of a GCaMP calcium indicator for neural activity imaging. J Neurosci*, 2012. 32(40): pp. 13819–13840.
324. Peters, J.H., et al., *Cooperative activation of cultured vagal afferent neurons by leptin and cholecystokinin. Endocrinology*, 2004. 145(8): pp. 3652–3657.
325. Simasko, S.M., et al., *Cholecystokinin increases cytosolic calcium in a subpopulation of cultured vagal afferent neurons. Am J Phys Regul Integr Comp Phys*, 2002. 283(6): pp. R1303–R1313.
326. Tan, H.E., et al., *The gut-brain axis mediates sugar preference. Nature*, 2020. 580(7804): pp. 511–516.

11 Neuronal Regulation of Adipose Tissue Biology

Wenwen Zeng and Xinmin Qian
Tsinghua University, China

CONTENTS

11.1 ADIPOSE TISSUE DIVERSITY

The adipose tissues were initially regarded as wandering or generic connective tissues but were gradually recognized as a distinct entity critical for metabolic homeostasis. They have gained much attention for their quality of being versatile, changing in tissue appearance and cellular morphology in response to nutritional fluctuation, environmental temperature variations, or during lactation. They are composed of a diverse array of cell types other than adipocytes, including precursor cells, vascular endothelial cells, immune cells, fibroblasts, and nerve tissues, which communicate intensively to form an intricate network (Figure 11.1). Our knowledge of the metabolic network together with adipose tissue plasticity has been greatly enhanced by studies made over the past few decades, revealing molecular and cellular insights in depth.

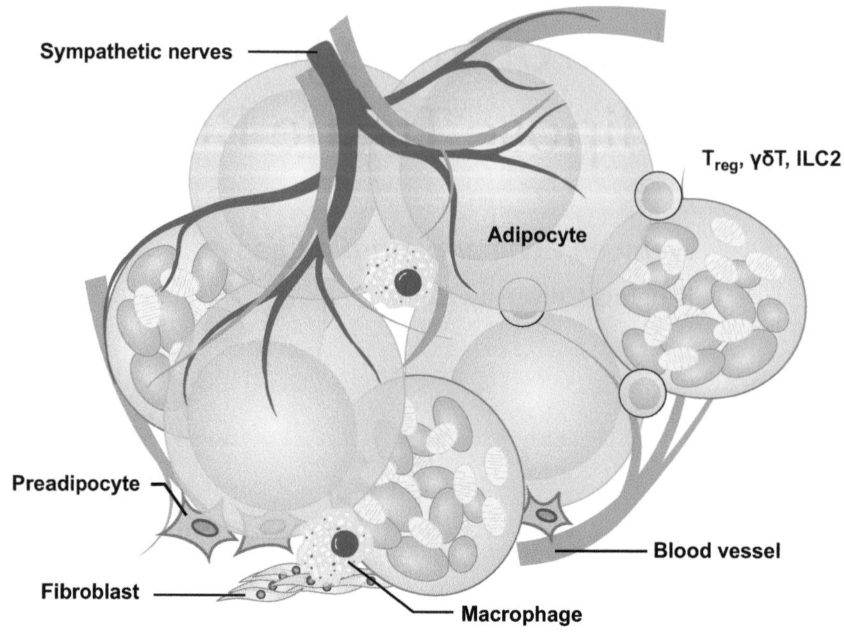

FIGURE 11.1 Adipose tissue composition. The adipose tissues are comprised of an interactive cellular network, including adipocytes, precursor cells (such as the preadipocyte), vascular endothelial cells (as in blood vessels), fibroblasts, immune cell subsets (such as macrophages, T_{reg}s, $\gamma\delta$T cells, and ILC2s), and nerve tissues (such as sympathetic nerves). T_{reg}: regulatory T cells; ILC2: group 2 innate lymphoid cells.

The white adipose tissues are abundantly present in mammals and are in charge of lipid storage and energy supply (Figure 11.2). Measured by diameter in hundreds of micrometers, the white adipocytes are well equipped with the molecular machinery to store and dispense a large amount of energy as triglycerides. With one large lipid droplet occupying most of the intracellular space, the white adipocyte is highly specialized for lipid synthesis and hydrolysis, and lipid and glucose uptake, for coping with the dynamic metabolic states of energy deficiency or excess.

The brown adipose tissues are morphologically distinguishable from the white adipose tissues and are the major site for adaptive thermogenesis (Figure 11.2). The color of brown adipose tissues is attributed to the richness of mitochondria and vasculatures, which empower the tissues with great capacity for heat generation and dissipation. These tissues have been extensively studied in rodents, functions of which confer the small mammal with a survival advantage when facing environmental challenges such as a rapid drop in the surrounding temperature.

Divergent from the dichotomic view of brown versus white adipose tissues, the brown-like adipocytes appear within the white fat depots in low environmental temperature-acclimated animals, which shifts the predominant metabolic capacity from energy storage to consumption (Figure 11.2). The process is called browning or beiging, and the brown-like cells are termed "brite" (brown-in-white) or beige adipocytes. The past decade has witnessed intensive examination of the process, together with adipocyte

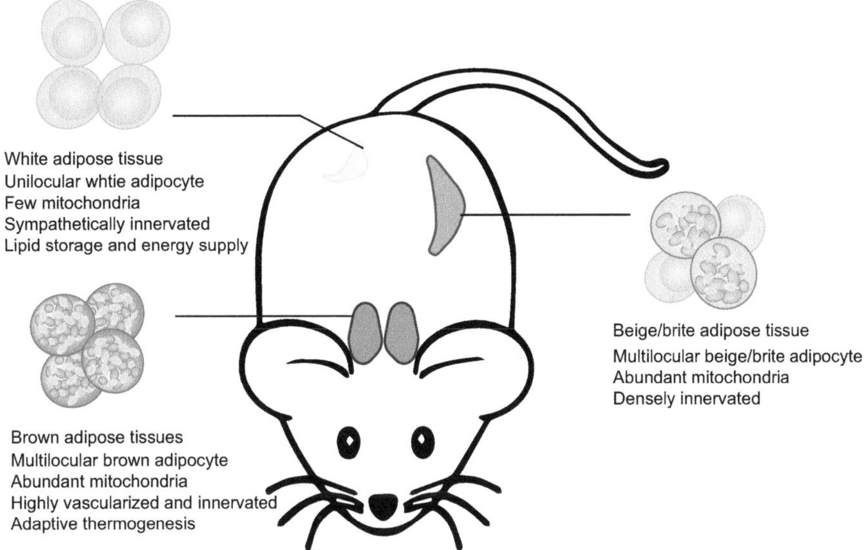

FIGURE 11.2 Adipose tissue diversity. The adipose tissues can be categorized into multiple types including white, brown, and beige/brite. The white adipose tissues are innervated by sympathetic nerves, and the white adipocytes contain a single lipid droplet and are specialized for lipid storage and hydrolysis. The brown adipose tissues are highly innervated and vascularized, and the brown adipocytes have multiple lipid droplets, contain abundant mitochondria, and mediate adaptive thermogenesis. The beige adipose tissues are densely innervated by sympathetic nerves, and the beige adipocytes share similar morphological and functional characteristics of brown adipocytes and can be found in various white adipose depots or induced by stimuli such as environmental cold.

biology. The beige adipocytes exhibit a large number of mitochondria and highly express the uncoupling protein-1 (UCP1), two defining features of thermogenic brown adipocytes. Of particular interest for therapeutic exploitation, the beige cells show a wide spectrum of plasticity, with the number of cells and the extent of resemblance to the brown adipocytes altering dynamically within the fat pads, in adaptation to external and internal cues such as environmental temperature or nutritional status.

Adult humans contain mainly white adipose tissues with unilocular morphology, which typically comprise ~20–30% of the total body weight in the non-obese population. At infancy, the brown adipose tissues are abundant in the neck and back regions. In contrast to the conspicuous presence of brown adipose tissue in rodents, human adults lose the classical morphology of brown adipocytes during development. The typical brown adipose tissue appears to be rare in the interscapular region, according to biopsies and autopsies, which is the dominant brown adipose tissue depot in rodents. However, human studies indicate that functional brown or beige-like adipose tissues persist into adulthood. Fluorodeoxyglucose (FDG) positron emission tomography and computed tomography (PET/CT) detect active glucose uptake into fat depots residing in locations such as the cervical, supraclavicular, axillary, mediastinal, paravertebral, and abdominal regions in cancerous patients and in healthy adults. Expression profiling (such as UCP1) and cellular characterization uncover the fact that adult adipose tissues contain adipocytes with beige-like or classical brown signatures. Their mass and activity are correlated with metabolic health and with less activated depots in obese than lean subjects. The recent appreciation of the inducible and recruitable natures of UCP1-expressing beige adipose tissues in rodents has inspired new efforts to harness the metabolic plasticity of the adipose tissues in humans, particularly the potential to engineer their biological capabilities to promote energy expenditure.

11.2 NEURONAL CONTROL OF ADAPTIVE THERMOGENESIS IN BROWN ADIPOSE TISSUES

The brown adipose tissues function as the primary site for consuming lipids and generating heat, a non-shivering thermogenic process also called adaptive thermogenesis, which occurs in response to cold exposure, internal thermo-sensation, arousal from hibernation, pathogen infection or inflammation, as well as controlled conditions of dietary intake (Figure 11.3). The brown adipocytes present with multilocular morphology, enclosing multiple lipid droplets and enriched with mitochondria. When activated, the fatty acids,

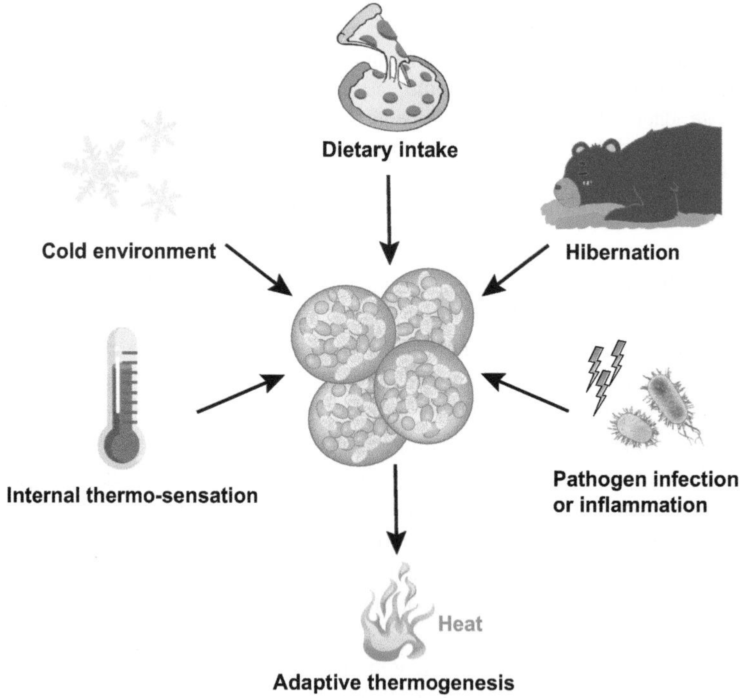

FIGURE 11.3 Adaptive thermogenesis in brown adipose tissues. Adaptive thermogenesis by brown adipose tissues is affected by various factors including environmental cold, internal thermo-sensation, arousal from hibernation, pathogen infection or inflammation, and possibly dietary intake.

derived from the hydrolysis of intracellular triglyceride, plasma lipoproteins, or directly from circulation, undergo β-oxidation to produce acetyl-CoA, which enters the tricarboxylic acid cycle and further drives the electron transport chain. Instead of producing adenosine triphosphate (ATP) as the energy currency, the brown adipocytes are wired into a thermogenic program, engaging UCP1, an inner-membrane mitochondrial protein to shuttle protons back into the mitochondria matrix and uncouple the electron transport chain from ATP production. During adaptive thermogenesis, the glucose uptake into brown adipose tissues is enhanced, which enables the visualization by PET/CT when combined with a radioactive glucose tracer (^{18}F-FDG) or oxygen ($^{15}O\text{-}O_2$).

The abundant distribution of sympathetic nerve fibers has been documented in brown adipose tissues and characterized in many species including mice, rats, and hamsters. Electron microscopy, histochemical staining, immunohistochemical staining, and measurement of the amount of sympathetic neurotransmitter norepinephrine have together demonstrated sympathetic innervation and activity. Neuronal tracing agents including the retrograde tract tracer horseradish peroxide and the retrograde trans-neuronal viral tract tracer pseudorabies virus (PRV) have assisted the delineation of the neuroanatomy of the nerve supply to interscapular brown adipose tissues. The sympathetic preganglionic neurons reside in the intermediolateral cell column (IML) of the spinal cord, and the postganglionic neurons are located in the paravertebral ganglia, with predominant presence in the stellate ganglion, though a significant number of postganglionic neurons are found in the upper thoracic chain ganglia of mice but not of rats or Siberian hamsters. The efferent nerves enter the brown fat pad at its ventral surface, and in addition to the densely innervated blood vessels, numerous fibers project into the parenchyma and run in close proximity to brown adipocytes.

The interscapular brown adipose tissues are composed of a pair of lobules in rodents, innervated by a separate nerve supply from the sympathetic ganglia. The symmetrical position on either side of the midline offers ease of access for denervation by surgical or chemical means and subsequent analysis (Figure 11.4). The nerves on one side can be kept intact as a control and the other side surgically transected, removed, or chemically disrupted. Blockage of the sympathetic outflow unilaterally by surgical denervation results in a transient effect of glycogen deposition, and a prolonged period of denervation leads to lipid accumulation and an increased size of the lipid droplet when compared with the contralateral side in rats and mice. Early observations provided a key insight into the regulatory role of locally distributed nerve innervations in lipid and glucose metabolism.

Adaptive thermogenesis elicited by environmental cold which consumes lipids is a process tightly regulated by sympathetic activity (Figure 11.5). Skin cooling is perceived by the cutaneous sensory nerve endings, which convey thermal information to the central nervous system. The afferent information is processed and integrated into brain regions particularly involving the hypothalamus. The central origins of the sympathetic outflow from the brain to brown adipose tissues are revealed through tract tracers such as trans-neuronal viruses. The efferent pathway descends from the hypothalamus to the rostral ventromedial medulla (RVM), including the rostral raphe nucleus (rRPa) in the brainstem, which contain neurons projecting to the IML of the spinal cord, where they innervate the sympathetic preganglionic neurons and further provide neuronal input to the brown adipose

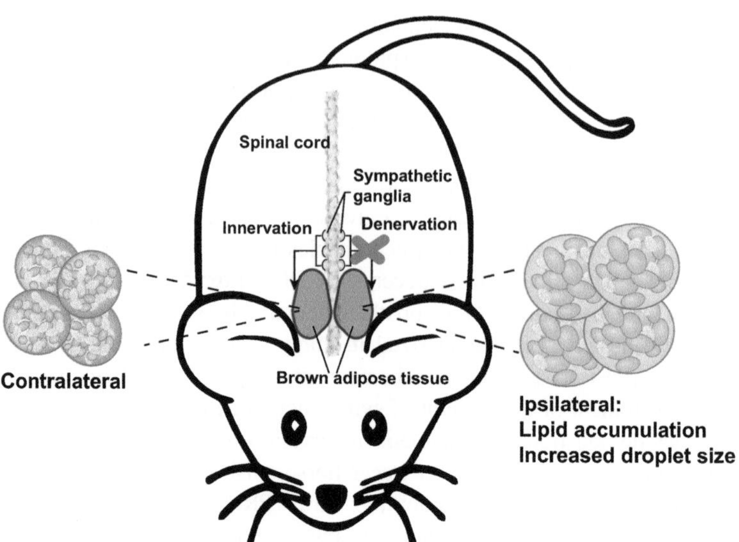

FIGURE 11.4 Experimental denervation of sympathetic input in brown adipose tissue. The interscapular brown adipose tissues are composed of a pair of lobules in rodents, innervated by a separate nerve supply from the sympathetic ganglia. Blockage of the sympathetic outflow can be achieved unilaterally by surgical or chemical approaches. Sidman and Fawcett (1954) showed that surgical denervation of the sympathetic outflow unilaterally for a prolonged period led to lipid accumulation and an increased size of the lipid droplet when compared with the contralateral side in rats and mice.

tissues via postganglionic neurons. Stimulated by skin cooling, the sympathetic nerve activity is readily detected by the electrophysiological recording of the nerve bundle beneath the interscapular brown fat, accompanied with an increased turnover rate of norepinephrine in the fat pad. In this process, the sympathetic activity mobilizes the lipid reservoir in the brown adipose tissues as the immediate energy source for combustion to combat cold. Unilateral denervation largely impairs lipid mobilization in the brown adipocytes but does not affect the intact side, and occurs within hours in a cold environment and deprived of food, presumably mimicking the natural challenge the animals likely encounter in the wild. In addition to the immediate thermogenic reaction, sympathetic stimulation promotes signaling events for the transcriptional increase of thermogenic genes and the expansion of the brown adipose tissues through proliferation and differentiation from the precursor cells, all of which lead to an increased thermogenic capacity.

On the cellular level, the effect of sympathetic activity on brown adipocytes is mediated through binding to β-adrenergic receptors on the cell membrane by norepinephrine (Figure 11.6). Nine adrenergic receptors are identified in mammals belonging to the 7-transmembrane G protein-coupled receptor (GPCR) family: α1-subtypes (α1A, α1B, and α1D), β-subtypes (β1, β 2, and β 3) that activate adenylate cyclase (AC) with a consequent increase of intracellular cyclic adenosine monophosphate (cAMP) and which are the predominant subtypes in adipocytes, and α2-subtypes (α2A, α2B, and

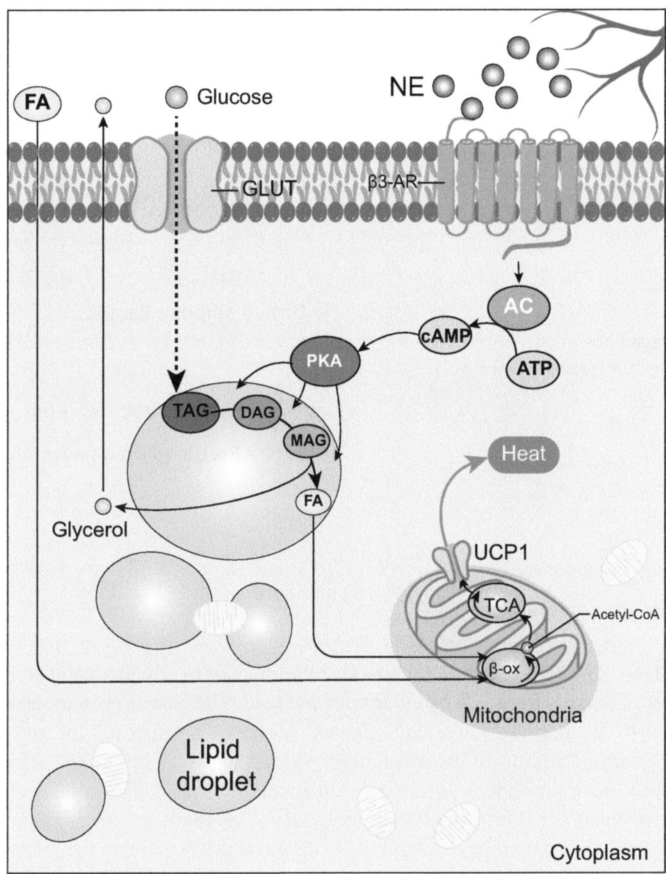

FIGURE 11.5 Adrenergic stimulation of adaptive thermogenesis in brown adipocytes. β3 adrenergic signaling engages adaptive thermogenesis in the brown adipocytes. When activated by norepinephrine (NE) stimulation, the fatty acids derived intracellularly via lipolysis or from circulation undergo beta-oxidation to produce acetyl-CoA, which enters the tricarboxylic acid cycle and further drives the electron transport chain. UCP1, an inner-membrane mitochondrial protein, shuttles protons back into the mitochondria matrix and uncouples the electron transport chain from ATP production, resulting in heat production. AC: adenylate cyclase; cAMP: cyclic adenosine monophosphate; PKA: protein kinase A; TAG: triacylglycerol; DAG: diacylglycerol; MAG: monoacylglycerol; FA: fatty acid; UCP1: uncoupling protein 1; NE: norepinephrine; GLUT: glucose transporter (GLUT4 and GLUT1); β3-AR: β3-adrenergic receptor; β-ox: beta-oxidation; TCA: tricarboxylic acid cycle.

α2C) that could counteract with the β adrenergic pathway. The mature brown adipocytes highly express the β3 adrenergic receptor, and the agonistic stimulation triggers the signaling cascade leading to the hydrolysis of triglyceride, β-oxidation of fatty acids, and activation of UCP1 to coordinate a thermogenic program.

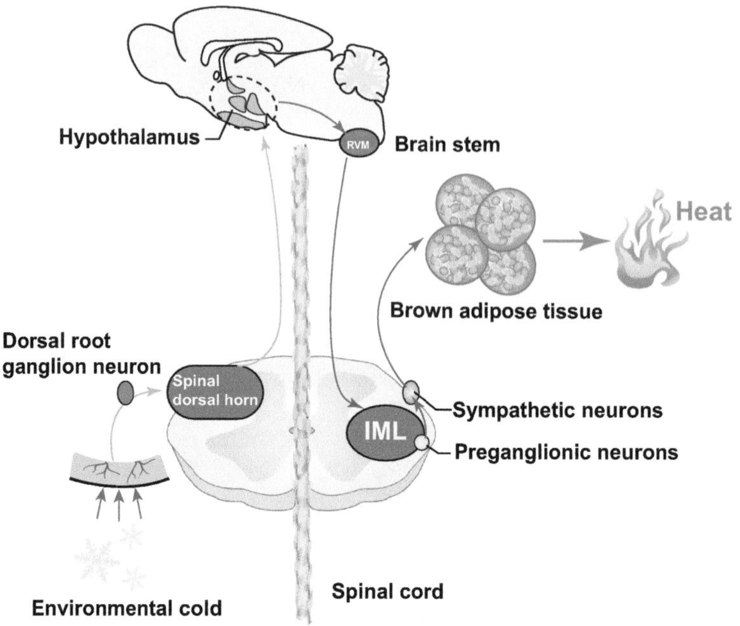

FIGURE 11.6 The neuronal axis for adaptive thermogenesis. Sympathetic activity controls adaptive thermogenesis triggered by environmental cold. The cutaneous temperature drop can be perceived by the sensory nerve endings, which convey the thermal information through dorsal root ganglion neurons to the spinal cord, and further to the brain. The afferent signal is integrated into the brain regions particularly involving the hypothalamus. The efferent signal descends from the brain via the brain stem (at the RVM), and further to the spinal cord (at the IML) where they innervate the preganglionic neurons, which then relay the information to the sympathetic neurons which stimulate adaptive thermogenesis. RVM: rostral ventromedial medulla; IML: intermediolateral cell column.

11.3 NEURONAL REGULATION OF LIPOLYSIS IN WHITE ADIPOSE TISSUES

One fundamental function of white adipose tissues is to maintain an energy reservoir. White adipocytes take up fatty acid and glucose from the circulation and convert them into triglycerides. Conversely, a constant lipolytic process occurs to break down the triglycerides into free fatty acid and glycerol. In the conditions of nutritional scarcity or sufficient lipid reserve indicated by a rise in leptin levels, the lipolysis is favored to either provide the energy sources to other organs or consume the surplus.

The revelation of the sympathetic innervation in white adipose tissues has been advanced mainly by progress in experimental approaches. Early histochemical staining and electron microscopy on tissue sections displayed the presence of nerve fibers, which were determined to be active sympathetic inputs, evidenced by catecholamine granules in nerve terminals, and the norepinephrine turnover in response to cold in rats or short photoperiod exposure in Siberian hamsters. Immunohistochemical studies based on tissue sections consolidated the findings by providing details on the nerve fiber subtype using specific molecular markers such as tyrosine hydroxylase (TH) for sympathetic nerves. Further, the holistic view of the nerve arborization in the intact fat pad is revealed by the whole-mount immunostaining and volume fluorescence-imaging technique, which combines the immunolabeling of specific molecules, tissue clearing, and light-sheet microscopic imaging. Visualization of the nerve arborization in its entirety illustrates that the white adipose tissues are densely innervated, and the majority of the adipocytes are in close apposition with the sympathetic fibers exemplified in the inguinal fat pad in mice, indicating a potentially profound and direct control by the sympathetic input. Three-dimensional adipose tissue imaging also reveals that the tissue architecture and sympathetic innervation differ significantly between subcutaneous and visceral depots, and that the subcutaneous fat demonstrates a regional variation in beige fat biogenesis with localization of UCP1-expressing beige adipocytes to areas with dense sympathetic neurites.

The neuroanatomy, from the central nervous system to the sympathetic ganglia and further to the white adipose tissues, has been constructed based on various neuronal tract tracing techniques. The peripheral administration of PRV labels the central regions, including the paraventricular hypothalamic nucleus (PVH), the dorsomedial hypothalamic nucleus (DMH), the preoptic areas, the arcuate nucleus of the hypothalamus, and the nucleus of the solitary tract, among others, when injected into the inguinal and epididymal fat pads of Siberian hamsters, domestic swine, and laboratory rats. The descending neurons project to the brainstem and IML in the spinal cord. A fluorescence tract tracer (Fluoro-Gold or indocarbocyanine perchlorate) and PRV show that sympathetic thoracolumbar ganglia relay the efferent signal to the perigonadal and the inguinal fat pads in Siberian hamsters and rats. Notably, the sympathetic outflow is not equal between the anatomically different fat pads. Variations in labeling are noticed in the sympathetic chain, spinal cord, and the brain regions when isogenic strains of PRV are used to retrogradely trace the neural axis to the inguinal and mesenteric fat pads of Siberian hamsters, or to the intraabdominal and subcutaneous fat pads of rats. The degree of viral labeling also differs in brain regions between epididymal and inguinal injections. In addition, the sympathetic drive shows differences between fat depots, collectively suggesting a fat pad-specific sympathetic circuitry. Much work is needed to fully reconstruct the anatomical map of the sympathetic innervations, which could be of importance in dissecting the functional neuronal circuitry from the brain to the individual white adipose tissue, optimally at single-fiber resolution.

Direct sympathetic innervation plays important roles in mediating the lipolytic process. Electrical stimulation of the nerves with isolated white adipose tissues or optogenetic nerve stimulation *in vivo* enhances the lipolysis and the liberation of free fatty acids. The extirpation of the individual sympathetic ganglion results in fat accumulation in the innervated fat pads. Unilateral surgical denervation of the splanchnic nerves in rats, cats, and rabbits leads to slowed fat mobilization and deposition to a lesser degree in the perirenal fat, indicated by impaired accumulation of Sudan III from the diet. Unilateral extirpation of the stellate and superior cervical ganglia affects the amount of pericardial fat, and unilateral extirpation of the lumbar and sacral ganglia results in a significant change of abdominal and subcutaneous fat. The effect on the molecular pathway of lipolysis is also validated with surgical denervation of the nerve branch in the epididymal fat in mice.

Sympathetic activity could elicit the lipolytic pathway in adipocytes through engaging β-adrenergic receptors by norepinephrine (Figure 11.7). An increase in AC activity results in an elevation in the second messenger of cAMP. The protein kinase A (PKA)

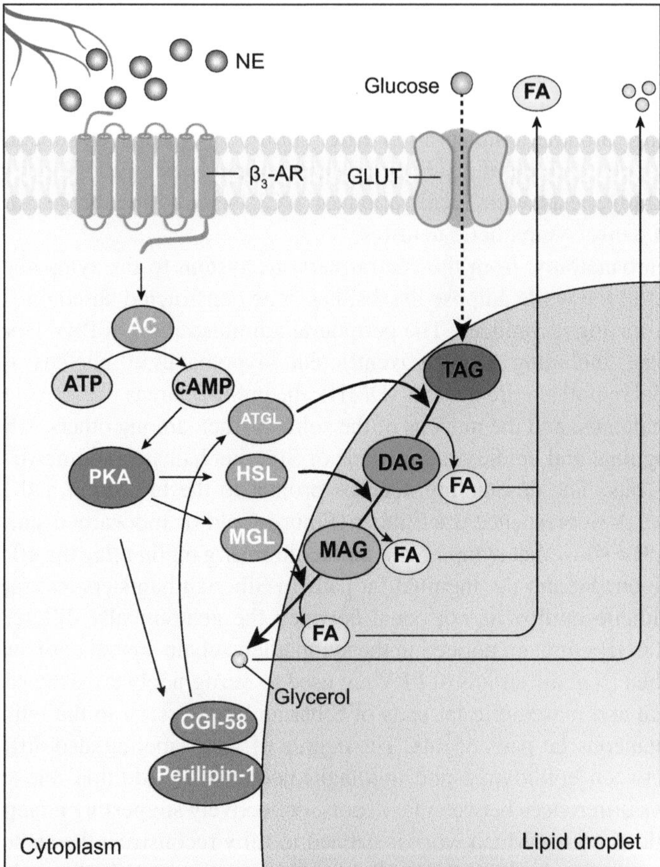

FIGURE 11.7 Sympathetic regulation of lipolysis in white adipocytes. Adrenergic signaling elicits lipolysis of triacylglycerol (TAG) in white adipocytes. β3-adrenergic stimulation by norepinephrine (NE) promotes an elevation in intracellular cAMP levels, which activates PKA. PKA-dependent activation of lipase cascade, including adipose triglyceride lipase (ATGL), hormone-sensitive lipase (HSL), and monoglyceride lipase (MGL), is critical for breaking down TAG into fatty acid and glycerol. Additional proteins are critically involved in mediating lipolysis, such that perilipin-1 and comparative gene identification-58 (CGI-58) are responsive to NE stimulation and facilitate the lipolytic pathway. AC: adenylate cyclase; cAMP: cyclic adenosine monophosphate; PKA: protein kinase A; TAG: triacylglycerol; DAG: diacylglycerol; MAG: monoacylglycerol; FA: fatty acid; ATGL: adipose triglyceride lipase; HSL: hormone-sensitive lipase; MGL: monoglyceride lipase; CGI-58: comparative gene identification-58; NE: norepinephrine; GLUT: glucose transporter; β3-AR: β3-adrenergic receptor.

is subsequently activated and further transduces the signal to lipolytic enzymes and accessory proteins. The enzymatic reactions mediated by the lipases, particularly the adipose triglyceride lipase (ATGL), hormone-sensitive lipase (HSL) and monoglyceride lipase (MGL), break the triglyceride into free fatty acid and glycerol. To facilitate the lipolytic process, the accessory proteins located on the surface of the lipid droplet, in the organelles, or in the cytosol, are also responsive to PKA activation and participate in streamlining the reaction. For instance, the protein cofactor CGI-58 is crucial for activating ATGL. Other than the monoamine neurotransmitter, a diverse list of paracrine, autocrine, or endocrine factors induce intracellular lipolysis, which signal to the variable receptors but generally converge on the shared enzymatic cascade.

In addition to predominant sympathetic innervation, the afferent sensory nerves are observed in selected fat depots. Immunohistochemical analysis detects calcitonin gene-related peptide (CGRP) and substance P (SP), molecular markers expressed in sensory subtypes in the periphery, in the white and brown adipose tissues in Siberian hamsters and rats. Denervation of the sensory nerves in the inguinal white adipose tissues with the local application of capsaicin results in increased average fat cell size, and the treatment of the epididymal white adipose tissues with capsaicin leads to an increased fat mass of retroperitoneal white adipose tissues in Siberian hamsters. Also, the fluorescent tract tracer and the antegrade trans-neuronal viral tract tracer (herpes simplex virus-1 H129 strain) label the neurons in the dorsal root ganglia where the cell bodies of sensory neurons are located. And the direct injection of β3 adrenergic receptor agonist CL316, 243 into an inguinal fat pad increases neuronal activation in dorsal root ganglion neurons, activation of which is subject to blockage by an antilipolytic agent in Siberian hamsters. These findings urge further investigations to show the potential crosstalk between energy sensation, informational integration, and execution of metabolic events.

11.4 NEURONAL CONTROL OF THE BROWNING/BEIGING PROCESS OF WHITE ADIPOSE TISSUES

Prolonged cold exposure promotes the formation of UCP1 positive, brown-fat-like cells designated as brown-in-white (brite) or beige cells in the white adipose tissues through a process called browning or beiging. The induction of beige cells expands the thermogenic capacity for defense against hypothermia and also confers the animals with improved energy metabolism, protecting mice from diet-induced obesity and insulin resistance. Those inducible beige adipocytes are derived via differentiation from precursor cells, or reprograming from mature adipocytes. Resembling brown adipocytes, the beige cells acquire a multilocular morphology with high mitochondrial content, and highly express the thermogenic gene of UCP1. Additional genes are also elevated in the process of beiging to coordinate the thermogenic program: PPARγ coactivator 1α (PGC1α) for regulating mitochondria biogenesis, and type 2 iodothyronine deiodinase (DIO2) for generating triiodothyronine (T3) from thyroxine (T4) and enhancing mRNA synthesis, including UCP1.

The sympathetic input in white adipose tissues is critically involved in the beiging process during cold acclimation (Figure 11.8). The fat pads at different anatomical locations have various propensities to undergo beiging, which is positively correlated

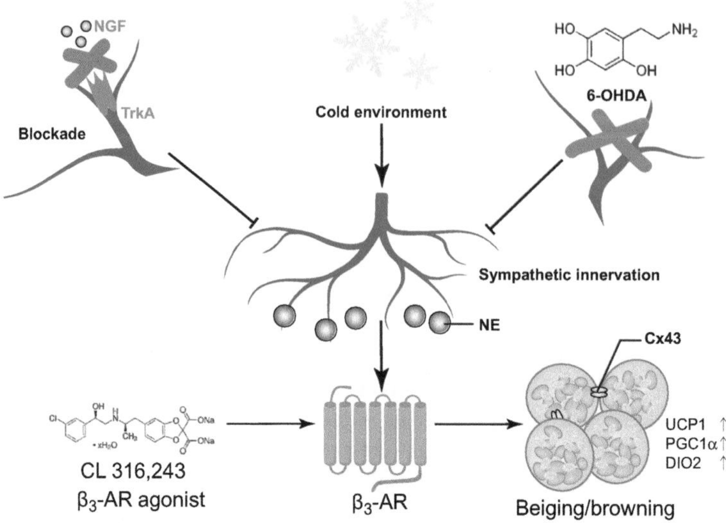

FIGURE 11.8 Neuronal control of the browning/beiging process of white adipose tissues. Sympathetic input in the white adipose tissues is critically involved in the beiging process during cold acclimation. Genetic ablation of neurotrophic receptor tyrosine kinase 1 (TrkA) in the sympathetic neurons causes reduced parenchymal nerve density together with compromised beiging. Locally, disruption of the nerve fibers in the fat pad by treatment with 6-hydroxydopamine (6-OHDA) significantly impairs beiging. Administration of a β3-adrenergic receptor agonist, such as CL 316,243, could mimic the effect of sympathetic stimulation and promote beiging. Additional mechanisms could be involved in modulating the sympathetic outflow, such as cell-to-cell coupling via connexin 43, which could enhance sympathetic input through signal amplification. NE: norepinephrine; TrkA: neurotrophic receptor tyrosine kinase 1; β3-AR: β3-adrenergic receptor; 6-OHDA: 6-hydroxydopamine; UCP1: uncoupling protein 1; PGC1α: peroxisome proliferator-activated receptor-γ coactivator (PGC)-1α; DIO2: type 2 iodothyronine deiodinase; Cx43: connexin 43.

with the density of sympathetic nerve fibers in mice. A large number of beige cells are readily detected in the subcutaneous adipose tissues, though much less in perigonadal adipose tissues. Genetic abrogation of the sympathetic nerves through deleting the neurotrophic receptor tyrosine kinase 1 (TrkA) in the sympathetic neurons, and the receptor for the nerve growth factor (NGF) which is required for sympathetic neuron survival and early development, causes reduced parenchymal nerve density together with compromised beiging. Treatment with 6-hydroxydopamine (6-OHDA), a specific catecholaminergic neurotoxin that ablates the nerve fibers in the fat pad when applied locally, also impairs beiging. The signaling events in the adipocytes are mainly mediated through β adrenergic receptors, predominantly the β3 subtype; administration of a β3 adrenergic receptor agonist, such as CL 316,243, could mimic the effect of sympathetic stimulation and promote beiging. Additional mechanisms exist to enhance the sympathetic input, e.g. cell-to-cell coupling via connexin 43 (Cx43) could contribute to signal amplification through gap junction channels.

Other than cold exposure, a number of catabolic or pathological stimuli are also associated with beiging and brown adipose tissue activation, such as leptin stimulation, cancer cachexia, and tissue injury. However, the possible involvement of sympathetic activity is largely understudied for most of those conditions, though in-depth analysis could be of significant value from the translational perspective. For instance, the sympathetic activation of brown adipose tissues is observed in cachexia. Surgical ablation of sympathetic innervations in the brown adipose tissues compromises the induction of the thermogenic program, and blockade of the β adrenergic receptor impairs the beiging process, hinting at a therapeutic possibility of targeting sympathetic activity in ameliorating a fatally metabolic imbalance.

11.5 NEURONAL MEDIATION OF THE ADIPOSE TISSUE ENDOCRINE FUNCTION

The adipose tissues produce hundreds of secreting molecules such as proteins and bioactive lipids, which function as autocrine, paracrine, or endocrine mediators and act on organs including the brain, liver, pancreas, muscle, and heart. The individual factors in the category of adipocyte secretome (the collection of secreting molecules produced by adipocytes), also referred to as adipokines, influence a broad range of metabolic activities such as appetite control, glucose homeostasis, and lipid metabolism.

Leptin, identified in 1994, has established the adipose tissues as a key endocrine organ. Leptin is mostly produced by white adipocytes, and the plasma level is highly proportional to the fat mass reservoir. The circulating leptin serves as a measure of body fat storage, and regulates appetite and energy expenditure. The rapid decline of leptin occurs in response to cold exposure, β-3 adrenergic receptor agonist treatment, or fasting. On the other hand, the adrenergic signaling mediated by a2A subtype positively regulates leptin synthesis in visceral fat upon starvation, suggesting a complex role of sympathetic activity in leptin production. Besides leptin, a repertoire of secreting molecules derived from adipocytes, such as adiponectin, and from a variety of other residential cell types such as immune cells, change dynamically and play crucial roles in metabolic activities. Though the underlying biological process is far from what we can fathom now, an open question remains as to whether the neuronal activity might constantly reshape the secreting profile, thereby influencing the biological activities of adipose tissues and distant organs as a whole (Figure 11.9).

11.6 NEURONAL MODULATION OF VASCULATURES IN ADIPOSE TISSUES

Adipose tissues are highly vascularized, which enables an effective response to organismal metabolic adaptations of lipid storage, mobilization, and heat dissipation. Around 14 meters and 1 meter in length of vasculatures are packed into the volume of 1 cubic millimeter of the interscapular brown and inguinal white fat pads in mice, respectively, visualized by whole-mount immunostaining and volume-fluorescence imaging in the entirety. Electrical stimulation of sympathetic innervation in canine subcutaneous white adipose tissues increases vascular permeability involving the signaling of adrenergic receptors, leading to the enhanced dispensation of free fatty acid. Also, the vascular network undergoes remodeling in response to metabolic demands, and cold acclimation increases vascularization in the brown and white

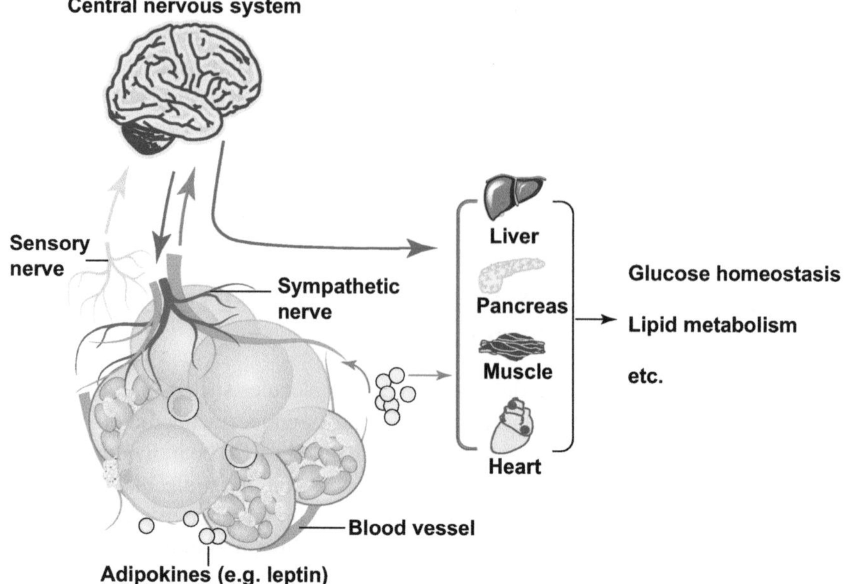

FIGURE 11.9 Neuronal mediation of the adipose tissue endocrine function. Neuronal activity could play a variety of roles in regulating adipose tissue biology, through bidirectional communication with the central nervous system, involving both sympathetic and sensory divisions, and through changing the endocrine factors. A collection of secreting factors derived from adipose tissues, including adipokines produced from adipocytes, regulate a wide range of metabolic activities such as appetite control, glucose homeostasis, lipid metabolism, and energy expenditure, through actions in other organs and tissues including the brain, liver, pancreas, muscle, and heart. Leptin is a key endocrine molecule in suppressing food intake and promoting energy expenditure, which could be regulated by sympathetic activity.

adipose tissues. Within the white adipose tissues, the sympathetic nerves are spatially engaged with the vasculatures to a large extent. Mechanistic investigation shows that cold exposure induces angiogenesis via increasing the expression of proangiogenic factor vascular endothelial growth factor a (VEGFα), which is promoted by sympathetic activity. As a result, the endothelial cells proliferate and form numerous new capillaries and the relative proportion of brown adipocytes/endothelial cells is kept largely consistent during cold-induced brown fat hyperplasia.

11.7 SYMPATHETIC INNERVATION AND PLASTICITY

Sympathetic nerve arborization is established during late embryogenesis and early postnatal development. NGF is a neurotrophin supporting the survival and differentiation of sympathetic neurons and mediating axonal innervation and dendritic growth. The target-derived NGF signals are translocated retrogradely from the distal axons to the somata of sympathetic neurons via the receptor TrkA signaling endosomes. Genetic ablation of TrkA in the sympathetic neurons leads to impaired sympathetic innervation, especially in the white adipose tissue parenchyma. In addition, sympathetic innervation could be shaped during the developmental stage. Rats reared in a cool environment exhibit increased sympathetic innervation with augmented sympathetic outflow and higher norepinephrine content and turnover rates in brown adipose tissue in comparison with rats kept in a warm environment.

Sympathetic arborization also responds to dynamic cues, either from adipose tissues or other organs, during adulthood. The sympathetic density increases significantly in the cold-acclimated animals, but decreases in thermoneutrality assessed by whole-mount immunostaining and volume-fluorescence imaging. The target-derived NGF is elevated and plays a crucial role in regulating axonal outgrowth in response to cold. In addition, an increasing list of candidates has recently been identified which either promotes or inhibits sympathetic innervations in adipose tissues. Genetic deletion of calsyntenin 3b or interleukin 17 receptor C in adipocytes reduces functional sympathetic innervations in thermogenic adipose tissues. Conversely, the ablation of fatty acid synthase (FASN) in adipocytes increases the sympathetic innervation of inguinal adipose tissues. Further, deletion of FASN in adipocytes but not selectively in thermogenic adipocytes results in increased sympathetic innervation in brown adipose tissues, and deficiency of Tsukushi, a liver-derived secreted factor, results in increased sympathetic innervation in adipose tissues, implying a layer of inter-organ regulatory mechanism on neuronal control. Also, overexpression of bone morphogenetic protein 8 in adipocytes increases sympathetic innervation via action on neuregulin 4, a member of the epidermal growth factor family of extracellular ligands, which is highly produced by brown adipocytes and can induce sympathetic neurite outgrowth *in vitro*. Also, the immune cell subsets play their parts in modulating the sympathetic activity, such as macrophages in regulating the turnover of norepinephrine. The quickly evolving field is projected to resolve these intricate findings and provide a coherent picture of how the intercellular dialogue is exchanged between sympathetic innervation and those variable molecular components.

11.8 THE PATHOPHYSIOLOGY OF SYMPATHETIC INNERVATIONS

Obesity and aging are the two prominent factors closely associated with dysfunctional sympathetic outflow. Multiple lines of evidence suggest that sympathetic activity is chronically elevated in the obese and elderly populations. For instance, muscle sympathetic nerve traffic measurement detects sympathetic overdrive in overweight and obese subjects across multiple studies. The heightened sympathetic activity is postulated to primarily function as a compensatory mechanism to increase energy expenditure, although the long-term sympathetic overactivation leads to negative consequences, such as desensitization of stimulatory adrenergic signaling and detrimental effects on the cardiovascular system.

The distribution and composition of adipose tissues change drastically during the development of obesity: a substantial amount of fat is deposited in visceral and subcutaneous depots; lipid accumulation and decreased thermogenic functions are evident in the brown adipose tissues. In contrast to systemic sympathetic overexcitation, adipose tissues show less innervation. Visualization with whole-mount immunostaining and volume-fluorescence imaging reveals the greatly decreased density of sympathetic arborization in the inguinal fat pad of obese mice, including genetically obese (*ob* and *db* mice) and diet-induced obese animals, indicating an impaired local neuronal control. Though the underlying mechanism awaits to be elucidated, the adverse conditions associated with obesity, such as hypoxia and maladaptive lipid and glucose metabolism, could inevitably influence neuron homeostasis, ultimately contributing to the pathological change. Further, the malfunction of local neural control could affect the crucial processes of lipolysis, browning/beiging, and thermogenesis, thereby precipitating the vicious cycle of metabolic abnormalities.

11.9 CONCLUDING REMARKS

The nervous system has been proven to be a crucial nexus in the integrative network of energy balance. The barely digested knowledge of sympathetic activity in metabolic homeostasis could pave a way to probe its crosstalk with the rest of the nervous system, such as sensory and parasympathetic divisions. Also, a plethora of signals originating in the periphery impact adipose tissue activity may or may not involve local innervation directly. Construction of neuronal organization will benefit the endeavor to understand how neuronal activity may act in concert with the endocrine or paracrine branches. Further, the neuronal innervation of fat depots varies with the anatomical locations, and illustrations of the precise structural and functional circuitry will inform possible undertakings in human counterparts. The therapeutic potential to manipulate neuronal control in improving the metabolism in obesity, type 2 diabetes, and cardiovascular diseases has been reinforced as an appealing opportunity.

REFERENCES

Adler, E. S., J. H. Hollis, I. J. Clarke, D. R. Grattan, and B. J. Oldfield. "Neurochemical Characterization and Sexual Dimorphism of Projections from the Brain to Abdominal and Subcutaneous White Adipose Tissue in the Rat." *J Neurosci* 32, no. 45 (Nov 7 2012): 15913–15921.

Ahima, R. S., C. B. Saper, J. S. Flier, and J. K. Elmquist. "Leptin Regulation of Neuroendocrine Systems." *Front Neuroendocrinol* 21, no. 3 (Jul 2000): 263–307.

Bachman, E. S., H. Dhillon, C. Y. Zhang, S. Cinti, A. C. Bianco, B. K. Kobilka, and B. B. Lowell. "Betaar Signaling Required for Diet-Induced Thermogenesis and Obesity Resistance." *Science* 297, no. 5582 (Aug 2 2002): 843–845.

Bamshad, M., V. T. Aoki, M. G. Adkison, W. S. Warren, and T. J. Bartness. "Central Nervous System Origins of the Sympathetic Nervous System Outflow to White Adipose Tissue." *Am J Phys* 275, no. 1 (Jul 1998): R291–R299.

Bamshad, M., C. K. Song, and T. J. Bartness. "Cns Origins of the Sympathetic Nervous System Outflow to Brown Adipose Tissue." *Am J Phys* 276, no. 6 (Jun 1999): R1569–R1578.

Barbatelli, G., I. Murano, L. Madsen, Q. Hao, M. Jimenez, K. Kristiansen, J. P. Giacobino, R. De Matteis, and S. Cinti. "The Emergence of Cold-Induced Brown Adipocytes in Mouse White Fat Depots Is Determined Predominantly by White to Brown Adipocyte Transdifferentiation." *Am J Physiol Endocrinol Metab* 298, no. 6 (Jun 2010): E1244–E1253.

Bargmann, W., G. von Hehn, and E. Lindner. "[On the Cells of the Brown Fatty Tissue and Their Innervation]." *Z Zellforsch Mikrosk Anat* 85, no. 4 (1968): 601–613.

Bartness, T. J., and M. Bamshad. "Innervation of Mammalian White Adipose Tissue: Implications for the Regulation of Total Body Fat." *Am J Phys* 275, no. 5 (Nov 1998): R1399–R1411.

Bartness, T. J., C. Kay Song, H. Shi, R. R. Bowers, and M. T. Foster. "Brain-Adipose Tissue Cross Talk." *Proc Nutr Soc* 64, no. 1 (Feb 2005): 53–64.

Bartness, T. J., Y. Liu, Y. B. Shrestha, and V. Ryu. "Neural Innervation of White Adipose Tissue and the Control of Lipolysis." *Front Neuroendocrinol* 35, no. 4 (Oct 2014): 473–493.

Bartness, T. J., and V. Ryu. "Neural Control of White, Beige and Brown Adipocytes." *Int J Obes Suppl* 5, no. Suppl 1 (Aug 2015): S35–S39.

Bartness, T. J., Y. B. Shrestha, C. H. Vaughan, G. J. Schwartz, and C. K. Song. "Sensory and Sympathetic Nervous System Control of White Adipose Tissue Lipolysis." *Mol Cell Endocrinol* 318, no. 1-2 (Apr 29 2010a): 34–43.

Bartness, T. J., C. H. Vaughan, and C. K. Song. "Sympathetic and Sensory Innervation of Brown Adipose Tissue." *Int J Obes* 34 Suppl 1 (Oct 2010b): S36–S42.

Berry, D. C., Y. Jiang, and J. M. Graff. "Mouse Strains to Study Cold-Inducible Beige Progenitors and Beige Adipocyte Formation and Function." *Nat Commun* 7 (Jan 5 2016): 10184.

Bertin, R., I. Mouroux, F. De Marco, and R. Portet. "Norepinephrine Turnover in Brown Adipose Tissue of Young Rats: Effects of Rearing Temperature." *Am J Phys* 259, no. 1 Pt 2 (Jul 1990): R90-6.

Beznak, ABL, and Z Hasch. "The Effect of Sympathectomy on the Fatty Deposit in Connective Tissue." *Q J Exp Physio: Trans Integr* 27, no. 1 (1937): 1–15.

Blaszkiewicz, M., J. W. Willows, A. L. Dubois, S. Waible, K. DiBello, L. L. Lyons, C. P. Johnson, et al. "Neuropathy and Neural Plasticity in the Subcutaneous White Adipose Depot." *PLoS One* 14, no. 9 (2019): e0221766.

Bowers, R. R., W. T. Festuccia, C. K. Song, H. Shi, R. H. Migliorini, and T. J. Bartness. "Sympathetic Innervation of White Adipose Tissue and Its Regulation of Fat Cell Number." *Am J Phys Regul Integr Comp Phys* 286, no. 6 (Jun 2004): R1167–R1175.

Brito, M. N., N. A. Brito, D. J. Baro, C. K. Song, and T. J. Bartness. "Differential Activation of the Sympathetic Innervation of Adipose Tissues by Melanocortin Receptor Stimulation." *Endocrinology* 148, no. 11 (Nov 2007): 5339–5347.

Brito, N. A., M. N. Brito, and T. J. Bartness. "Differential Sympathetic Drive to Adipose Tissues after Food Deprivation, Cold Exposure or Glucoprivation." *Am J Phys Regul Integr Comp Phys* 294, no. 5 (May 2008): R1445–R1452.

Brooks, S. L., A. M. Neville, N. J. Rothwell, M. J. Stock, and S. Wilson. "Sympathetic Activation of Brown-Adipose-Tissue Thermogenesis in Cachexia." *Biosci Rep* 1, no. 6 (Jun 1981): 509–517.

Bukowiecki, L., N. Follea, J. Vallieres, and J. Leblanc. "Beta-Adrenergic Receptors in Brown-Adipose Tissue. Characterization and Alterations During Acclimation of Rats to Cold." *Eur J Biochem* 92, no. 1 (Dec 1 1978): 189–196.

Bukowiecki, L. J., A. Geloen, and A. J. Collet. "Proliferation and Differentiation of Brown Adipocytes from Interstitial Cells During Cold Acclimation." *Am J Phys* 250, no. 6 Pt 1 (Jun 1986): C880-7.

Camell, C. D., J. Sander, O. Spadaro, A. Lee, K. Y. Nguyen, A. Wing, E. L. Goldberg, et al. "Inflammasome-Driven Catecholamine Catabolism in Macrophages Blunts Lipolysis During Ageing." *Nature* 550, no. 7674 (Oct 5 2017): 119–123.

Cannon, B., and J. Nedergaard. "Brown Adipose Tissue: Function and Physiological Significance." *Physiol Rev* 84, no. 1 (Jan 2004): 277–359.

Cano, G., A. M. Passerin, J. C. Schiltz, J. P. Card, S. F. Morrison, and A. F. Sved. "Anatomical Substrates for the Central Control of Sympathetic Outflow to Interscapular Adipose Tissue During Cold Exposure." *J Comp Neurol* 460, no. 3 (Jun 2 2003): 303–326.

Cao, W. H., W. Fan, and S. F. Morrison. "Medullary Pathways Mediating Specific Sympathetic Responses to Activation of Dorsomedial Hypothalamus." *Neuroscience* 126, no. 1 (2004): 229–240.

Cao, Y. "Angiogenesis and Vascular Functions in Modulation of Obesity, Adipose Metabolism, and Insulin Sensitivity." *Cell Metab* 18, no. 4 (Oct 1 2013): 478–489.

Cao, Y., H. Wang, Q. Wang, X. Han, and W. Zeng. "Three-Dimensional Volume Fluorescence-Imaging of Vascular Plasticity in Adipose Tissues." *Mol Metab* 14 (Aug 2018a): 71–81.

Cao, Y., H. Wang, and W. Zeng. "Whole-Tissue 3d Imaging Reveals Intra-Adipose Sympathetic Plasticity Regulated by Ngf-Trka Signal in Cold-Induced Beiging." *Protein Cell* 9, no. 6 (Jun 2018b): 527–539.

Caron, A., H. M. Dungan Lemko, C. M. Castorena, T. Fujikawa, S. Lee, C. C. Lord, N. Ahmed, et al. "Pomc Neurons Expressing Leptin Receptors Coordinate Metabolic Responses to Fasting Via Suppression of Leptin Levels." *elife* 7 (Mar 12 2018a).

Caron, A., S. Lee, J. K. Elmquist, and L. Gautron. "Leptin and Brain-Adipose Crosstalks." *Nat Rev Neurosci* 19, no. 3 (Feb 16 2018b): 153–165.

Caron, A., R. P. Reynolds, C. M. Castorena, N. J. Michael, C. E. Lee, S. Lee, R. Berdeaux, P. E. Scherer, and J. K. Elmquist. "Adipocyte Gs but Not Gi Signaling Regulates Whole-Body Glucose Homeostasis." *Mol Metab* 27 (Sep 2019): 11–21.

Chi, J., Z. Wu, C. H. J. Choi, L. Nguyen, S. Tegegne, S. E. Ackerman, A. Crane, et al. "Three-Dimensional Adipose Tissue Imaging Reveals Regional Variation in Beige Fat Biogenesis and Prdm16-Dependent Sympathetic Neurite Density." *Cell Metab* 27, no. 1 (Jan 9 2018): 226–36 e3.

Chouchani, E. T., L. Kazak, and B. M. Spiegelman. "New Advances in Adaptive Thermogenesis: Ucp1 and Beyond." *Cell Metab* 29, no. 1 (Jan 8 2019): 27–37.

Christensen, C. R., P. B. Clark, and K. A. Morton. "Reversal of Hypermetabolic Brown Adipose Tissue in F-18 Fdg Pet Imaging." *Clin Nucl Med* 31, no. 4 (Apr 2006): 193–196.

Cinti, S. "Adipose Organ Development and Remodeling." *Compr Physiol* 8, no. 4 (Sep 14 2018): 1357–1431.

———. "Anatomy and Physiology of the Nutritional System." *Mol Asp Med* 68 (Aug 2019): 101–107.

———. "Transdifferentiation Properties of Adipocytes in the Adipose Organ." *Am J Physiol Endocrinol Metab* 297, no. 5 (Nov 2009): E977–E986.

Collins, S. "Beta-Adrenoceptor Signaling Networks in Adipocytes for Recruiting Stored Fat and Energy Expenditure." *Front Endocrinol (Lausanne)* 2 (2011): 102.

Commins, S. P., P. M. Watson, N. Levin, R. J. Beiler, and T. W. Gettys. "Central Leptin Regulates the Ucp1 and Ob Genes in Brown and White Adipose Tissue Via Different Beta-Adrenoceptor Subtypes." *J Biol Chem* 275, no. 42 (Oct 20 2000): 33059–33067.

Commins, S. P., P. M. Watson, M. A. Padgett, A. Dudley, G. Argyropoulos, and T. W. Gettys. "Induction of Uncoupling Protein Expression in Brown and White Adipose Tissue by Leptin." *Endocrinology* 140, no. 1 (Jan 1999): 292–300.

Correll, J. W. "Adipose Tissue: Ability to Respond to Nerve Stimulation in Vitro." *Science* 140, no. 3565 (Apr 26 1963): 387–388.

Cousin, B., S. Cinti, M. Morroni, S. Raimbault, D. Ricquier, L. Penicaud, and L. Casteilla. "Occurrence of Brown Adipocytes in Rat White Adipose Tissue: Molecular and Morphological Characterization." *J Cell Sci* 103 (Pt 4) (Dec 1992): 931–942.

Crowley, C., S. D. Spencer, M. C. Nishimura, K. S. Chen, S. Pitts-Meek, M. P. Armanini, L. H. Ling, et al. "Mice Lacking Nerve Growth Factor Display Perinatal Loss of Sensory and Sympathetic Neurons yet Develop Basal Forebrain Cholinergic Neurons." *Cell* 76, no. 6 (Mar 25 1994): 1001–1011.

Cypess, A. M., S. Lehman, G. Williams, I. Tal, D. Rodman, A. B. Goldfine, F. C. Kuo, et al. "Identification and Importance of Brown Adipose Tissue in Adult Humans." *N Engl J Med* 360, no. 15 (Apr 9 2009): 1509–1517.

Cypess, A. M., A. P. White, C. Vernochet, T. J. Schulz, R. Xue, C. A. Sass, T. L. Huang, et al. "Anatomical Localization, Gene Expression Profiling and Functional Characterization of Adult Human Neck Brown Fat." *Nat Med* 19, no. 5 (May 2013): 635–639.

Czaja, K., C. R. Barb, and R. R. Kraeling. "Hypothalamic Neurons Innervating Fat Tissue in the Pig Express Leptin Receptor Immunoreactivity." *Neurosci Lett* 425, no. 1 (Sep 20 2007): 6–11.

Czaja, K., R. R. Kraeling, and C. R. Barb. "Are Hypothalamic Neurons Transsynaptically Connected to Porcine Adipose Tissue?". *Biochem Biophys Res Commun* 311, no. 2 (Nov 14 2003): 482–485.

De Matteis, R., D. Ricquier, and S. Cinti. "Th-, Npy-, Sp-, and Cgrp-Immunoreactive Nerves in Interscapular Brown Adipose Tissue of Adult Rats Acclimated at Different Temperatures: An Immunohistochemical Study." *J Neurocytol* 27, no. 12 (Dec 1998): 877–886.

Demas, G. E., and T. J. Bartness. "Direct Innervation of White Fat and Adrenal Medullary Catecholamines Mediate Photoperiodic Changes in Body Fat." *Am J Phys Regul Integr Comp Phys* 281, no. 5 (Nov 2001): R1499–R1505.

Deng, C., M. Moinat, L. Curtis, A. Nadakal, F. Preitner, O. Boss, F. Assimacopoulos-Jeannet, J. Seydoux, and J. P. Giacobino. "Effects of Beta-Adrenoceptor Subtype Stimulation on Obese Gene Messenger Ribonucleic Acid and on Leptin Secretion in Mouse Brown Adipocytes Differentiated in Culture." *Endocrinology* 138, no. 2 (Feb 1997): 548–552.

Diculescu, I., and M. Stoica. "Fluorescence Histochemical Investigation on the Adrenergic Innervation of the White Adipose Tissue in the Rat." *J Neurovisc Relat* 32, no. 1 (1970): 25–36.

Dodd, G. T., S. Decherf, K. Loh, S. E. Simonds, F. Wiede, E. Balland, T. L. Merry, et al. "Leptin and Insulin Act on Pomc Neurons to Promote the Browning of White Fat." *Cell* 160, no. 1–2 (Jan 15 2015): 88–104.

Fain, J. N., and J. A. Garcija-Sainz. "Adrenergic Regulation of Adipocyte Metabolism." *J Lipid Res* 24, no. 8 (Aug 1983): 945–966.

Feldmann, H. M., V. Golozoubova, B. Cannon, and J. Nedergaard. "Ucp1 Ablation Induces Obesity and Abolishes Diet-Induced Thermogenesis in Mice Exempt from Thermal Stress by Living at Thermoneutrality." *Cell Metab* 9, no. 2 (Feb 2009): 203–209.

Fishman, R. B., and J. Dark. "Sensory Innervation of White Adipose Tissue." *Am J Phys* 253, no. 6 Pt 2 (Dec 1987): R942–R944.

Foster, M. T., and T. J. Bartness. "Sympathetic but Not Sensory Denervation Stimulates White Adipocyte Proliferation." *Am J Phys Regul Integr Comp Phys* 291, no. 6 (Dec 2006): R1630–R1637.

Francois, M., H. Torres, C. Huesing, R. Zhang, C. Saurage, N. Lee, E. Qualls-Creekmore, et al. "Sympathetic Innervation of the Interscapular Brown Adipose Tissue in Mouse." *Ann N Y Acad Sci* 1454, no. 1 (Oct 2019): 3–13.

Friedman, J. "Leptin and the Regulation of Food Intake and Body Weight." *J Nutr Sci Vitaminol (Tokyo)* 61 Suppl (2015): S202.

———. "The Long Road to Leptin." *J Clin Invest* 126, no. 12 (Dec 1 2016): 4727–4734.

Funcke, J. B., and P. E. Scherer. "Beyond Adiponectin and Leptin: Adipose Tissue-Derived Mediators of Inter-Organ Communication." *J Lipid Res* 60, no. 10 (Oct 2019): 1648–1684.

Gao, M., X. Huang, B. L. Song, and H. Yang. "The Biogenesis of Lipid Droplets: Lipids Take Center Stage." *Prog Lipid Res* 75 (Jul 2019): 100989.

Garofalo, M. A., I. C. Kettelhut, J. E. Roselino, and R. H. Migliorini. "Effect of Acute Cold Exposure on Norepinephrine Turnover Rates in Rat White Adipose Tissue." *J Auton Nerv Syst* 60, no. 3 (Sep 12 1996): 206–208.

Garretson, J. T., L. A. Szymanski, G. J. Schwartz, B. Xue, V. Ryu, and T. J. Bartness. "Lipolysis Sensation by White Fat Afferent Nerves Triggers Brown Fat Thermogenesis." *Mol Metab* 5, no. 8 (Aug 2016): 626–634.

Geloen, A., A. J. Collet, and L. J. Bukowiecki. "Role of Sympathetic Innervation in Brown Adipocyte Proliferation." *Am J Phys* 263, no. 6 Pt 2 (Dec 1992): R1176–R1181.

Gettys, T. W., P. J. Harkness, and P. M. Watson. "The Beta 3-Adrenergic Receptor Inhibits Insulin-Stimulated Leptin Secretion from Isolated Rat Adipocytes." *Endocrinology* 137, no. 9 (Sep 1996): 4054–4057.

Ghaben, A. L., and P. E. Scherer. "Adipogenesis and Metabolic Health." *Nat Rev Mol Cell Biol* 20, no. 4 (Apr 2019): 242–258.

Ghorbani, M., and J. Himms-Hagen. "Appearance of Brown Adipocytes in White Adipose Tissue During Cl 316,243-Induced Reversal of Obesity and Diabetes in Zucker Fa/Fa Rats." *Int J Obes Relat Metab Disord* 21, no. 6 (Jun 1997): 465–475.

Giordano, A., A. Frontini, and S. Cinti. "Convertible Visceral Fat as a Therapeutic Target to Curb Obesity." *Nat Rev Drug Discov* 15, no. 6 (Jun 2016): 405–424.

Giordano, A., A. Frontini, I. Murano, C. Tonello, M. A. Marino, M. O. Carruba, E. Nisoli, and S. Cinti. "Regional-Dependent Increase of Sympathetic Innervation in Rat White Adipose Tissue During Prolonged Fasting." *J Histochem Cytochem* 53, no. 6 (Jun 2005): 679–687.

Giordano, A., M. Morroni, F. Carle, R. Gesuita, G. F. Marchesi, and S. Cinti. "Sensory Nerves Affect the Recruitment and Differentiation of Rat Periovarian Brown Adipocytes During Cold Acclimation." *J Cell Sci* 111 (Pt 17) (Sep 1998): 2587–2594.

Giordano, A., M. Morroni, G. Santone, G. F. Marchesi, and S. Cinti. "Tyrosine Hydroxylase, Neuropeptide Y, Substance P, Calcitonin Gene-Related Peptide and Vasoactive Intestinal Peptide in Nerves of Rat Periovarian Adipose Tissue: An Immunohistochemical and Ultrastructural Investigation." *J Neurocytol* 25, no. 2 (Feb 1996): 125–136.

Giordano, A., C. K. Song, R. R. Bowers, J. C. Ehlen, A. Frontini, S. Cinti, and T. J. Bartness. "White Adipose Tissue Lacks Significant Vagal Innervation and Immunohistochemical Evidence of Parasympathetic Innervation." *Am J Phys Regul Integr Comp Phys* 291, no. 5 (Nov 2006): R1243–R1255.

Glebova, N. O., and D. D. Ginty. "Heterogeneous Requirement of Ngf for Sympathetic Target Innervation in Vivo." *J Neurosci* 24, no. 3 (Jan 21 2004): 743–751.

Golozoubova, V., B. Cannon, and J. Nedergaard. "Ucp1 Is Essential for Adaptive Adrenergic Nonshivering Thermogenesis." *Am J Physiol Endocrinol Metab* 291, no. 2 (Aug 2006): E350–E357.

Grassi, G., A. Biffi, G. Seravalle, F. Q. Trevano, R. Dell'Oro, G. Corrao, and G. Mancia. "Sympathetic Neural Overdrive in the Obese and Overweight State." *Hypertension* 74, no. 2 (Aug 2019): 349–358.

Guilherme, A., F. Henriques, A. H. Bedard, and M. P. Czech. "Molecular Pathways Linking Adipose Innervation to Insulin Action in Obesity and Diabetes Mellitus." *Nat Rev Endocrinol* 15, no. 4 (Apr 2019): 207–225.

Guilherme, A., D. J. Pedersen, E. Henchey, F. S. Henriques, L. V. Danai, Y. Shen, B. Yenilmez, et al. "Adipocyte Lipid Synthesis Coupled to Neuronal Control of Thermogenic Programming." *Mol Metab* 6, no. 8 (Aug 2017): 781–796.

Guilherme, A., D. J. Pedersen, F. Henriques, A. H. Bedard, E. Henchey, M. Kelly, D. A. Morgan, K. Rahmouni, and M. P. Czech. "Neuronal Modulation of Brown Adipose Activity through Perturbation of White Adipocyte Lipogenesis." *Mol Metab* 16 (Oct 2018): 116–125.

Guilherme, A., J. V. Virbasius, V. Puri, and M. P. Czech. "Adipocyte Dysfunctions Linking Obesity to Insulin Resistance and Type 2 Diabetes." *Nat Rev Mol Cell Biol* 9, no. 5 (May 2008): 367–377.

Haemmerle, G., A. Lass, R. Zimmermann, G. Gorkiewicz, C. Meyer, J. Rozman, G. Heldmaier, et al. "Defective Lipolysis and Altered Energy Metabolism in Mice Lacking Adipose Triglyceride Lipase." *Science* 312, no. 5774 (May 5 2006): 734–737.

Hanssen, M. J., A. A. van der Lans, B. Brans, J. Hoeks, K. M. Jardon, G. Schaart, F. M. Mottaghy, P. Schrauwen, and W. D. van Marken Lichtenbelt. "Short-Term Cold Acclimation Recruits Brown Adipose Tissue in Obese Humans." *Diabetes* 65, no. 5 (May 2016): 1179–1189.

Harms, M., and P. Seale. "Brown and Beige Fat: Development, Function and Therapeutic Potential." *Nat Med* 19, no. 10 (Oct 2013): 1252–1263.

Haynes, W. G., D. A. Morgan, A. Djalali, W. I. Sivitz, and A. L. Mark. "Interactions between the Melanocortin System and Leptin in Control of Sympathetic Nerve Traffic." *Hypertension* 33, no. 1 Pt 2 (Jan 1999): 542–547.

Hu, B., C. Jin, X. Zeng, J. M. Resch, M. P. Jedrychowski, Z. Yang, B. N. Desai, et al. "Gammadelta T Cells and Adipocyte Il-17rc Control Fat Innervation and Thermogenesis." *Nature* 578, no. 7796 (Feb 2020): 610–614.

Ikeda, K., P. Maretich, and S. Kajimura. "The Common and Distinct Features of Brown and Beige Adipocytes." *Trends Endocrinol Metab* 29, no. 3 (Mar 2018): 191–200.

Intaglietta, M., and S. Rosell. "Capillary Permeability and Sympathetic Activity in Canine Subcutaneous Adipose Tissue." *Nature* 249, no. 456 (May 31 1974): 481–482.

Jenkins, C. M., D. J. Mancuso, W. Yan, H. F. Sims, B. Gibson, and R. W. Gross. "Identification, Cloning, Expression, and Purification of Three Novel Human Calcium-Independent Phospholipase A2 Family Members Possessing Triacylglycerol Lipase and Acylglycerol Transacylase Activities." *J Biol Chem* 279, no. 47 (Nov 19 2004): 48968–48975.

Jiang, H., X. Ding, Y. Cao, H. Wang, and W. Zeng. "Dense Intra-Adipose Sympathetic Arborizations Are Essential for Cold-Induced Beiging of Mouse White Adipose Tissue." *Cell Metab* 26, no. 4 (Oct 3 2017): 686–692.

Jimenez, M., G. Barbatelli, R. Allevi, S. Cinti, J. Seydoux, J. P. Giacobino, P. Muzzin, and F. Preitner. "Beta 3-Adrenoceptor Knockout in C57bl/6j Mice Depresses the Occurrence of Brown Adipocytes in White Fat." *Eur J Biochem* 270, no. 4 (Feb 2003): 699–705.

Kajimura, S., and M. Saito. "A New Era in Brown Adipose Tissue Biology: Molecular Control of Brown Fat Development and Energy Homeostasis." *Annu Rev Physiol* 76 (2014): 225–249.

Kajimura, S., B. M. Spiegelman, and P. Seale. "Brown and Beige Fat: Physiological Roles Beyond Heat Generation." *Cell Metab* 22, no. 4 (Oct 6 2015): 546–559.

Kershaw, E. E., and J. S. Flier. "Adipose Tissue as an Endocrine Organ." *J Clin Endocrinol Metab* 89, no. 6 (Jun 2004): 2548–2556.

Kir, S., J. P. White, S. Kleiner, L. Kazak, P. Cohen, V. E. Baracos, and B. M. Spiegelman. "Tumour-Derived Pth-Related Protein Triggers Adipose Tissue Browning and Cancer Cachexia." *Nature* 513, no. 7516 (Sep 4 2014): 100–104.

Kreier, F., Y. S. Kap, T. C. Mettenleiter, C. van Heijningen, J. van der Vliet, A. Kalsbeek, H. P. Sauerwein, et al. "Tracing from Fat Tissue, Liver, and Pancreas: A Neuroanatomical Framework for the Role of the Brain in Type 2 Diabetes." *Endocrinology* 147, no. 3 (Mar 2006): 1140–1147.

Kuruvilla, R., L. S. Zweifel, N. O. Glebova, B. E. Lonze, G. Valdez, H. Ye, and D. D. Ginty. "A Neurotrophin Signaling Cascade Coordinates Sympathetic Neuron Development through Differential Control of Trka Trafficking and Retrograde Signaling." *Cell* 118, no. 2 (Jul 23 2004): 243–255.

Labbe, S. M., A. Caron, D. Lanfray, B. Monge-Rofarello, T. J. Bartness, and D. Richard. "Hypothalamic Control of Brown Adipose Tissue Thermogenesis." *Front Syst Neurosci* 9 (2015): 150.

Landsberg, L. "Feast or Famine: The Sympathetic Nervous System Response to Nutrient Intake." *Cell Mol Neurobiol* 26, no. 4–6 (Jul–Aug 2006): 497–508.

Landsberg, L., and J. B. Young. "Fasting, Feeding and Regulation of the Sympathetic Nervous System." *N Engl J Med* 298, no. 23 (Jun 8 1978): 1295–1301.

Lass, A., R. Zimmermann, G. Haemmerle, M. Riederer, G. Schoiswohl, M. Schweiger, P. Kienesberger, et al. "Adipose Triglyceride Lipase-Mediated Lipolysis of Cellular Fat Stores Is Activated by Cgi-58 and Defective in Chanarin-Dorfman Syndrome." *Cell Metab* 3, no. 5 (May 2006): 309–319.

Lean, M. E., W. P. James, G. Jennings, and P. Trayhurn. "Brown Adipose Tissue Uncoupling Protein Content in Human Infants, Children and Adults." *Clin Sci (Lond)* 71, no. 3 (Sep 1986): 291–297.

Lee, P., S. Smith, J. Linderman, A. B. Courville, R. J. Brychta, W. Dieckmann, C. D. Werner, K. Y. Chen, and F. S. Celi. "Temperature-Acclimated Brown Adipose Tissue Modulates Insulin Sensitivity in Humans." *Diabetes* 63, no. 11 (Nov 2014): 3686–3698.

Lee, Y. H., A. P. Petkova, A. A. Konkar, and J. G. Granneman. "Cellular Origins of Cold-Induced Brown Adipocytes in Adult Mice." *FASEB J* 29, no. 1 (Jan 2015): 286–299.

Leitner, B. P., S. Huang, R. J. Brychta, C. J. Duckworth, A. S. Baskin, S. McGehee, I. Tal, et al. "Mapping of Human Brown Adipose Tissue in Lean and Obese Young Men." *Proc Natl Acad Sci U S A* 114, no. 32 (Aug 8 2017): 8649–8654.

Lever, J. D., S. Mukherjee, D. Norman, D. Symons, and R. T. Jung. "Neuropeptide and Noradrenaline Distributions in Rat Interscapular Brown Fat and in Its Intact and Obstructed Nerves of Supply." *J Auton Nerv Syst* 25, no. 1 (Nov 1988): 15–25.

Lidell, M. E., M. J. Betz, O. Dahlqvist Leinhard, M. Heglind, L. Elander, M. Slawik, T. Mussack, et al. "Evidence for Two Types of Brown Adipose Tissue in Humans." *Nat Med* 19, no. 5 (May 2013): 631–634.

Loncar, D., B. A. Afzelius, and B. Cannon. "Epididymal White Adipose Tissue after Cold Stress in Rats. I. Nonmitochondrial Changes." *J Ultrastruct Mol Struct Res* 101, no. 2–3 (Nov–Dec 1988): 109–122.

Mantzoros, C. S., D. Qu, R. C. Frederich, V. S. Susulic, B. B. Lowell, E. Maratos-Flier, and J. S. Flier. "Activation of Beta(3) Adrenergic Receptors Suppresses Leptin Expression and Mediates a Leptin-Independent Inhibition of Food Intake in Mice." *Diabetes* 45, no. 7 (Jul 1996): 909–914.

Moinat, M., C. Deng, P. Muzzin, F. Assimacopoulos-Jeannet, J. Seydoux, A. G. Dulloo, and J. P. Giacobino. "Modulation of Obese Gene Expression in Rat Brown and White Adipose Tissues." *FEBS Lett* 373, no. 2 (Oct 9 1995): 131–134.

Morrison, S. F. "Central Neural Control of Thermoregulation and Brown Adipose Tissue." *Auton Neurosci* 196 (Apr 2016): 14–24.

Morrison, S. F., K. Nakamura, and C. J. Madden. "Central Control of Thermogenesis in Mammals." *Exp Physiol* 93, no. 7 (Jul 2008): 773–797.

Morrison, S. F., S. Ramamurthy, and J. B. Young. "Reduced Rearing Temperature Augments Responses in Sympathetic Outflow to Brown Adipose Tissue." *J Neurosci* 20, no. 24 (Dec 15 2000): 9264–9271.

Murano, I., G. Barbatelli, A. Giordano, and S. Cinti. "Noradrenergic Parenchymal Nerve Fiber Branching after Cold Acclimatisation Correlates with Brown Adipocyte Density in Mouse Adipose Organ." *J Anat* 214, no. 1 (Jan 2009): 171–178.

Nakamura, K., K. Matsumura, T. Hubschle, Y. Nakamura, H. Hioki, F. Fujiyama, Z. Boldogkoi, et al. "Identification of Sympathetic Premotor Neurons in Medullary Raphe Regions Mediating Fever and Other Thermoregulatory Functions." *J Neurosci* 24, no. 23 (Jun 9 2004): 5370–5380.

Nakamura, K., and S. F. Morrison. "Central Efferent Pathways Mediating Skin Cooling-Evoked Sympathetic Thermogenesis in Brown Adipose Tissue." *Am J Phys Regul Integr Comp Phys* 292, no. 1 (Jan 2007): R127–R136.

Nedergaard, J., T. Bengtsson, and B. Cannon. "Unexpected Evidence for Active Brown Adipose Tissue in Adult Humans." *Am J Physiol Endocrinol Metab* 293, no. 2 (Aug 2007): E444–E452.

Nguyen, N. L., C. L. Barr, V. Ryu, Q. Cao, B. Xue, and T. J. Bartness. "Separate and Shared Sympathetic Outflow to White and Brown Fat Coordinately Regulates Thermoregulation and Beige Adipocyte Recruitment." *Am J Phys Regul Integr Comp Phys* 312, no. 1 (Jan 1 2017): R132–RR45.

Nguyen, N. L., J. Randall, B. W. Banfield, and T. J. Bartness. "Central Sympathetic Innervations to Visceral and Subcutaneous White Adipose Tissue." *Am J Phys Regul Integr Comp Phys* 306, no. 6 (Mar 15 2014): R375–R386.

Nguyen, N. L. T., B. Xue, and T. J. Bartness. "Sensory Denervation of Inguinal White Fat Modifies Sympathetic Outflow to White and Brown Fat in Siberian Hamsters." *Physiol Behav* 190 (Jun 1 2018): 28–33.

Nishizawa, Y., and G. A. Bray. "Ventromedial Hypothalamic Lesions and the Mobilization of Fatty Acids." *J Clin Invest* 61, no. 3 (Mar 1978): 714–721.

Nnodim, J. O., and J. D. Lever. "Neural and Vascular Provisions of Rat Interscapular Brown Adipose Tissue." *Am J Anat* 182, no. 3 (Jul 1988): 283–293.

Norman, D., S. Mukherjee, D. Symons, R. T. Jung, and J. D. Lever. "Neuropeptides in Interscapular and Perirenal Brown Adipose Tissue in the Rat: A Plurality of Innervation." *J Neurocytol* 17, no. 3 (Jun 1988): 305–311.

Oberg, B., and S. Rosell. "Sympathetic Control of Consecutive Vascular Sections in Canine Subcutaneous Adipose Tissue." *Acta Physiol Scand* 71, no. 1 (Sep 1967): 47–56.

Oldfield, B. J., M. E. Giles, A. Watson, C. Anderson, L. M. Colvill, and M. J. McKinley. "The Neurochemical Characterisation of Hypothalamic Pathways Projecting Polysynaptically to Brown Adipose Tissue in the Rat." *Neuroscience* 110, no. 3 (2002): 515–526.

Ouchi, N., J. L. Parker, J. J. Lugus, and K. Walsh. "Adipokines in Inflammation and Metabolic Disease." *Nat Rev Immunol* 11, no. 2 (Feb 2011): 85–97.

Pellegrinelli, V., V. J. Peirce, L. Howard, S. Virtue, D. Turei, M. Senzacqua, A. Frontini, et al. "Adipocyte-Secreted Bmp8b Mediates Adrenergic-Induced Remodeling of the Neuro-Vascular Network in Adipose Tissue." *Nat Commun* 9, no. 1 (Nov 26 2018): 4974.

Petrovic, N., T. B. Walden, I. G. Shabalina, J. A. Timmons, B. Cannon, and J. Nedergaard. "Chronic Peroxisome Proliferator-Activated Receptor Gamma (Ppargamma) Activation of Epididymally Derived White Adipocyte Cultures Reveals a Population of Thermogenically Competent, Ucp1-Containing Adipocytes Molecularly Distinct from Classic Brown Adipocytes." *J Biol Chem* 285, no. 10 (Mar 5 2010): 7153–7164.

Petruzzelli, M., M. Schweiger, R. Schreiber, R. Campos-Olivas, M. Tsoli, J. Allen, M. Swarbrick, et al. "A Switch from White to Brown Fat Increases Energy Expenditure in Cancer-Associated Cachexia." *Cell Metab* 20, no. 3 (Sep 2 2014): 433–447.

Pirzgalska, R. M., E. Seixas, J. S. Seidman, V. M. Link, N. M. Sanchez, I. Mahu, R. Mendes, et al. "Sympathetic Neuron-Associated Macrophages Contribute to Obesity by Importing and Metabolizing Norepinephrine." *Nat Med* 23, no. 11 (Nov 2017): 1309–1318.

Rosell, S. "Release of Free Fatty Acids from Subcutaneous Adipose Tissue in Dogs Following Sympathetic Nerve Stimulation." *Acta Physiol Scand* 67, no. 3 (Jul–Aug 1966): 343–351.

Rosell, S., and E. Belfrage. "Blood Circulation in Adipose Tissue." *Physiol Rev* 59, no. 4 (Oct 1979): 1078–1104.

Rosen, E. D., and B. M. Spiegelman. "What We Talk About When We Talk About Fat." *Cell* 156, no. 1–2 (Jan 16 2014): 20–44.

Rothwell, N. J., and M. J. Stock. "A Role for Brown Adipose Tissue in Diet-Induced Thermogenesis." *Nature* 281, no. 5726 (Sep 6 1979): 31–35.

Rousset, S., M. C. Alves-Guerra, J. Mozo, B. Miroux, A. M. Cassard-Doulcier, F. Bouillaud, and D. Ricquier. "The Biology of Mitochondrial Uncoupling Proteins." *Diabetes* 53 Suppl 1 (Feb 2004): S130–S135.

Rutkowski, J. M., K. E. Davis, and P. E. Scherer. "Mechanisms of Obesity and Related Pathologies: The Macro- and Microcirculation of Adipose Tissue." *FEBS J* 276, no. 20 (Oct 2009): 5738–5746.

Ryu, V., J. T. Garretson, Y. Liu, C. H. Vaughan, and T. J. Bartness. "Brown Adipose Tissue Has Sympathetic-Sensory Feedback Circuits." *J Neurosci* 35, no. 5 (Feb 4 2015): 2181–2190.

Saito, M., Y. Okamatsu-Ogura, M. Matsushita, K. Watanabe, T. Yoneshiro, J. Nio-Kobayashi, T. Iwanaga, et al. "High Incidence of Metabolically Active Brown Adipose Tissue in Healthy Adult Humans: Effects of Cold Exposure and Adiposity." *Diabetes* 58, no. 7 (Jul 2009): 1526–1531.

Satoh, N., Y. Ogawa, G. Katsuura, Y. Numata, T. Tsuji, M. Hayase, K. Ebihara, et al. "Sympathetic Activation of Leptin Via the Ventromedial Hypothalamus: Leptin-Induced Increase in Catecholamine Secretion." *Diabetes* 48, no. 9 (Sep 1999): 1787–1793.

Scarpace, P. J., and M. Matheny. "Leptin Induction of Ucp1 Gene Expression Is Dependent on Sympathetic Innervation." *Am J Phys* 275, no. 2 (Aug 1998): E259–E264.

Seale, P., H. M. Conroe, J. Estall, S. Kajimura, A. Frontini, J. Ishibashi, P. Cohen, S. Cinti, and B. M. Spiegelman. "Prdm16 Determines the Thermogenic Program of Subcutaneous White Adipose Tissue in Mice." *J Clin Invest* 121, no. 1 (Jan 2011): 96–105.

Sharp, L. Z., K. Shinoda, H. Ohno, D. W. Scheel, E. Tomoda, L. Ruiz, H. Hu, et al. "Human Bat Possesses Molecular Signatures That Resemble Beige/Brite Cells." *PLoS One* 7, no. 11 (2012): e49452.

Shi, H., and T. J. Bartness. "Neurochemical Phenotype of Sympathetic Nervous System Outflow from Brain to White Fat." *Brain Res Bull* 54, no. 4 (Mar 1 2001): 375–385.

Shi, H.. "White Adipose Tissue Sensory Nerve Denervation Mimics Lipectomy-Induced Compensatory Increases in Adiposity." *Am J Phys Regul Integr Comp Phys* 289, no. 2 (Aug 2005): R514–RR20.

Shi, H., C. K. Song, A. Giordano, S. Cinti, and T. J. Bartness. "Sensory or Sympathetic White Adipose Tissue Denervation Differentially Affects Depot Growth and Cellularity." *Am J Phys Regul Integr Comp Phys* 288, no. 4 (Apr 2005): R1028–R1037.

Shinoda, K., I. H. Luijten, Y. Hasegawa, H. Hong, S. B. Sonne, M. Kim, R. Xue, et al. "Genetic and Functional Characterization of Clonally Derived Adult Human Brown Adipocytes." *Nat Med* 21, no. 4 (Apr 2015): 389–394.

Sidman, R. L., and D. W. Fawcett. "The Effect of Peripheral Nerve Section on Some Metabolic Responses of Brown Adipose Tissue in Mice." *Anat Rec* 118, no. 3 (Mar 1954): 487–507.

Slavin, B. G., and K. W. Ballard. "Morphological Studies on the Adrenergic Innervation of White Adipose Tissue." *Anat Rec* 191, no. 3 (Jul 1978): 377–389.

Smalley, R. L., and R. L. Dryer. "Brown Fat: Thermogenic Effect During Arousal from Hibernation in the Bat." *Science* 140, no. 3573 (Jun 21 1963): 1333–1334.

Smith, R. E., and R. J. Hock. "Brown Fat: Thermogenic Effector of Arousal in Hibernators." *Science* 140, no. 3563 (Apr 12 1963): 199–200.

Soderlund, V., S. A. Larsson, and H. Jacobsson. "Reduction of Fdg Uptake in Brown Adipose Tissue in Clinical Patients by a Single Dose of Propranolol." *Eur J Nucl Med Mol Imaging* 34, no. 7 (Jul 2007): 1018–1022.

Song, C. K., and T. J. Bartness. "Cns Sympathetic Outflow Neurons to White Fat That Express Mel Receptors May Mediate Seasonal Adiposity." *Am J Phys Regul Integr Comp Phys* 281, no. 2 (Aug 2001): R666–R672.

Song, C. K., R. M. Jackson, R. B. Harris, D. Richard, and T. J. Bartness. "Melanocortin-4 Receptor Mrna Is Expressed in Sympathetic Nervous System Outflow Neurons to White Adipose Tissue." *Am J Phys Regul Integr Comp Phys* 289, no. 5 (Nov 2005): R1467–R1476.

Song, C. K., G. J. Schwartz, and T. J. Bartness. "Anterograde Transneuronal Viral Tract Tracing Reveals Central Sensory Circuits from White Adipose Tissue." *Am J Phys Regul Integr Comp Phys* 296, no. 3 (Mar 2009): R501–R511.

Song, C. K., C. H. Vaughan, E. Keen-Rhinehart, R. B. Harris, D. Richard, and T. J. Bartness. "Melanocortin-4 Receptor Mrna Expressed in Sympathetic Outflow Neurons to Brown Adipose Tissue: Neuroanatomical and Functional Evidence." *Am J Phys Regul Integr Comp Phys* 295, no. 2 (Aug 2008): R417–R428.

Stanley, S., S. Pinto, J. Segal, C. A. Perez, A. Viale, J. DeFalco, X. Cai, L. K. Heisler, and J. M. Friedman. "Identification of Neuronal Subpopulations That Project from Hypothalamus to Both Liver and Adipose Tissue Polysynaptically." *Proc Natl Acad Sci U S A* 107, no. 15 (Apr 13 2010): 7024–7029.

Stern, J. H., J. M. Rutkowski, and P. E. Scherer. "Adiponectin, Leptin, and Fatty Acids in the Maintenance of Metabolic Homeostasis through Adipose Tissue Crosstalk." *Cell Metab* 23, no. 5 (May 10 2016): 770–784.

Stock, K., and E. O. Westermann. "Concentration of Norepinephrine, Serotonin, and Histamine, and of Amine-Metabolizing Enzymes in Mammalian Adipose Tissue." *J Lipid Res* 4 (Jul 1963): 297–304.

Stornetta, R. L., D. L. Rosin, J. R. Simmons, T. J. McQuiston, N. Vujovic, M. C. Weston, and P. G. Guyenet. "Coexpression of Vesicular Glutamate Transporter-3 and Gamma-Aminobutyric Acidergic Markers in Rat Rostral Medullary Raphe and Intermediolateral Cell Column." *J Comp Neurol* 492, no. 4 (Nov 28 2005): 477–494.

Straub, L. G., and P. E. Scherer. "Metabolic Messengers: Adiponectin." [In English]. *Nat Meta* 1, no. 3 (Mar 2019): 334–339.

Takahashi, A., and T. Shimazu. "Hypothalamic Regulation of Lipid Metabolism in the Rat: Effect of Hypothalamic Stimulation on Lipolysis." *J Auton Nerv Syst* 4, no. 3 (Sep 1981): 195–205.

Trayhurn, P., J. S. Duncan, D. V. Rayner, and L. J. Hardie. "Rapid Inhibition of Ob Gene Expression and Circulating Leptin Levels in Lean Mice by the Beta 3-Adrenoceptor Agonists Brl 35135a and Zd2079." *Biochem Biophys Res Commun* 228, no. 2 (Nov 12 1996): 605–610.

Tsoli, M., M. Moore, D. Burg, A. Painter, R. Taylor, S. H. Lockie, N. Turner, et al. "Activation of Thermogenesis in Brown Adipose Tissue and Dysregulated Lipid Metabolism Associated with Cancer Cachexia in Mice." *Cancer Res* 72, no. 17 (Sep 1 2012): 4372–4382.

van der Lans, A. A., J. Hoeks, B. Brans, G. H. Vijgen, M. G. Visser, M. J. Vosselman, J. Hansen, et al. "Cold Acclimation Recruits Human Brown Fat and Increases Nonshivering Thermogenesis." *J Clin Invest* 123, no. 8 (Aug 2013): 3395–3403.

van Marken Lichtenbelt, W. D., J. W. Vanhommerig, N. M. Smulders, J. M. Drossaerts, G. J. Kemerink, N. D. Bouvy, P. Schrauwen, and G. J. Teule. "Cold-Activated Brown Adipose Tissue in Healthy Men." *N Engl J Med* 360, no. 15 (Apr 9 2009): 1500–1508.

Vaughan, M., J. E. Berger, and D. Steinberg. "Hormone-Sensitive Lipase and Monoglyceride Lipase Activities in Adipose Tissue." *J Biol Chem* 239 (Feb 1964): 401–409.

Villarroya, F., R. Cereijo, J. Villarroya, and M. Giralt. "Brown Adipose Tissue as a Secretory Organ." *Nat Rev Endocrinol* 13, no. 1 (Jan 2017): 26–35.

Villena, J. A., S. Roy, E. Sarkadi-Nagy, K. H. Kim, and H. S. Sul. "Desnutrin, an Adipocyte Gene Encoding a Novel Patatin Domain-Containing Protein, Is Induced by Fasting and Glucocorticoids: Ectopic Expression of Desnutrin Increases Triglyceride Hydrolysis." *J Biol Chem* 279, no. 45 (Nov 5 2004): 47066–47075.

Virtanen, K. A., M. E. Lidell, J. Orava, M. Heglind, R. Westergren, T. Niemi, M. Taittonen, et al. "Functional Brown Adipose Tissue in Healthy Adults." *N Engl J Med* 360, no. 15 (Apr 9 2009): 1518–1525.

Walther, T. C., J. Chung, and R. V. Farese, Jr. "Lipid Droplet Biogenesis." *Annu Rev Cell Dev Biol* 33 (Oct 6 2017): 491–510.

Wang, G. X., X. Y. Zhao, Z. X. Meng, M. Kern, A. Dietrich, Z. Chen, Z. Cozacov, et al. "The Brown Fat-Enriched Secreted Factor Nrg4 Preserves Metabolic Homeostasis through Attenuation of Hepatic Lipogenesis." *Nat Med* 20, no. 12 (Dec 2014): 1436–1443.

Wang, Q. A., C. Tao, R. K. Gupta, and P. E. Scherer. "Tracking Adipogenesis During White Adipose Tissue Development, Expansion and Regeneration." *Nat Med* 19, no. 10 (Oct 2013): 1338–1344.

Wang, Q., V. P. Sharma, H. Shen, Y. Xiao, Q. Zhu, X. Xiong, L. Guo, et al. "The Hepatokine Tsukushi Gates Energy Expenditure Via Brown Fat Sympathetic Innervation." *Nat Metab* 1, no. 2 (Feb 2019): 251–260.

Wang, W. S., and P. Seale. "Control of Brown and Beige Fat Development." [In English]. *Nat Rev Mol Cell Biol* 17, no. 11 (Nov 2016): 691–702.

Weiner, N., M. Perkins, and R. L. Sidman. "Effect of Reserpine on Noradrenaline Content of Innervated and Denervated Brown Adipose Tissue of the Rat." *Nature* 193 (Jan 13 1962): 137–138.

Wirsen, C. "Distribution of Adrenergic Nerve Fibers in Brown and White Adipose Tissue." *Comp Physiol* (2010): 197–199.

Wirsén, Claes. "*Studies in Lipid Mobilization: With Special Reference to Morphological and Histochemical Aspects*." *Acta Physiol Scand* 65 (1965): 146.

Wu, J., P. Bostrom, L. M. Sparks, L. Ye, J. H. Choi, A. H. Giang, M. Khandekar, et al. "Beige Adipocytes Are a Distinct Type of Thermogenic Fat Cell in Mouse and Human." *Cell* 150, no. 2 (Jul 20 2012): 366–376.

Wu, Z., P. Puigserver, U. Andersson, C. Zhang, G. Adelmant, V. Mootha, A. Troy, et al. "Mechanisms Controlling Mitochondrial Biogenesis and Respiration through the Thermogenic Coactivator Pgc-1." *Cell* 98, no. 1 (Jul 9 1999): 115–124.

Xue, Y., N. Petrovic, R. Cao, O. Larsson, S. Lim, S. Chen, H. M. Feldmann, et al. "Hypoxia-Independent Angiogenesis in Adipose Tissues During Cold Acclimation." *Cell Metab* 9, no. 1 (Jan 7 2009): 99–109.

Yoneshiro, T., S. Aita, M. Matsushita, T. Kayahara, T. Kameya, Y. Kawai, T. Iwanaga, and M. Saito. "Recruited Brown Adipose Tissue as an Antiobesity Agent in Humans." *J Clin Invest* 123, no. 8 (Aug 2013): 3404–3408.

Yoshida, K., K. Nakamura, K. Matsumura, K. Kanosue, M. Konig, H. J. Thiel, Z. Boldogkoi, et al. "Neurons of the Rat Preoptic Area and the Raphe Pallidus Nucleus Innervating the Brown Adipose Tissue Express the Prostaglandin E Receptor Subtype Ep3." *Eur J Neurosci* 18, no. 7 (Oct 2003): 1848–1860.

Young, J. B., and L. Landsberg. "Stimulation of the Sympathetic Nervous System During Sucrose Feeding." *Nature* 269, no. 5629 (Oct 13 1977): 615–617.

Young, J. B.. "Suppression of Sympathetic Nervous System During Fasting." *Science* 196, no. 4297 (Jun 24 1977): 1473–1475.

Young, P., J. R. Arch, and M. Ashwell. "Brown Adipose Tissue in the Parametrial Fat Pad of the Mouse." *FEBS Lett* 167, no. 1 (Feb 13 1984): 10–14.

Young, S. G., and R. Zechner. "Biochemistry and Pathophysiology of Intravascular and Intracellular Lipolysis." *Genes Dev* 27, no. 5 (Mar 1 2013): 459–484.

Youngstrom, T. G., and T. J. Bartness. "Catecholaminergic Innervation of White Adipose Tissue in Siberian Hamsters." *Am J Phys* 268, no. 3 Pt 2 (Mar 1995): R744–R751.

Zeng, W., R. M. Pirzgalska, M. M. Pereira, N. Kubasova, A. Barateiro, E. Seixas, Y. H. Lu, et al. "Sympathetic Neuro-Adipose Connections Mediate Leptin-Driven Lipolysis." *Cell* 163, no. 1 (Sep 24 2015): 84–94.

Zeng, X., M. Ye, J. M. Resch, M. P. Jedrychowski, B. Hu, B. B. Lowell, D. D. Ginty, and B. M. Spiegelman. "Innervation of Thermogenic Adipose Tissue Via a Calsyntenin 3beta-S100b Axis." *Nature* 569, no. 7755 (May 2019): 229–235.

Zhang, Y., R. Proenca, M. Maffei, M. Barone, L. Leopold, and J. M. Friedman. "Positional Cloning of the Mouse Obese Gene and Its Human Homologue." *Nature* 372, no. 6505 (Dec 1 1994): 425–432.

Zhu, Y., Y. Gao, C. Tao, M. Shao, S. Zhao, W. Huang, T. Yao, et al. "Connexin 43 Mediates White Adipose Tissue Beiging by Facilitating the Propagation of Sympathetic Neuronal Signals." *Cell Metab* 24, no. 3 (Sep 13 2016): 420–433.

Zimmermann, R., J. G. Strauss, G. Haemmerle, G. Schoiswohl, R. Birner-Gruenberger, M. Riederer, A. Lass, et al. "Fat Mobilization in Adipose Tissue Is Promoted by Adipose Triglyceride Lipase." *Science* 306, no. 5700 (Nov 19 2004): 1383–1386.

Zingaretti, M. C., F. Crosta, A. Vitali, M. Guerrieri, A. Frontini, B. Cannon, J. Nedergaard, and S. Cinti. "The Presence of Ucp1 Demonstrates That Metabolically Active Adipose Tissue in the Neck of Adult Humans Truly Represents Brown Adipose Tissue." *FASEB J* 23, no. 9 (Sep 2009): 3113–3120.

12 Sex Differences in Feeding Regulated by Estrogen

Crosstalk between Dopaminergic Reward Circuitry and Adiposity Signals

Kristen N. Krolick, Danielle N. Tapp, Matthew S. McMurray and Haifei Shi
Miami University, USA

CONTENTS

12.1 INTRODUCTION

12.1.1 Feeding Behavior

Feeding behavior and homeostasis of energy metabolism are critical for survival. Accordingly, the neurobiology underlying these processes is constantly adapting to reflect the homeostatic needs of individual organisms, food availability and demands, and food wanting and value. Feeding is not only guided by the homeostatic energy needs that determine the number of calories ingested, but is also regulated by rewarding the value of food, which is associated with the sensory inputs of food such as smell and taste and is modulated by hunger and satiety states (Rolls 2012). This chapter discusses homeostatic and reward-associated brain regions underlying the behaviors of feeding pattern and food choice.

The term "feeding pattern" indicates various aspects of meals, such as meal size, timing, frequency, spacing, duration, rate, and regularity (Leech et al. 2015). The term "food choice" refers to which food individuals choose to eat when given a choice of two or more types of foods with different energy contents, caloric density, palatability, and nutrient composition. Individuals also assess metabolic consequences of the meal after consumption, learn the association between its sensory properties and metabolic consequences, and are motivated to select foods with favorable consequences for maintaining homeostasis (Day, Kyriazakis, and Rogers 1998). Thus, food choice is not only determined by metabolic signals, but is also regulated by motivation and learning (Anderson and Petrovich 2015, Day, Kyriazakis, and Rogers 1998). Altered feeding pattern and food choice, as observed in eating disorders, is driven in part by changes in the neural activity of reward circuits and homeostatic circuits that regulate "hedonic" and "homeostatic" feeding respectively (Morton et al. 2006).

While in this chapter we separate "hedonic" and "homeostatic" feeding for the sake of simplicity, it is important to note that the circuitries responsible for both are interconnected and have dynamic influence over each other (Hoebel and Teitelbaum 1962, Liu and Kanoski 2018, Margules and Olds 1962, Rossi and Stuber 2018). Homeostatic circuitry, mainly located in the hypothalamic and brainstem regions, is modulated by circulating signals such as adiposity hormones related to energy storage and gastrointestinal hormones associated with hunger, satiety, and related meal status (Woods 2009). Reward circuitry determines motivation and appetitive desire that occur before feeding and during a meal, both of which are modulated dynamically by the reward system and integrated with learning and memories associated with the food (Berridge 2009, Clark, Hollon, and Phillips 2012, Meneses and Liy-Salmeron 2012). The reward circuitry includes various brain anatomical structures, along with multiple neurotransmitters and neurohormones, such as dopamine (DA), serotonin, endocannabinoids, and many others. Effective regulation of feeding behavior requires appropriate integration of hedonic reward and homeostatic feeding circuitries with various brain regions that are important for emotional regulation, learning, and executive function. Although we limit the scope of this chapter to the DA system and circulating adiposity hormones, differential regulation of feeding by other neurotransmitters and circulating factors also exist between males and females (Asarian and Geary 2013, Chowen, Freire-Regatillo, and Argente 2019, Liu et al. 2019, Soriano-Guillén et al. 2016) and are in need of further study. Motivation to obtain food and homeostatic regulation of feeding can be increased or decreased depending on physiological energy status and meal-related signals, and could be associated with the presence of a reward, such as palatable and energy-dense foods. Therefore, various factors integrate and change neural activity, receptor expression, and function of reward and homeostatic circuitries to ultimately determine feeding behavior.

Dysfunction of the balance between metabolic regulation and motivation can lead to devastating consequences, as seen in the current obesity epidemic, with approximate 40% of adults and 20% of youth in the USA meeting the criterion for obesity (Hales et al. 2017). With obesity and its related metabolic disorders increasing in prevalence, hundreds of billions of US dollars are being spent each year to treat and prevent obesity and its related conditions (Friedrich 2017). Fundamental to our clinical and biological understanding of these diseases, sex differences are apparent in this crisis, with women demonstrating a higher prevalence of obesity than men (Friedrich 2017, Lovejoy, Sainsbury, and the Stock Conference Working 2009), but also with a higher percentage of women suggested to have metabolically healthy obesity compared to men (Palmer and Clegg 2015). Sex differences are also apparent in eating disorder symptoms and types, with more women than men exhibiting eating disorders (Hudson et al. 2007, Kinasz et al. 2016). It is thus imperative that we better understand the role of sex differences in the neural circuits involved in satiety and motivation, which underlie the sex differences seen in eating disorders and obesity, and reinforce the established need for sex-specific medicine (Clayton and Collins 2014).

12.1.2 Sex Differences in Eating Behaviors

Food choice and feeding pattern are the main determinants of feeding behaviors (Meule and Vögele 2013, Strubbe and Woods 2004), both of which could be influenced by sensory cues such as taste and caloric content. Brain neural circuitry activation in response to tastants differs between the sexes, dependent on physiological energy status and the specific properties of the tastants (Haase, Green, and Murphy 2011). Human brain imaging studies using functional magnetic resonance imaging (fMRI) have reported that viewing palatable, high-calorie foods stimulates brain activation to a greater extent than low-calorie foods, and these brain activation sites differ between the sexes (Killgore and Yurgelun-Todd 2010), indicating that men and women respond differentially to sensory cues associated with high-calorie food. Specifically, women show greater activation within cortical regions involved in cognition, food evaluation, and self-control, including the prefrontal cortex, cingulate, and insula (D'Argembeau et al. 2010, Pochon et al. 2001); while men show greater activation in regions associated with stress and emotional responses to environmental cues for detecting palatability and determining appetitive value of food, including limbic structures and the amygdala (Killgore and Yurgelun-Todd 2010, Piech et al. 2009). These neuroimaging studies support the existence of sex differences in food choice. In line with this, some data suggest that women are more concerned about diet and nutrition than men (Ek 2015, Rolls, Fedoroff, and Guthrie 1991) and consume more low-energy-content food such as fruits and vegetables than men (Arganini et al. 2012, Beer-Borst et al. 2000, Bere, Brug, and Klepp 2008, Grimm et al. 2010, Prättälä et al. 2007, Shiferaw et al. 2012, Wardle et al. 2004), while men tend to consume higher energy-content food such as meat and protein than women (Aparicio et al. 2017, Ledikwe et al. 2005, Shiferaw et al. 2012, Wansink, Cheney, and Chan 2003). To summarize, women tend to choose lower energy-content foods than men.

Although women choose healthy foods more often than men in general (Arganini et al. 2012), women could be more impulsive and susceptible to food reward than men, however. For many men and women, stress alters food choice towards increasing intake of palatable comfort food typically containing high amounts of carbohydrates and fats (Dallman et al. 2003). Eating a comfort food reduces stress responses in male rats; as well as diminishes stress, alleviates adverse feelings, and improves mood in people (Ulrich-Lai et al. 2015). A longitudinal study examining food choice has found that women choose mainly snack-related comfort foods generally thought of as less healthy, while men choose mainly meal-related comfort foods generally considered more nutritious (Wansink, Cheney, and Chan 2003). Further, more women than men report overeating when being stressed (Zellner et al. 2006, Zellner, Saito, and Gonzalez 2007). When stressed (Kandiah et al. 2006) or food with greater energy density is present (Aparicio et al. 2017, Ledikwe et al. 2005, Shiferaw et al. 2012, Wansink, Cheney, and Chan 2003), women prefer unhealthy sweet snacks and are more likely to choose mainly high-energy foods to increase their food intake. Related to sex differences in behavioral aspects of feeding and stress regulation, sex differences are also pervasive in metabolic regulation (Shi, Seeley, and Clegg 2009, Mauvais-Jarvis 2015, Xu and López 2018). It is noteworthy that understanding feeding behavior in humans is complex, as it is also influenced by many non-biological factors such as cultural influence, individual experience, and socioeconomic variables, which are not discussed in this chapter.

12.1.3 General Effects of Estrogen on Eating Behaviors

Estrogen is a major biological factor that differentiates in its levels and functions, and underlies many differences in feeding between males and females. Besides regulating reproduction, estrogen accounts for sex differences in energy balance via regulating feeding behavior and energy metabolism (Xu and López 2018). The prevalence of obesity among women varies significantly by age, which increases after menopause. Specifically, the incidence of obesity increases from 37.0% in women at age 20–39 to 44.6% in women at age 40–59, most of whom are menopausal (Flegal et al. 2016). Similarly, ovariectomized (OVX) rodents significantly increase their food intake and body weight gain (Asarian and Geary 2013). Additionally, in many species including humans, caloric intake changes across the estrous cycle due to changes in meal size, with females eating the most calories when estrogen levels are low (metestrous), and eating the fewest calories when estrogen levels are high immediately prior to ovulation (Asarian and Geary 2013).

Interestingly, suppression of caloric intake by estrogen ceases when palatable food choices are offered alongside the regular diet in female rhesus monkeys (Johnson et al. 2013). Following estrogen treatment, rhesus monkeys prefer a more palatable diet over the regular diet (Johnson et al. 2013). Furthermore, estrogen increases "snacking" behavior outside of regularly scheduled meals for both palatable and regular diet choices (Johnson et al. 2013). It is noteworthy that, in this study, dominance ranks were formed among rhesus monkeys as a social stressor. The effect of estrogen treatment on feeding behavior was not significantly impacted by social status in either dietary condition, suggesting that estrogen's effect on feeding behavior is primarily modulated by diet composition rather than exposure to social stress of subordination in female macaques (Johnson et al. 2013). Therefore, self-regulation of caloric intake in an obesogenic environment could be disturbed to a greater extent in females with higher levels of estrogen on average than males.

Phases of the estrous cycle not only affect quantity of food consumed, but also affect food choice, although reported findings of nutrient selection are not consistent between studies in either humans or rats (Geary 2004). For example, increased food cravings associated with protein intake during the luteal phase have been reported in women (Gorczyca et al. 2016), while a separate study has reported decreased protein intake during the luteal phase (Barbosa et al. 2015). Possible explanations for the inconsistencies in human studies could be due to a number of factors, including individual histories of food consumption, culture and ethnicity, and how food selection and intake are assessed. In animal studies, changes in macronutrient selection can be observed across phases of the estrous cycle, but also following administration of exogenous estrogen. However, even with this added control, disagreements still remain. One study in rats reported increased intake of carbohydrates during estrus, but decreased consumption of fat (Geiselman et al. 1981); while other studies reported increased intake of fat during estrus, but decreased intake of carbohydrate (Bartness and Waldbillig 1984, Heisler, Kanarek, and Homoleski 1999, Wurtman and Baum 1980). Such inconsistent findings in rodent studies are likely due to different properties of macronutrients being used for testing. Variation in fat or carbohydrate content among experimental choices may not be detectable by rodents or may be too exaggerated, causing aversion. Although the particular changes in macronutrient selection are inconsistent among different studies, most of the studies that compare macronutrient selection across the estrous cycle have indeed reported cycle-related fluctuation, even though the direction of such fluctuation varies. It is possible that cyclic changes of estrogen affect rewarding values of fat or carbohydrate, contributing to estrous cycle-related changes in macronutrient selection.

To summarize, the estrous cycle and associated changes in levels of estrogen appear to affect caloric intake based on energy status via homeostatic regulation, but affect macronutrient selection with the presence of an obesogenic diet via modifying reward processing that regulates pleasurable aspects associated with food reward. We propose that the hormone estrogen modulates reward circuitry to drive sex differences in both feeding pattern and food choice. In support of this, the remainder of this chapter explores human and animal studies regarding sex differences in dopaminergic (DA) reward circuitry that regulate feeding-related motivation and satiety. We primarily review the influences of estrogen and estrogen receptors in major DA pathways as an underlying mechanism for sex differences (Section 12.2); discuss interactions among these processes with homeostatic brain regions that regulate feeding behavior (Section 12.3); and discuss how dysfunction of these processes contribute to the development of obesity and eating disorders in men and women, and future research direction (Section 12.4).

12.2 ROLE OF DOPAMINERGIC SIGNALING IN SEX DIFFERENCES IN FEEDING BEHAVIORS

12.2.1 Dopamine Determines Feeding Pattern and Food Choice

The DA system is the most well-studied component of the reward and motivation system, and is involved in the processing of both the "rewarding" nature of foods during consumption and the sensory aspects of food predictive cues such as smell and taste (Baldo and Kelley 2007, Norgren, Hajnal, and Mungarndee 2006, Sclafani and Ackroff 2012). Among the key DA pathways is the mesocorticolimbic system, with DA cell bodies originating in the ventral tegmental area (VTA) and projecting to numerous brain regions including the nucleus accumbens (NAc), hippocampus, amygdala, lateral hypothalamus (LH), and multiple regions of the prefrontal cortex (Dichter, Damiano, and Allen 2012). The nigrostriatal system is a second major DA pathway, with DA cell bodies in the substantia nigra (SN) projecting to the caudate (dorsomedial) and putamen (dorsolateral) nuclei of the dorsal striatum. These two systems have overlapping, but also distinct, roles in reward processing, learning, and motivation related to both food and non-food rewards (Ilango et al. 2014) (Figure 12.1).

Among all the target regions of DA neurons, DA release into the striatum has been the most extensively studied in the context of reward seeking and learning related to food. As a reward becomes paired with a previously neutral stimulus, the predictive stimulus generates DA release and subsequent increases in NAc activity. The NAc (ventral striatum) is typically divided into two subregions, the shell and the core. Specifically, NAc core neurons display peak activity during unexpected reward delivery and show a predictable shift to peak activity upon repeated pairing with reward predictive cues, supporting the roles of the NAc core in encoding information related to reward outcomes (Brown et al. 2011). Additionally, pairing a reward with predictive cues can generate incentive salience and the extent of DA release reflects inherent motivational value for the subject. Rewards that are more valued by individuals generate stronger DA release into the NAc core (Brown et al. 2011). While the NAc core is responsible for cue-dependent DA increases, the role of the NAc shell is somewhat less defined. Enhanced DA release into the NAc shell occurs during the consumption phase of feeding, but also during unpredicted reward delivery (Bassareo and Di Chiara 1999). However, DA release into the shell is attenuated during the consumption phase once rewards become paired with

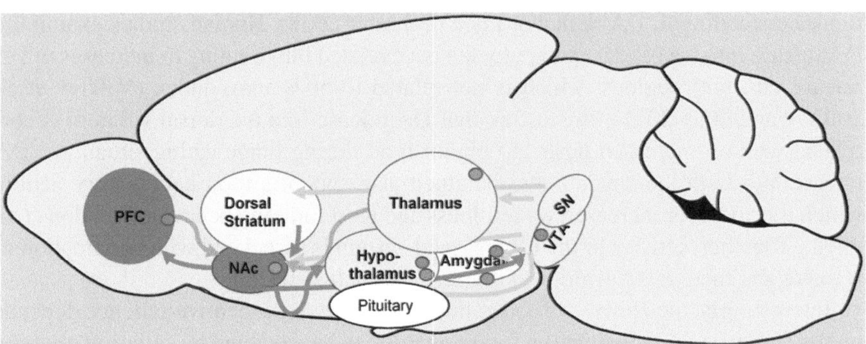

FIGURE 12.1 Dopaminergic system and expression of hormone receptors in the brain. The diagram indicates projections among various brain regions. Projections in yellow are primarily dopaminergic, in red are primarily gamma-aminobutyric acid (GABA)-ergic, and in green are primarily glutamatergic. This chapter focuses on the roles of dopamine pathways in feeding regulation. Many reward regions also express estrogen receptors. Estrogen receptor α (indicated by pink circles) are expressed in the ventral tegmental area (VTA), amygdala, many subregions of the hypothalamus, and the prefrontal cortex (PFC). Estrogen receptor β (indicated by purple circles) are expressed in subregions of the hypothalamus, thalamus, amygdala, and nucleus accumbens (NAc). Receptors of adiposity signal leptin (indicated by blue circles) are expressed in various nuclei at the hypothalamus projecting to the VTA and NAc. Receptors of adiposity signal insulin (indicated by green circles) are expressed in hypothalamic subregions and at the VTA and the substantia nigra (SN). By acting on hormone receptors, estrogen and adiposity signals can modulate reward activity through a variety of mechanisms.

reward-predictive cues. These results suggest that the NAc shell is only responsible for the reward-encoding when rewards are delivered in an unpredicted manner (Bassareo and Di Chiara 1999). Contrastingly, other studies have found the opposite, showing that cues paired with sucrose reward evoke sustained DA release into the NAc shell compared to the core (Cacciapaglia et al. 2012). Furthermore, recent studies have added complexity to this story, showing a role for the NAc shell in reward "value" encoding (Sackett, Saddoris, and Carelli 2017). Despite differences between the NAc core and shell in terms of process, both subregions produce critical signals for learning about food rewards and mediate food-seeking behaviors.

The nigrostriatal pathway is also involved in food-seeking behaviors. Both the caudate (dorsomedial striatum) and the putamen (dorsolateral striatum) modulate reward seeking and decision making (Hamid et al. 2016) that contribute to feeding. In operant tasks for food rewards, dorsolateral striatum DA exhibits sustained peaks immediately prior to food approach actions, which terminates as soon as action begins, suggesting that the putamen and DA release at the dorsolateral striatum guide upcoming actions for food rewards, including food-seeking and approach (London et al. 2018). In DA-deficient mice, restoration of DA into the dorsolateral striatum via administration of a precursor for DA synthesis L-DOPA is sufficient to restore food-seeking in an operant setting, although their motivation for rewards is reduced, likely due to partial restoration of the DA system function (Palmiter 2008). Similarly, restoring DA synthesis in the dorsolateral striatum and DA cell bodies in the SN reinstates feeding in DA-deficient mice (Palmiter 2008). Human studies examining DA release into the caudate and putamen have related binge eating to increases in DA release into both regions, which is not related to body mass index (Volkow et al. 2002, Wang et al. 2011), suggesting that DA release into the dorsal striatum is correlated with an increased desire to obtain food during binge eating situations. DA release into both the caudate and putamen also supports food anticipatory action, which is critical for increased wakefulness and food foraging behavior (London et al. 2018). Together, activity of the nigrostriatal system is associated with anticipation of rewards and increases reward-seeking actions, such as feeding.

Interestingly, the ability of food-related cues to evoke incentive salience depends on the energy state. Specifically, food rewards can be devalued by satiation, thereby reducing DA release into the NAc shell (West and Carelli 2016). In contrast, hunger (due to either food restriction or deprivation) and satiety modulate the activity of the DA system to increase and decrease food-seeking respectively. Indeed, activity in the DA system changes dynamically as animals shift between these states. For example, DA release into the NAc core is greater when animals are in a hungry state than in a sated state, and greater increases in DA release occur for higher calorie foods when animals are hungry (Aitken, Greenfield, and Wassum 2016, McCutcheon et al. 2012). The need-dependent ability of food cues to increase DA release into the NAc core drives enhanced motivation to obtain food, illustrated by the positive correlation between the degree of DA release into the NAc core and increased energy investment of animals to obtain rewards (McCutcheon et al. 2012). Additionally, hunger determines specific structures downstream of the VTA to be activated. For example, hunger in food-restricted rats can alter the projection of certain mesolimbic pathways to the LH to increase the rewarding potency of food (Cabeza De Vaca, Holiman, and Carr 1998, Legrand et al. 2015).

Considering the literature reviewed above, there are clear roles for the DA system in universal physiological conditions that help to restore energy homeostasis. However, DA also plays a clear role in obesity and anorexia, two disease conditions characterized by dysregulation of energy homeostasis (discussed in Section 12.4 of this chapter). The use of specialized diets can induce obese states and experimental food restriction can induce anorectic states in animals, allowing for the examination of the effects of these conditions on DA function. Feeding animals an obesogenic diet generally dampens the activity of the DA system, whereas food restriction generally enhances DA system activity (Jones et al. 2017). However, there are complexities to this statement. For example, both obesity-promoting high-fat diet feeding and food restriction can reduce DA transporter reactivity and expression in the caudate and putamen, but not in the NAc. Diet treatments also affect insulin-induced enhancement of DA uptake, with high-fat diet feeding decreasing DA release into the NAc while food restriction increases DA release into both ventral and dorsal regions of the striatum. This is likely mediated by diet-induced changes in insulin receptor expression causing downstream effects on DA D2 receptor expression (Jones et al. 2017, Johnson and Kenny 2010). The findings reviewed here establish a strong role of the DA system in determining both feeding pattern and food choice.

12.2.2 Dopamine-Mediated Behavioral Effects of Estrogen on Feeding

While elevated estrogen level is associated with increased motivation to obtain sex and drugs, it is paradoxically associated with decreased motivation for food (Yoest, Cummings, and Becker 2014). Motivation to obtain food in animals can be assessed using a progressive ratio task, in which operant requirements increase after each reward delivery. In this context, motivation to obtain food is lowest during estrus, the phase immediately following peak estrogen levels and therefore the highest relative estrogen signaling (Richard et al. 2017). This effect appears to be DA-mediated, as estradiol injection directly into the VTA reduces food-seeking independent of satiety state (Richard et al. 2017), suggesting that estrogen may act directly on the mesolimbic pathway to cause this effect.

In addition to regulating motivation for food (feeding pattern), estrogen also regulates food choice. However, while high levels of estrogen decrease motivation to obtain food, it also increases preference for highly palatable foods when subjects can choose (Richard et al. 2017). Estrogen of cycling females and hormone-treated OVX females increases the activity of VTA DA projections to the NAc, enhancing the motivation to obtain highly palatable foods, and similarly intensifies the "value" of that food (Afonso et al. 2009). Illustrating this, female rats have a higher preference than males for a location previously paired with high-fat and high-sugar diets (Sinclair et al. 2017). This result is consistent with human studies showing greater DA activity after food reward in women than men (Van Vugt and Reid 2014). Additionally, females demonstrate greater expression of Fos, an immediate early gene and commonly used marker of neuronal activation in mesocorticolimbic regions, providing neurobiological evidence for sex differences in response to palatable food by mesocorticolimbic reward circuits (Sinclair et al. 2017).

12.2.3 Estrogen-Mediated Feeding Effects on Dopamine

On an anatomical level, estrogen interacts with the DA system at multiple sites. Estrogen receptors exist widely throughout the mesolimbic and nigrostriatal systems (Creutz and Kritzer 2002, Milner et al. 2010) (Figure 12.1), leading to diverse effects on DA activity. The action of estrogen in the reward process can occur via direct or indirect modulation of the five known DA receptor subtypes. DA receptors can be classified as D1-like receptors, including D1 and D5 receptors that enhance postsynaptic activity; and D2-like receptors including D2, D3, and D4 receptors that suppress postsynaptic activity (Beaulieu, Espinoza, and Gainetdinov 2015), whose actions will be discussed in later sections of this chapter. In general, elevated circulating levels of estrogen increase mesolimbic responses to food via enhancing food value and increasing motivation (Zhang et al. 2008, Calipari et al. 2017, Proaño et al. 2018). This general pattern is apparent in both gonadally intact cycling females, as well as OVX females following super-physiological estrogen administration. Given this pattern, functional differences in reward processing and related motivational behavior between the sexes are likely due to estrogen-enhanced DA signaling (Greenberg and Trainor 2016), contributing to many meaningful differences in feeding pattern and food choice.

Estrogen directly alters mesolimbic DA transmission pre- and post-synaptically by stimulating DA synthesis and release (Joyce, Smith, and van Hartesveldt 1982, Becker 1990, Chiodo and Caggiula 1980, Ramirez and Zheng 1996, Thompson and Moss 1994), DA reuptake (Thompson, Bridges, and Weirs 2001), changing DA receptor expression (Gordon and Fields 1989) and activity (Febo et al. 2003), and increasing DA receptor binding by slowing DA metabolism (Shimizu and Bray 1993). Opposite to estrogen-stimulated increases in DA signaling, lowered levels of estrogen following OVX reduce DA release at the VTA and NAc measured in brain punches of the VTA and NA by high-performance liquid chromatography (Russo et al. 2003), which can be reversed by estrogen replacement in OVX rats (Afonso et al. 2009). Additionally, the density of DA neurons in the SN is greater in cycling female African green monkeys than both males and female OVX monkeys (Leranth et al. 2000). It is noteworthy that estrogen can upregulate D1 receptors that enhance post-synaptic activity but downregulate D2 receptors that suppress postsynaptic activity. In particular, administration of estrogen increases the density of D1 receptors in the striatum of rats (Hruska and Nowak 1988). In contrast, D2 receptor expression in the caudate and putamen nuclei of cynomolgus monkeys (Czoty et al. 2008) and in the striatum of rats (Bazzett and Becker 1994) is higher during the luteal phase of the estrous cycle when endogenous estrogen is low, compared to the follicular phase when endogenous estrogen is high. Likewise, reducing estrogen levels via OVX increases, while estradiol treatment reduces, D2 receptors in the striatum of rats (Bazzett and Becker 1994, Lammers et al. 1999). Estrogen also indirectly elevates DA neuron activity by reducing the activity of connected inhibitory gamma-amino-butyric acid (GABA)-ergic neurons to elevate DA neuron activity (McGinnis, Gordon, and Gorski 1980). All these effects of estrogen lead to enhanced responsiveness to DA neurotransmission and likely account for the sex differences in feeding pattern and food choice, as both are dictated by the DA system.

It is noteworthy that although estrogen facilitates DA neurotransmission in general (Becker 1990, Thompson and Moss 1994), inhibitory effects of estrogen on DA neurotransmission have also been reported (Morel et al. 2009, Disshon, Boja, and Dluzen 1998). For example, Dupont et al. reported reduced DA concentrations in the NAc following daily treatment of estrogen for two weeks (Dupont et al. 1981). Zhou et al. reported an increase in the expression of D3 receptors that suppress DA neuron activity in the VTA following estrogen replacement in OVX rats (Zhou, Cunningham, and Thomas 2002). There are also some discrepancies regarding the regulatory effects of estrogen on the DA transporters. DA transporter concentrations in the mesolimbic system are decreased by high estrogen levels (Disshon, Boja, and Dluzen 1998, Rehavi et al. 1998, Bazzett and Becker 1994). Such effects would delay DA reuptake and increase the duration of DA neurotransmission. However, some reports suggest that DA transporter concentrations are increased by exogenous estrogen treatment in OVX rats or when endogenous estrogen levels are high during proestrus of naturally cycling rats (Bossé, Rivest, and Di Paolo 1997, Chavez et al. 2010), or not changed by high estrogen levels (Morissette and Di Paolo 1993).

While the general pattern of estrogen-enhanced DA signaling may be well-supported, clearly more research regarding the specific molecular mechanisms of this process is needed. The inconsistent effects of estrogen on DA signaling is not surprising considering the different methods utilized across studies, such as the different ages of subjects and dissimilar methods of estrogen treatment/modulation, including administration route, dose and duration, and testing time following estrogen administration. While there are discrepancies in the exact mechanisms by which estrogen affects the DA system, estrogen remains a particularly potent modulator of the DA system, thus affecting feeding pattern and food choice, and thus likely relates to the higher risk of obesity and eating disorders in females.

It is important to note that most studies of the mesocortical and nigrostriatal systems have used food rewards paired with some form of food deprivation. The studies cited above focus on the processing of food rewards themselves, but may be confounded by the significant deprivation and/or types of foods used. Other reward types, such as drugs and sex, also have confounds of their own (e.g. drug tolerance). Thus, the magnitude and effects of DA reward circuitry activation observed in animal models may be artificially inflated or altered, and may not reflect naturalistic activity patterns. Regardless, the findings reviewed here establish a strong role of interaction between estrogen and the DA system in determining both feeding pattern and food choice.

12.3 CROSSTALK BETWEEN CIRCULATING ADIPOSITY SIGNALS AND REWARD CIRCUITRY

12.3.1 Circulating Factors Regulate Feeding Behavior Via Dopamine

Estrogen modulates neural pathways (Anderson and Petrovich 2015) to suppress caloric intake (Asarian and Geary 2013) via two primary mechanisms: (1) activating anorexigenic neurons in homeostatic brain regions expressing estrogen receptors (Gao et al. 2007) at the arcuate nucleus (ARC) and paraventricular nucleus (PVN) of the hypothalamus (Thammacharoen et al. 2009) and the nucleus tractus solitarius of the hindbrain (Thammacharoen et al. 2008); and (2) acting on multiple neurotransmitter signaling systems in reward-associated brain regions (Xu and López 2018). Thus, estrogen affects both homeostatic and hedonic regulation of feeding. An emphasis on the effects of estrogen on the DA system and in the hypothalamus will be discussed in this chapter.

Feeding behavior is not only influenced by metabolic states and energy needs necessary for survival and metabolism, but also influenced by response to satiety and hunger signals in neural networks. Circulating signals include adiposity hormones that provide information about long-term accumulated energy stores and gastrointestinal hormones that provide information about short-term meal-related hunger and satiety status (Woods 2009). Additionally, meal-related information is transmitted from the gastrointestinal tract via meal-related signals and afferent fibers of the vagus nerve to the nucleus tractus solitarius in the brainstem, and are further relayed to the feeding center in the hypothalamic ARC, PVN, and LH where integration with adiposity and gastrointestinal signals occur (Morton et al. 2006). Furthermore, receptors for adiposity and gastrointestinal hormones exist in brain regions involved in DA reward circuitry. Therefore, circulating signals regulate feeding via crosstalk between homeostatic circuitry and reward circuitry (Gautron and Elmquist 2011, Farooqi et al. 2007). In general, orexigenic hormones such as ghrelin and orexin enhance, whereas anorexigenic hormones such as adiposity hormones and most gastrointestinal hormones suppress, DA signaling and reward-related activity including feeding behavior. It is possible that food restriction enhances orexigenic hormone levels and subsequently activates reward circuitry. Importantly, adiposity hormones and gastrointestinal hormones regulate feeding behavior in a sex-different manner. We focus on how circulating adiposity hormones regulate sex-specific feeding behaviors via affecting homeostatic and hedonic reward circuitry involving DA. Other mechanisms that are unrelated to DA reward circuitry have been discussed elsewhere (Asarian and Geary 2013) and are beyond the scope of this chapter.

12.3.2 Overview of Adiposity Signals Leptin and Insulin

Adiposity hormones, such as leptin mostly secreted by white adipocytes (Gautron and Elmquist 2011) and insulin secreted by pancreatic β cells (Plum, Belgardt, and Brüning 2006), function as long-term peripheral signals to monitor the amount of energy stored within the body, as their levels are correlated with the body fat stores in both males and females. It is noteworthy that temporary macronutrient consumption and dietary intake also influence the levels of leptin and insulin (Havel 2001). Adiposity hormones act directly on their receptors in neurons of the hypothalamus to inform the brain of adiposity status and to regulate energy balance (Woods 2009). Leptin plays critical roles in suppressing food intake and enhancing energy expenditure (Friedman 2009), predominately through its long-form receptors expressed in many brain nuclei (de Luca et al. 2005), including DA neurons in the hypothalamus and reward circuitry (Elmquist et al. 1998). Similarly, insulin receptors are expressed in both homeostatic hypothalamic regions (Woods 2009) and DA neurons at the VTA and the SN of motivation/reward regions that relay signals linked to feeding (Figlewicz et al. 2003). In the hypothalamus, adiposity hormones leptin and insulin modulate a number of orexigenic and anorexigenic neurohormones and neurotransmitters to suppress energy intake, via directly targeting hypothalamic nuclei including the ARC, PVN, LH, ventromedial nucleus, and dorsomedial nucleus (Friedman 2009). The ARC is one of the most researched hypothalamic nuclei. Leptin and insulin modulate feeding via interaction with two primary groups of peptidergic ARC neurons that directly inhibit each other to control hunger and satiety. Specifically, proopiomelanocortin (POMC) neurons and cocaine and amphetamine related transcription factor (CART) neurons are classified as satiety neurons and receive GABAergic connections from pro-hunger neuropeptide Y (NPY) neurons and agouti-related peptide (AgRP) neurons that directly inhibit the satiety. Both POMC/CART and NPY/AgRP neurons express receptors for both leptin and insulin to regulate feeding and energy expenditure (Woods 2009).

Besides playing critical roles in the long-term regulation of energy homeostasis, leptin and insulin exhibit short-term regulation of the amount of food ingested and related feeding behavior (Friedman 2009). Indeed, hedonic reward behavior and motivation are also affected by leptin and insulin (Davis et al. 2011). Elevated leptin levels due to positive energy balance suppress reward behaviors; conversely, lowered leptin levels due to negative energy balance increase reward behaviors in rats (Davis, Choi, and Benoit 2010). The ARC of the hypothalamus sends direct projections to the DA system by POMC neurons to modulate VTA (Qu et al. 2020) and NAc (van

Zessen, van der Plasse, and Adan 2012), and subsequently interacts with the reward system. Both leptin and insulin suppress DA reward activation. Leptin and insulin levels, along with leptin and insulin sensitivity, are associated with brain responses to images of palatable food (Jastreboff et al. 2014, Jastreboff et al. 2013). Leptin modifies reward pathways and food motivation by decreasing striatal brain activation. Specifically, leptin treatment suppresses activity of the NAc in patients with congenital leptin deficiency (Farooqi et al. 2007). Additionally, obesity patients report higher liking ratings for food due to leptin resistance (Farooqi et al. 2007). In both men and women, disease states of leptin resistance and insulin resistance, as seen in obese and diabetic patients respectively, are associated with an increased craving for palatable food with positive correlation to neural activity in the VTA and exaggerated responses to images of palatable food in various reward circuits involving striatum, including the cortical region for integration and interoception, the striatal region for reward and motivation, and the limbic region for emotion and memory (Jastreboff et al. 2013). Thus, leptin and insulin are satiety activating hormones and critical in food reward regulation, via modulating the hypothalamus to control feeding and downregulating DA reward circuitry.

12.3.3 Behavioral Effects of Estrogen on Feeding Mediated by Leptin and Insulin

12.3.3.1 Hypothalamus-Mediated Effects of Adiposity Signals on Feeding

Hypothalamic ventricular cells express receptors for feeding-related circulating signals more densely than at other brain regions (Hill et al. 1986, Scott, Mason, and Sharpe 2009, Zigman et al. 2006). These hypothalamic ventricular cells also function specifically in the regulation of feeding behavior (Rossi and Stuber 2018). The ARC of the hypothalamus is located in an area particularly well-suited for sensing circulating nutritional and adiposity signals due to its location adjacent to the median eminence, a circumventricular organ with proximity to the hypothalamus (Haddad-Tóvolli et al. 2017). Thus, ventricular neurons act as mediators for circulating signals to impact on brain circuitry. Specifically, when the level of adiposity signals leptin and insulin are lower than normal ranges, which indicates depleted energy stores, subjects are motivated to increase feeding.

Besides the ARC, the LH is another important component of the reward circuit, connecting the hypothalamus and mesolimbic reward pathways that assess the incentive values of food (Stuber and Wise 2016). Neurons in the LH integrate information from a network of neurons including the cortical regions and amygdala, and project integrated information to reward circuits to regulate feeding (Stuber and Wise 2016). Stimulation of the LH leads to increased reward and feeding (Stuber and Wise 2016). It is noteworthy that the LH comprises various groups of neurons expressing distinct types of neurotransmitters including glutamate and GABA and neurohormones including orexin and melanin-concentrating hormone (DiLeone, Georgescu, and Nestler 2003, Harris, Wimmer, and Aston-Jones 2005). For example, orexins expressing neurons at the LH project to the VTA and regulate reward and motivational behavior such as feeding (Harris, Wimmer, and Aston-Jones 2005, Borgland et al. 2006). The orexin neurons at the LH are activated in the presence of palatable food, leading to increased release of orexin that further activates VTA DA neurons (Zheng, Patterson, and Berthoud 2007). Sex-different feeding responses in orexin neurons have been reported, with female, but not male, rats, increasing orexin expression in response to fasting, leading to sex different responses in food intake (Funabashi et al. 2009). An interesting sex difference in the regulation of feeding has been reported across species. Male mice that are acutely food-deprived (Nohara et al. 2011) or chronically food-restricted (Shi et al. 2007) compensate the negative energy balance state by overeating; whereas similarly challenged female mice compensate negative energy balance by decreasing energy expenditure. Comparable sex differences are seen in rats (Valle et al. 2005) and humans (Zandian et al. 2011). These sex differences could be attributed to the crosstalk between peripheral metabolic signals and sex hormones, and central reward and hypothalamic circuitry.

Sex differences have been reported in the regulation of feeding by leptin and insulin. Intracerebroventricular administration of leptin inhibits feeding to a greater extent in female rats than male rats (Ainslie et al. 2001, Clegg et al. 2003, Clegg et al. 2006), a sex difference related to the activational effects of estrogen. In OVX rats, estrogen treatment upregulates leptin receptor expression in the hypothalamus (Meli et al. 2004, Rocha et al. 2004) and increases the eating-inhibitory potency of leptin (Ainslie et al. 2001, Clegg et al. 2003, Clegg et al. 2006). Sex differences in insulin-inhibited eating has also been reported. Specifically, intracerebroventricular administration of insulin inhibits eating more in male rats than in their female counterparts with matched ages or body weights (Clegg et al. 2003, Clegg et al. 2006). Similar sex differences in the anorexic effects of insulin have been reported in humans where insulin treatment decreases food intake and body fat in men but not in women (Hallschmid et al. 2004, Benedict et al. 2008).

It has been accepted that leptin and insulin exert their effects on energy balance mainly through hypothalamic neuronal populations including POMC/CART and NPY/AgRP neurons at the ARC (Balthasar et al. 2004, Coppari et al. 2005, Könner et al. 2007, Hill et al. 2010) and steroidogenic factor 1 neurons at the ventromedial nucleus (Dhillon et al. 2006). It is noteworthy that leptin- and insulin-responsive POMC neurons represent two distinct populations (Williams et al. 2010). Importantly, a single-cell RNA sequencing study has reported that leptin receptors are expressed in 58% of AgRP neurons, but only 12% of POMC neurons, in the ARC (Lam et al. 2017). Leptin receptor expressing POMC neurons in the ARC have been traditionally but wrongly associated with producing anorexigenic effects by leptin (Caron et al. 2018), mainly due to earlier transgenic mouse studies in which specific deletion of leptin receptors in POMC neurons produced confounding developmental compensation of NPY/AgRP neurons that share common developmental origins with POMC neurons (Padilla, Carmody, and Zeltser 2010). Furthermore, a recent groundbreaking study with leptin receptor knockdown in ARC POMC neurons initiated during adulthood without mice showing any developmental confounds has revealed these POMC neurons as indispensable for hepatic glucose production and a fasting-induced fall in leptin levels, but not as responsible for decreasing food intake (Caron et al. 2018). Thus, anorexigenic effects of leptin could be administered mainly through its suppression of AgRP neurons expressing leptin receptors in the hypothalamus and reward regions, rather than POMC neurons in the ARC.

12.3.3.2 Dopaminergic Effects of Adiposity Signals on Feeding

Leptin receptors are detected in homeostatic hypothalamic regions (Schwartz et al. 2000) and reward regions, including the VTA, SN, and LH (Figlewicz et al. 2003, Fulton et al. 2006, Hommel et al. 2006, Leinninger et al. 2009, Opland, Leinninger, and Myers 2010), some of which are DA and GABA neurons in the VTA (Fulton et al. 2006, Hommel et al. 2006). Supra-physiological doses of leptin directly reduce firing of the DA neurons in the VTA in anesthetized rats (Hommel et al. 2006). Leptin also acts on neurons expressing leptin receptors in the LH projecting to the VTA (Leinninger et al. 2009) and in the ARC projecting to the VTA (Qu et al. 2020) and NAc (van Zessen, van der Plasse, and Adan 2012), which subsequently diminishes DA release and decreases the activity of the VTA and NAc, key reward regions of the mesolimbic DA system, and consequently reduces the motivation for feeding and food consumption (Opland, Leinninger, and Myers 2010). Additionally, leptin suppresses neurons in the LH expressing orexigenic hormones, including orexin and melanin-concentrating hormone, reduces expression of these neurohormones, and ultimately inhibits reward responses to food (Leinninger et al. 2009). Leptin also suppresses fasting-induced activation of orexin neurons (Yamanaka et al. 2003, Segal-Lieberman et al. 2003). As stated in Section 12.3.3.1 that females are more sensitive to leptin than males, sex difference in feeding could occur at the level of the LH, involving suppression of orexin neurons by leptin.

Similar to leptin, expression of insulin receptors has been detected in the DA neurons in the VTA (Figlewicz et al. 2003). Insulin dose-dependently decreases DA concentration in the VTA via upregulating the number and activity of DA transporters and increasing DA reuptake to reduce DA concentration in the VTA (Mebel et al. 2012), and ultimately attenuates the feeding of palatable food (Mebel et al. 2012). Both leptin and insulin act on the DA system to reduce the incentive value of food reward and suppress motivated performance (Figlewicz et al. 2006, Fulton et al. 2006). Taken together, adiposity signals leptin and insulin operate both homeostatically, involving multiple hypothalamic regions, and hedonically, involving the DA system to regulate feeding.

12.4 CLINICAL IMPLICATIONS AND FUTURE RESEARCH

12.4.1 Sex Differences in Eating Disorders and Obesity Due to Dysfunction of the Dopamine System

Obesity and eating disorders such as anorexia show extremes in feeding behavior, and are associated with alterations to the reward nature of food involving the DA system and adiposity hormones, revealed by studies using human and animal models of these conditions. More women are obese than men globally (Kanter and Caballero 2012). In the United States, according to the recent CDC release, women have a higher prevalence of obesity than men (Hales et al. 2017). The prevalence of eating disorders is two to six times higher in women than in men across lifetime (Hudson et al. 2007, Kinasz et al. 2016), including adolescence (Croll et al. 2002), midlife (Baker et al. 2017), and old age (Hilbert, de Zwaan, and Braehler 2012). Likewise, animal studies using a binge-eating model showed that intermittently exposes rats to palatable food have shown that female rats display binge-eating behavior two-to-six-fold higher than male rats (Klump et al. 2013). Anorexia is an eating disorder defined by a conscious reduction or refusal to consume food due to a fear of weight gain, accompanied by severe body dysmorphia. Individuals with anorexia are often anhedonic and experience several severe physiological consequences associated with dramatic weight loss, including loss of menstrual cycle, severe muscle weakness, and a loss of bone density. Despite these consequences, individuals with anorexia compulsively over exercise in order to contribute to weight loss. Two of the most common eating disorders associated with disturbance of reward regulation are anorexia nervosa and bulimia nervosa. Patients with anorexia nervosa are generally characterized by restriction in food intake, compulsory exercise, and weight loss; whereas patients with bulimia nervosa are generally characterized by a cycle of episodes of binge eating followed by compensatory behaviors such as purging and fasting to avoid weight gain (American Psychiatric Association 2013). It is noteworthy that the incidence of eating disorders increases dramatically in early adolescent girls during puberty (Klump et al. 2012, Swanson et al. 2011), suggesting elevated estrogen level as a risk factor for being vulnerable to eating disorders. Similarly, female rats display increased vulnerability for binge eating at the onset of puberty (Klump et al. 2011). Therefore, the sex hormone estrogen could considerably influence various aspects of feeding behavior and reward processing.

Of particular importance to feeding behavior, the organization and structure of neural circuits regulating food-related reward processing show extensive and complex sex differences (Del Parigi et al. 2002, Haase, Green, and Murphy 2011, Smeets et al. 2006). The activation of reward circuitry to palatable food in women fluctuate over the course of the menstrual cycle and depend on the phases (Van Vugt and Reid 2014). It has been accepted that the menstrual cycle of women and associated changes in ovarian hormone levels are critical biological regulators to study caloric intake, food choice, meal pattern, and other feeding-related physiology and behavior. Additionally, it is known that estrogen enhances anorexigenic gene expression involved in leptin signaling (Gao et al. 2007). Furthermore, estrogen could interact with reward circuitry to regulate feeding via enhancing the effects of the mesolimbic DA system on appetite, as discussed in Section 12.2.

Our understanding of the neurobiology of anorexia has been greatly enhanced by the development of the activity-based anorexia animal model. When rodents are food restricted to 40% of their *ad libitum* food intake and given access to running wheels, animals voluntarily become extremely hypophagic and over-exercise, leading to extreme weight loss that would otherwise lead to death if not allowed to recover (Klenotich and Dulawa 2012, Schalla and Stengel 2019). This over-exercising associated with anorexia occurs in both sexes but females accelerate weight loss faster. Thus, female rodents are overwhelmingly utilized to model the patient demographic seen in anorexia. This activity-based anorexia rodent model provides a strong basis for the establishment of voluntary starvation that is completely absent from previous animal models (Schalla and Stengel 2019). It is noteworthy that, unlike what is seen in humans, animals recover quickly after the removal of the running wheel and returning to an *ad libitum* feeding schedule, indicating gaps exist between basic animal research and human clinical studies. Further, activating the VTA-NAc pathway using DREADDs in an animal study prevents the development of an activity-based anorexia-like phenotype (Foldi, Milton, and Oldfield 2017). Exposure to a palatable high-fat diet substantially reduces the likelihood of developing activity-based anorexia in rodents (Brown, Avena, and Hoebel 2008), suggesting that a metabolic factor can be protective and reduce anorexia susceptibility. The activity-based anorexia model is relatively new and examination of the subsequent activity of the DA system has yet to be explored, particularly as related to pharmacological and specific neuroanatomical interventions of reward circuitry.

Opposite to anorexia, overeating due to exposure to highly palatable foods with rewarding and reinforcing properties and the resultant obesity that usually involves altered interaction between DA reward circuitry and adiposity hormones, which drives the addiction-like behavior of hedonic feeding and consequently increases the incidence of excess food consumption. Such hedonic feeding via activating the reward system is similar to enacting the addictive behaviors of consuming substances, and therefore has been termed "food addiction" (Leigh and Morris 2018). Animal studies have explored alterations to the DA system in obesity, utilizing various animal models with differential diet exposure to induce obesity, and have detected similarities in the underlying mechanisms between food addiction and substance addiction. The mesolimbic DA system is a common reward pathway that is changed by palatable food and short-term exposure to addictive substances (Johnson and Kenny 2010). For example, rats fed a high-fat cafeteria diet exhibit greater evoked DA release to cues associated with higher caloric content related rewards, compared to a lower DA release to a low-fat diet (Geiger et al. 2009). Additionally, these rats exposed to a high-fat cafeteria diet demonstrate accelerated compulsive sucrose seeking behavior by silencing DA D2 receptor expression in the NAc (Johnson and Kenny 2010), suggesting that an obesogenic diet induces upregulated DA activity to promote feeding. DA D2 receptors in striatum are also reduced in obese rats compared with lean rats (Johnson and Kenny 2010), which triggers hedonic eating behavior. Overall, studies have suggested a powerfully evoked DA release to food rewards with an under-functioning of the DA system involving lowered D2 receptor in the NAc in an obese state, leading to anhedonia, increased impulsive choice, and enhanced feeding behavior, similar to the changes observed in drug addiction (Kenny 2011). In support of the findings from animal studies, human studies have reported that body mass index is negatively correlated with striatal D2 receptor in obese individuals. Human neuroimaging studies using a positron emission tomography scan with DA D2 receptor radioligand [C-11]raclopride for indicating D2 receptor availability in obese and normal-weight individuals have found reduced availability of striatal D2 receptor in obese individuals (Wang et al. 2001). Palatable foods stimulate more brain activation than low-caloric food in both normal-weight and obese individuals. Neuroimaging studies reveal increased activity of brain reward circuits and emotion regions with greater activations in prefrontal and limbic regions, as well as enhanced motivational responses to food images in obese individuals compared to normal-weight individuals (Martin et al. 2010). It is noteworthy that greater activation of DA signaling in response to images of high energy density foods, especially in the mesolimbic DA system involving the VTA-NAc pathway and projecting to the anterior insular cortex, anterior cingulate cortex, orbitofrontal cortex, and amygdala, has been detected in obese individuals than in normal-weight individuals (Carnell et al. 2012, Stice et al. 2011, Stoeckel et al. 2008, Van Vugt and Reid 2014). These findings indicate activation of the DA reward system as a potential mechanism for enhancing the hedonic value of food and increasing motivational and rewarding behaviors for eating palatable food in obese individuals.

Human neuroimaging studies also detect similarities between using addictive substances and compulsively consuming palatable food. Specifically, there are overlapping brain regions and pathways involved in learning, reward, and motivation that are activated by both drugs and palatable food (Volkow, Wise, and Baler 2017). A meta-analysis that has compared blood oxygen level-dependent (BOLD) fMRI response to reward among participants with substance addiction, non-substance (e.g. gambling) addiction, and obesity has detected many commonalities in BOLD activations between obesity and substance addiction, but not non-substance addiction (García-García et al. 2014). This study provides neurological evidence that obese and substance addictive individuals share overlapping dysfunctions in reward circuits.

Adiposity hormones affect both homeostatic and hedonic pathways to regulate feeding (Kowalska, Karczewska-Kupczewska, and Strączkowski 2011). As discussed in Section 12.3.2, leptin regulates homeostatic feeding in a sexually dimorphic manner and influences the reward process. A low level of leptin is one of the characteristics of anorexia nervosa patients, but leptin levels in bulimia nervosa patients are inconsistent, as leptin levels could change across different stages and could be dependent on the severity of the symptoms of the eating disorders (Monteleone and Maj 2013). Additionally, leptin resistance accompanying obesity and related metabolic diseases influences eating disorders (Misra and Klibanski 2014). Current research focuses on the importance of leptin in the regulation of appetite, body weight, and lean body mass in eating disorders (Yilmaz et al. 2014), and increasing circulating leptin levels has been proposed as a therapy for anorexia nervosa patients (Rybakowski, Slopien, and Tyszkiewicz-Nwafor 2014).

12.4.2 Gaps between Animal and Human Studies

The incidence of obesity (Friedrich 2017) and eating disorders (Hoek 2006, Striegel-Moore et al. 2009) is universally higher in women than in men. While gender and societal influences play obvious roles in feeding behaviors including food choice and meal pattern (CIHR Institute of Gender and Health 2012), biological factors, such as neural circuits, hormones, energy state, and meal status, also modulate homeostatic feeding and hedonic reward circuits between the sexes, leading to the differences witnessed in eating disorders, obesity, and metabolic diseases, all of which are recognized public health threats due to their increased prevalence and high cost in treatment and prevention. Although some of the brain reward circuitry have known sex differences, these are unknown for many others. Such sex differences could be anatomical in morphology involving structures and pathways, could be physiological and functional in reward processing, and could be behavioral in reward responses.

Human imaging studies have begun analyzing brain regions involved in feeding, responding to different metabolic conditions (Gupta et al. 2018) and stressors (Goldstein et al. 2010) in men and women. Human studies are mostly limited to the below aspects. First, brain imaging studies do not actually measure neural activity, but indirectly assess neural functions using positron emission tomography to detect cerebral glucose metabolism or using fMRI to detect cerebral blood flow. Second, neural response is affected by various simultaneous factors influencing cognition, emotion, memories, and many others, which makes experimental design difficult to control between and within subjects. Third, changed brain regions are identified, but the underlying biochemical, cellular, or molecular mechanisms are not investigated. For example, altered brain glucose metabolism and blood flow may be due to excitation or inhibition of neural activity, and different neurotransmitters could be used for excitation or inhibition. While most of the literature is catching up, the molecular studies on sex differences in the reward circuits underlying feeding regulation remain indisputably lacking. Unfortunately, many findings of human studies in the literature are limited to studying association, instead of cause-and-effect mechanism.

Gaps exist between the basic research and clinical studies. Animal models of dysregulated eating behaviors provide powerful insights and serve as the basis for developing therapeutics for eating disorders or for understanding how various drugs modulate feeding. Investigations into feeding behavior in animals translating to humans have been unsuccessful, which is a bit surprising, considering the amount of data and successful animal studies that reveal feeding inhibition and weight loss induced by various manipulations, at least in the short term. What is missing from animal studies, yet is occurring in human studies, is the consequences of reward circuitry and hormones on food choice rather than food restriction or deprivation of a single type of diet. Further, food availability and subtle cues of foods with closely matched calories drive food choice. Additionally, socioeconomic factors such as habituation and cost and personal factors such as body image are key elements of human food intake. These factors determining how biological brain circuitry and hormones may drive subsequent food choice, especially when the calories are closely matched, have yet to be explored. Humans are making these choices regularly, with complex factors leading to one decision over another; and the metabolic consequences of these choices remain and interact with one another. Such complicated psychological and socioeconomic elements are challenging to model in animals.

12.4.3 Improvements Needed in Future Studies

Sex differences exist in various aspects of neural structures and various neurotransmitters. Morphological differences exist between sexes (Feis et al. 2013), which could lead to sex differences in feeding behavior. Most of the animal studies either use male subjects only, or use both male and female subjects, but findings are not analyzed separately, at the disregard of confounding variables due to sex. Albeit estrogen-induced sex differences in reward circuits are widely accepted knowledge, only a fraction of neuroimaging studies have compared and assessed reward responses to food across different phases of the menstrual cycle (Alonso-Alonso et al. 2011, Dreher et al. 2007, Frank et al. 2010, McVay et al. 2012). It is essential to account for sexes, sex hormones, and phases of the menstrual cycle as variables in human neuroimaging studies.

While many findings about how sex hormones and phases of the estrous cycle affects reward circuits and behaviors are being revealed, our understanding of the mechanisms of reward at the molecular level is still mostly limited to males. Mechanistic studies that include female subjects or examine sex differences are lacking, and understanding of the molecular mechanisms underlying feeding behaviors and responses is not actually an incredibly accurate representation for both sexes, with most of the mechanisms controlling the sexual divergence seen in behaviors remaining unknown. Therapeutic approaches based on current research findings that have used male animals only are likely not relevant to females and therefore not beneficial to women. With regard to preventing and treating eating disorders and related metabolic diseases, there is an urgent need to study both sexes. As having been advocated by the NIH, scientists need to consider sex in their studies to ensure that women get the same benefit as men from the findings of preclinical research (Clayton and Collins 2014). Therefore, more research including both male and female subjects in all aspects of neural and behavioral research is needed. Because sex as a biological factor is receiving more attention and more investigators are including both male and female subjects in their studies, more sex differences will be reported in future.

ACKNOWLEDGMENT

This work was supported by a Miami University Dissertation Scholarship to KNK and by the National Institutes of Health DK090823 to HS.

ABBREVIATIONS

AgRP agouti-related peptide
ARC arcuate nucleus
CART cocaine and amphetamine related transcription factor
DA dopamine or dopaminergic
fMRI functional magnetic resonance imaging
GABA gamma-aminobutyric acid
LH lateral hypothalamus
NAc nucleus accumbens
NPY neuropeptide Y
OFC orbitofrontal cortex
OVX ovariectomy or ovariectomized
POMC pro-opiomelanocortin
PVN paraventricular nucleus
SN substantia nigra
VTA ventral tegmental area

REFERENCES

Afonso, Veronica M., Samantha King, Diptendu Chatterjee, and Alison S. Fleming. 2009. "Hormones that increase maternal responsiveness affect accumbal dopaminergic responses to pup- and food-stimuli in the female rat." *Horm Behav* 56 (1):11–23.

Ainslie, D. A., M. J. Morris, G. Wittert, H. Turnbull, J. Proietto, and A. W. Thorburn. 2001. "Estrogen deficiency causes central leptin insensitivity and increased hypothalamic neuropeptide Y." *Int J Obes Relat Metab Disord* 25 (11):1680–1688.

Aitken, T. J., V. Y. Greenfield, and K. M. Wassum. 2016. "Nucleus accumbens core dopamine signaling tracks the need-based motivational value of food-paired cues." *J Neurochem* 136 (5):1026–1036.

Alonso-Alonso, Miguel, Florencia Ziemke, Faidon Magkos, Fernando A. Barrios, Mary Brinkoetter, Ingrid Boyd, Anne Rifkin-Graboi, Mary Yannakoulia, Rafael Rojas, Alvaro Pascual-Leone, et al. 2011. "Brain responses to food images during the early and late follicular phase of the menstrual cycle in healthy young women: relation to fasting and feeding." *Am J Clin Nutr* 94 (2):377–384.

American Psychiatric Association. 2013. *Diagnostic and statistical manual of mental disorders*. 5 ed: Washington, DC.

Anderson, Lauren C., and Gorica D. Petrovich. 2015. "Renewal of conditioned responding to food cues in rats: Sex differences and relevance of estradiol." *Physiol Behav* 151:338–344.

Aparicio, Aránzazu, Elena E. Rodríguez-Rodríguez, Javier Aranceta-Bartrina, Ángel Gil, Marcela González-Gross, Lluis Serra-Majem, Gregorio Varela-Moreiras, and Rosa Maria Ortega. 2017. "Differences in meal patterns and timing with regard to central obesity in the ANIBES ('Anthropometric data, macronutrients and micronutrients intake, practice of physical activity, socioeconomic data and lifestyles in Spain') Study." *Public Health Nutr* 20 (13):2364–2373.

Arganini, C., A. Turrini, A. Saba, F. Virgili, and R. Comitato. 2012. "Gender differences in food choice and dietary intake in modern western societies." In *Public Health—Social and Behavioral Health*, edited by J. Maddock, 85–102. Rijeka: InTech Open Access Publisher.

Asarian, Lori, and Nori Geary. 2013. "Sex differences in the physiology of eating." *Am J Physiol Regul Integr Comp Physiol* 305 (11):R1215–R1267.

Baker, Jessica H., Claire M. Peterson, Laura M. Thornton, Kimberly A. Brownley, Cynthia M. Bulik, Susan S. Girdler, Marsha D. Marcus, and Joyce T. Bromberger. 2017. "Reproductive and appetite hormones and bulimic symptoms during midlife." *Eur Eat Disord Rev* 25 (3):188–194.

Baldo, Brian A., and Ann E. Kelley. 2007. "Discrete neurochemical coding of distinguishable motivational processes: insights from nucleus accumbens control of feeding." *Psychopharmacology (Berl)* 191 (3):439–459.

Balthasar, Nina, Roberto Coppari, Julie McMinn, Shun M. Liu, Charlotte E. Lee, Vinsee Tang, Christopher D. Kenny, Robert A. McGovern, Streamson C. Chua Jr, Joel K. Elmquist, and Bradford B. Lowell. 2004. "Leptin receptor signaling in POMC neurons is required for normal body weight homeostasis." *Neuron* 42 (6):983–991.

Barbosa, Diane Eloy Chaves , Vanessa Rosse de Souza, Larissa Almenara Silva dos Santos, Claudete Corrêa de Jesus Chiappini, Solange Augusta de Sa, and Vilma Blondet de Azeredo. 2015. "Changes in taste and food intake during the menstrual cycle." *J Nutr Food Sci* 5 (383).

Bartness, Timothy J., and Robert J. Waldbillig. 1984. "Dietary self-selection in intact, ovariectomized, and estradiol-treated female rats." *Behav Neurosci* 98 (1):125–137.

Bassareo, V., and G. Di Chiara. 1999. "Differential responsiveness of dopamine transmission to food-stimuli in nucleus accumbens shell/core compartments." *Neuroscience* 89 (3):637–641.

Bazzett, Terence J., and Jill B. Becker. 1994. "Sex differences in the rapid and acute effects of estrogen on striatal D2 dopamine receptor binding." *Brain Res* 637 (1):163–172.

Beaulieu, J. M., S. Espinoza, and R. R. Gainetdinov. 2015. "Dopamine receptors - IUPHAR review 13." *Br J Pharmacol* 172 (1):1–23.

Becker, Jill B. 1990. "Estrogen rapidly potentiates amphetamine-induced striatal dopamine release and rotational behavior during microdialysis." *Neurosci Lett* 118 (2):169–171.

Beer-Borst, S., S. Hercberg, A. Morabia, M. S. Bernstein, P. Galan, R. Galasso, S. Giampaoli, E. McCrum, S. Panico, P. Preziosi, et al. 2000. "Dietary patterns in six european populations: results from EURALIM, a collaborative European data harmonization and information campaign." *Eur J Clin Nutr* 54:253.

Benedict, Christian, Werner Kern, Bernd Schultes, Jan Born, and Manfred Hallschmid. 2008. "Differential sensitivity of men and women to anorexigenic and memory-improving effects of intranasal insulin." *J Clin Endocrinol Metab* 93 (4):1339–1344.

Bere, Elling, Johannes Brug, and Knut-Inge Klepp. 2008. "Why do boys eat less fruit and vegetables than girls?" *Public Health Nutr* 11 (3):321–325.

Berridge, Kent C. 2009. "'Liking' and 'wanting' food rewards: brain substrates and roles in eating disorders." *Physiol Behav* 97 (5):537–550.

Borgland, Stephanie L., Sharif A. Taha, Federica Sarti, Howard L. Fields, and Antonello Bonci. 2006. "Orexin A in the VTA is critical for the induction of synaptic plasticity and behavioral sensitization to cocaine." *Neuron* 49 (4):589–601.

Bossé, R., R. Rivest, and T. Di Paolo. 1997. "Ovariectomy and estradiol treatment affect the dopamine transporter and its gene expression in the rat brain." *Brain Res Mol Brain Res* 46 (1–2):343–346.

Brown, A. J., N. M. Avena, and B. G. Hoebel. 2008. "A high-fat diet prevents and reverses the development of activity-based anorexia in rats." *Int J Eat Disord* 41 (5):383–389.

Brown, H. D., J. E. McCutcheon, J. J. Cone, M. E. Ragozzino, and M. F. Roitman. 2011. "Primary food reward and reward-predictive stimuli evoke different patterns of phasic dopamine signaling throughout the striatum." *Eur J Neurosci* 34 (12):1997–2006.

Cabeza De Vaca, S., S. Holiman, and K. D. Carr. 1998. "A search for the metabolic signal that sensitizes lateral hypothalamic self-stimulation in food-restricted rats." *Physiol Behav* 64 (3):251–260.

Cacciapaglia, F., M. P. Saddoris, R. M. Wightman, and R. M. Carelli. 2012. "Differential dopamine release dynamics in the nucleus accumbens core and shell track distinct aspects of goal-directed behavior for sucrose." *Neuropharmacology* 62 (5–6):2050–2056.

Calipari, E. S., B. Juarez, C. Morel, D. M. Walker, M. E. Cahill, E. Ribeiro, C. Roman-Ortiz, C. Ramakrishnan, K. Deisseroth, M. H. Han, et al. 2017. "Dopaminergic dynamics underlying sex-specific cocaine reward." *Nat Commun* 8:13877.

Carnell, S., C. Gibson, L. Benson, C. N. Ochner, and A. Geliebter. 2012. "Neuroimaging and obesity: current knowledge and future directions." *Obes Rev* 13 (1):43–56.

Caron, A., H. M. Dungan Lemko, C. M. Castorena, T. Fujikawa, S. Lee, C. C. Lord, N. Ahmed, C. E. Lee, W. L. Holland, C. Liu, et al. 2018. "POMC neurons expressing leptin receptors coordinate metabolic responses to fasting via suppression of leptin levels." *Elife* 7.

Chavez, Carolina, Marianne Hollaus, Elizabeth Scarr, Geoff Pavey, Andrea Gogos, and Maarten van den Buuse. 2010. "The effect of estrogen on dopamine and serotonin receptor and transporter levels in the brain: an autoradiography study." *Brain Res* 1321:51–59.

Chiodo, Louis A., and Anthony R. Caggiula. 1980. "Alterations in basal firing rate and autoreceptor sensitivity of dopamine neurons in the substantia nigra following acute and extended exposure to estrogen." *Eur J Pharmacol* 67 (1):165–166.

Chowen, J. A., A. Freire-Regatillo, and J. Argente. 2019. "Neurobiological characteristics underlying metabolic differences between males and females." *Prog Neurobiol* 176:18–32.

CIHR Institute of Gender and Health. 2012. "What a difference sex and gender make: a gender, sex and health research casebook." CIHR Institute of Gender and Health, accessed April 16. https://open.library.ubc.ca/collections/52383/items/1.0132684.

Clark, Jeremy J., Nick G. Hollon, and Paul E. M. Phillips. 2012. "Pavlovian valuation systems in learning and decision making." *Curr Opin Neurobiol* 22 (6):1054–1061.

Clayton, Janine A. , and Francis S. Collins. 2014. "Policy: NIH to balance sex in cell and animal studies." *Nature* 509 (7500):282–283.

Clegg, D. J., L. M. Brown, S. C. Woods, and S. C. Benoit. 2006. "Gonadal hormones determine sensitivity to central leptin and insulin." *Diabetes* 55 (4):978–987.

Clegg, Deborah J., Christine A. Riedy, Kathleen A. Blake Smith, Stephen C. Benoit, and Stephen C. Woods. 2003. "Differential sensitivity to central leptin and insulin in male and female rats." *Diabetes* 52 (3):682–687.

Coppari, Roberto, Masumi Ichinose, Charlotte E. Lee, Abigail E. Pullen, Christopher D. Kenny, Robert A. McGovern, Vinsee Tang, Shun M. Liu, Thomas Ludwig, Streamson C. Chua, et al. 2005. "The hypothalamic arcuate nucleus: A key site for mediating leptin's effects on glucose homeostasis and locomotor activity." *Cell Metab* 1 (1):63–72.

Creutz, L. M., and M. F. Kritzer. 2002. "Estrogen receptor-beta immunoreactivity in the midbrain of adult rats: regional, subregional, and cellular localization in the A10, A9, and A8 dopamine cell groups." *J Comp Neurol* 446 (3):288–300.

Croll, Jillian, Dianne Neumark-Sztainer, Mary Story, and Marjorie Ireland. 2002. "Prevalence and risk and protective factors related to disordered eating behaviors among adolescents: relationship to gender and ethnicity." *J Adolesc Health* 31 (2):166–175.

Czoty, Paul W., Natallia V. Riddick, H. Donald Gage, Mikki Sandridge, Susan H. Nader, Sudha Garg, Michael Bounds, Pradeep K. Garg, and Michael A. Nader. 2008. "Effect of menstrual cycle phase on dopamine D2 receptor availability in female cynomolgus monkeys." *Neuropsychopharmacol* 34:548.

D'Argembeau, Arnaud, David Stawarczyk, Steve Majerus, Fabienne Collette, Martial Van der Linden, Dorothée Feyers, Pierre Maquet, and Eric Salmon. 2010. "The neural basis of personal goal processing when envisioning future events." *J Cogn Neurosci* 22 (8):1701–1713.

Dallman, Mary F., Norman Pecoraro, Susan F. Akana, Susanne E. La Fleur, Francisca Gomez, Hani Houshyar, M. E. Bell, Seema Bhatnagar, Kevin D. Laugero, and Sotara Manalo. 2003. "Chronic stress and obesity: a new view of "comfort food"." *Proc Natl Acad Sci U S A* 100 (20):11696–11701.

Davis, Jon F., Derrick L. Choi, and Stephen C. Benoit. 2010. "Insulin, leptin and reward." *Trends Endocrinol Metab* 21 (2):68–74.

Davis, Jon F., Derrick L. Choi, Jennifer D. Schurdak, Maureen F. Fitzgerald, Debbie J. Clegg, Jack W. Lipton, Dianne P. Figlewicz, and Stephen C. Benoit. 2011. "Leptin regulates energy balance and motivation through action at distinct neural circuits." *Biol Psychiatry* 69 (7):668–674.

Day, Jon E. L., Ilias Kyriazakis, and Peter J. Rogers. 1998. "Food choice and intake: towards a unifying framework of learning and feeding motivation." *Nutr Res Rev* 11 (1):25–43.

Dhillon, Harveen, Jeffrey M. Zigman, Chianping Ye, Charlotte E. Lee, Robert A. McGovern, Vinsee Tang, Christopher D. Kenny, Lauryn M. Christiansen, Ryan D. White, Elisabeth A. Edelstein, et al. 2006. "Leptin directly activates SF1 neurons in the VMH, and this action by leptin is required for normal body-weight homeostasis." *Neuron* 49 (2):191–203.

Dichter, Gabriel S., Cara A. Damiano, and John A. Allen. 2012. "Reward circuitry dysfunction in psychiatric and neurodevelopmental disorders and genetic syndromes: animal models and clinical findings." *J Neurodev Disord* 4 (1):19.

DiLeone, Ralph J., Dan Georgescu, and Eric J. Nestler. 2003. "Lateral hypothalamic neuropeptides in reward and drug addiction." *Life Sci* 73 (6):759–768.

Disshon, Kimberly A., John W. Boja, and Dean E. Dluzen. 1998. "Inhibition of striatal dopamine transporter activity by 17β-estradiol." *Eur J Pharmacol* 345 (2):207–211.

Dreher, Jean-Claude, Peter J. Schmidt, Philip Kohn, Daniella Furman, David Rubinow, and Karen Faith Berman. 2007. "Menstrual cycle phase modulates reward-related neural function in women." *Proc Natl Acad Sci U S A* 104 (7):2465–2470.

Dupont, A., T. Di Paolo, B. Gagné, and N. Barden. 1981. "Effects of chronic estrogen treatment on dopamine concentrations and turnover in discrete brain nuclei of ovariectomized rats." *Neurosci Lett* 22 (1):69–74.

Ek, S. 2015. "Gender differences in health information behaviour: a Finnish population-based survey." *Health Promot Int* 30 (3):736–745.

Elmquist, Joel K. , Christian Bjørbæk, Rexford S. Ahima, Jeffrey S. Flier, and Clifford B. Saper. 1998. "Distributions of leptin receptor mRNA isoforms in the rat brain." *J Comp Neurol* 395 (4):535–547.

Farooqi, I. Sadaf, Edward Bullmore, Julia Keogh, Jonathan Gillard, Stephen O'Rahilly, and Paul C. Fletcher. 2007. "Leptin regulates striatal regions and human eating behavior." *Science* 317 (5843):1355–1355.

Febo, Marcelo, Loida A. González-Rodríguez, David E. Capó-Ramos, Naggai Y. González-Segarra, and Annabell C. Segarra. 2003. "Estrogen-dependent alterations in D2/D3-induced G protein activation in cocaine-sensitized female rats." *J Neurochem* 86 (2):405–412.

Feis, Delia-Lisa, Kay H. Brodersen, D. Yves von Cramon, Eileen Luders, and Marc Tittgemeyer. 2013. "Decoding gender dimorphism of the human brain using multimodal anatomical and diffusion MRI data." *NeuroImage* 70:250–257.

Figlewicz, Dianne P., Jennifer L. Bennett, Amy MacDonald Naleid, Charles Davis, and Jeffrey W. Grimm. 2006. "Intraventricular insulin and leptin decrease sucrose self-administration in rats." *Physiol Behav* 89 (4):611–616.

Figlewicz, D. P., S. B. Evans, J. Murphy, M. Hoen, and D. G. Baskin. 2003. "Expression of receptors for insulin and leptin in the ventral tegmental area/substantia nigra (VTA/SN) of the rat." *Brain Res* 964 (1):107–115.

Flegal, K. M., D. Kruszon-Moran, M. D. Carroll, C. D. Fryar, and C. L. Ogden. 2016. "Trends in obesity among adults in the united states, 2005 to 2014." *JAMA* 315 (21):2284–2291.

Foldi, C. J., L. K. Milton, and B. J. Oldfield. 2017. "The role of mesolimbic reward neurocircuitry in prevention and rescue of the activity-based anorexia (ABA) phenotype in rats." *Neuropsychopharmacol* 42 (12):2292–2300.

Frank, Sabine, Naima Laharnar, Stephanie Kullmann, Ralf Veit, Carlos Canova, Yiwen Li Hegner, Andreas Fritsche, and Hubert Preissl. 2010. "Processing of food pictures: Influence of hunger, gender and calorie content." *Brain Res* 1350:159–166.

Friedman, Jeffrey M. 2009. "Leptin at 14 y of age: an ongoing story." *Am J Clin Nutr* 89 (3):973S–979S.

Friedrich, M. J. 2017. "Global obesity epidemic worsening." *JAMA* 318 (7):603–603.

Fulton, Stephanie, Pavlos Pissios, Ramon Pinol Manchon, Linsey Stiles, Lauren Frank, Emmanuel N. Pothos, Eleftheria Maratos-Flier, and Jeffrey S. Flier. 2006. "Leptin regulation of the mesoaccumbens dopamine pathway." *Neuron* 51 (6):811–822.

Funabashi, Toshiya, Hiroko Hagiwara, Kazutaka Mogi, Dai Mitsushima, Kazuyuki Shinohara, and Fukuko Kimura. 2009. "Sex differences in the responses of orexin neurons in the lateral hypothalamic area and feeding behavior to fasting." *Neurosci Lett* 463 (1):31–34.

Gao, Qian, Gabor Mezei, Yongzhan Nie, Yan Rao, Cheol Soo Choi, Ingo Bechmann, Csaba Leranth, Dominique Toran-Allerand, Catherine A. Priest, James L. Roberts, et al. 2007. "Anorectic estrogen mimics leptin's effect on the rewiring of melanocortin cells and Stat3 signaling in obese animals." *Nat Med* 13 (1):89–94.

García-García, I., A. Horstmann, M. A. Jurado, M. Garolera, S. J. Chaudhry, D. S. Margulies, A. Villringer, and J. Neumann. 2014. "Reward processing in obesity, substance addiction and non-substance addiction." *Obesity Rev* 15 (11):853–869.

Gautron, Laurent, and Joel K. Elmquist. 2011. "Sixteen years and counting: an update on leptin in energy balance." *J Clin Invest* 121 (6):2087–2093.

Geary, Nori. 2004. "The estrogenic inhibition of eating." In *Neurobiology of food and fluid intake*, edited by Edward M. Stricker and Stephen C. Woods, 307–345. Springer US.

Geiger, B. M., M. Haburcak, N. M. Avena, M. C. Moyer, B. G. Hoebel, and E. N. Pothos. 2009. "Deficits of mesolimbic dopamine neurotransmission in rat dietary obesity." *Neuroscience* 159 (4):1193–1199.

Geiselman, Paula J., J. R. Martin, D. A. Vanderweele, and D. Novin. 1981. "Dietary self-selection in cycling and neonatally ovariectomized rats." *Appetite* 2 (2):87–101.

Goldstein, Jill M., Matthew Jerram, Brandon Abbs, Susan Whitfield-Gabrieli, and Nikos Makris. 2010. "Sex differences in stress response circuitry activation dependent on female hormonal cycle." *J Neurosci* 30 (2):431–438.

Gorczyca, Anna M., Lindsey A. Sjaarda, Emily M. Mitchell, Neil J. Perkins, Karen C. Schliep, Jean Wactawski-Wende, and Sunni L. Mumford. 2016. "Changes in macronutrient, micronutrient, and food group intakes throughout the menstrual cycle in healthy, premenopausal women." *Eur J Nutr* 55 (3):1181–1188.

Gordon, J. H., and J. Z. Fields. 1989. "A permanent dopamine receptor up-regulation in the ovariectomized rat." *Pharmacol Biochem Behav* 33 (1):123–125.

Greenberg, Gian D., and Brian C. Trainor. 2016. "Sex differences in the social behavior network and mesolimbic dopamine system." In *Sex differences in the central nervous system*, edited by Rebecca M Shansky, 77–106. San Diego: Academic Press.

Grimm, K.A., H.M. Blanck, K.S. Scanlon, L.V. Moore, L.M. Grummer-Strawn, and J.L. Foltz. 2010. "State-specific trends in fruit and vegetable consumption among adults - United States, 2000-2009." *Morb Mortal Wkly Rep* 59 (35):1125–1130.

Gupta, Arpana, Emeran A. Mayer, Jennifer S. Labus, Ravi R. Bhatt, Tiffany Ju, Aubrey Love, Amanat Bal, Kirsten Tillisch, Bruce Naliboff, Claudia P. Sanmiguel, et al. 2018. "Sex commonalities and differences in obesity-related alterations in intrinsic brain activity and connectivity." *Obesity* 26 (2):340–350.

Haase, Lori, Erin Green, and Claire Murphy. 2011. "Males and females show differential brain activation to taste when hungry and sated in gustatory and reward areas." *Appetite* 57 (2):421–434.

Haddad-Tóvolli, Roberta, Nathalia R. V. Dragano, Albina F. S. Ramalho, and Licio A. Velloso. 2017. "Development and function of the blood-brain barrier in the context of metabolic control." *Front neurosci* 11:224–224.

Hales, Craig M., Margaret D. Carroll, Cheryl D. Fryar, and Cynthia L. Ogden. 2017. "*Prevalence of obesity among adults and youth: United States, 2015–2016*." https://www.cdc.gov/nchs/products/databriefs/db288.htm.

Hallschmid, Manfred, Christian Benedict, Bernd Schultes, Horst-Lorenz Fehm, Jan Born, and Werner Kern. 2004. "Intranasal insulin reduces body fat in men but not in women." *Diabetes* 53 (11):3024–3029.

Hamid, A. A., J. R. Pettibone, O. S. Mabrouk, V. L. Hetrick, R. Schmidt, C. M. Vander Weele, R. T. Kennedy, B. J. Aragona, and J. D. Berke. 2016. "Mesolimbic dopamine signals the value of work." *Nat Neurosci* 19 (1):117–126.

Harris, Glenda C., Mathieu Wimmer, and Gary Aston-Jones. 2005. "A role for lateral hypothalamic orexin neurons in reward seeking." *Nature* 437:556.

Havel, P. J. 2001. "Peripheral signals conveying metabolic information to the brain: short-term and long-term regulation of food intake and energy homeostasis." *Exp Biol Med (Maywood)* 226 (11):963–977.

Heisler, Lora K., Robin B. Kanarek, and Brent Homoleski. 1999. "Reduction of fat and protein intakes but not carbohydrate intake following acute and chronic fluoxetine in female rats." *Pharmacol Biochem Behav* 63 (3):377–385.

Hilbert, Anja, Martina de Zwaan, and Elmar Braehler. 2012. "How frequent are eating disturbances in the population? Norms of the eating disorder examination-questionnaire." *PLoS One* 7 (1):e29125.

Hill, Jennifer W., Carol F. Elias, Makoto Fukuda, Kevin W. Williams, Eric D. Berglund, William L. Holland, You-Ree Cho, Jen-Chieh Chuang, Yong Xu, Michelle Choi, Danielle Lauzon, et al. 2010. "Direct insulin and leptin action on pro-opiomelanocortin neurons is required for normal glucose homeostasis and fertility." *Cell Metab* 11 (4):286–297.

Hill, J. M., M. A. Lesniak, C. B. Pert, and J. Roth. 1986. "Autoradiographic localization of insulin receptors in rat brain: prominence in olfactory and limbic areas." *Neuroscience* 17 (4):1127–1138.

Hoebel, Bartley G., and Philip Teitelbaum. 1962. "Hypothalamic control of feeding and self-stimulation." *Science* 135 (3501):375–377.

Hoek, Hans Wijbrand. 2006. "Incidence, prevalence and mortality of anorexia nervosa and other eating disorders." *Curr Opin Psychiatry* 19 (4):389–394.

Hommel, Jonathan D., Richard Trinko, Robert M. Sears, Dan Georgescu, Zong-Wu Liu, Xiao-Bing Gao, Jeremy J. Thurmon, Michela Marinelli, and Ralph J. DiLeone. 2006. "Leptin receptor signaling in midbrain dopamine neurons regulates feeding." *Neuron* 51 (6):801–810.

Hruska, Robert E., and Mark W. Nowak. 1988. "Estrogen treatment increases the density of D1 dopamine receptors in the rat striatum." *Brain Res* 442 (2):349–350.

Hudson, James I., Eva Hiripi, Harrison G. Pope, and Ronald C. Kessler. 2007. "The prevalence and correlates of eating disorders in the National Comorbidity Survey Replication." *Biol Psychiatry* 61 (3):348–358.

Ilango, Anton, Andrew J. Kesner, Kristine L. Keller, Garret D. Stuber, Antonello Bonci, and Satoshi Ikemoto. 2014. "Similar roles of substantia nigra and ventral tegmental dopamine neurons in reward and aversion." *J Neurosci* 34 (3):817–822.

Jastreboff, Ania M., Cheryl Lacadie, Dongju Seo, Jessica Kubat, Michelle A. Van Name, Cosimo Giannini, Mary Savoye, R. Todd Constable, Robert S. Sherwin, Sonia Caprio, et al. 2014. "Leptin is associated with exaggerated brain reward and emotion responses to food images in adolescent obesity." *Diabetes Care* 37 (11):3061–3068.

Jastreboff, Ania M., Rajita Sinha, Cheryl Lacadie, Dana M. Small, Robert S. Sherwin, and Marc N. Potenza. 2013. "Neural correlates of stress- and food cue-induced food craving in obesity: association with insulin levels." *Diabetes Care* 36 (2):394–402.

Johnson, Paul M., and Paul J. Kenny. 2010. "Dopamine D2 receptors in addiction-like reward dysfunction and compulsive eating in obese rats." *Nat Neurosci* 13 (5):635–641.

Johnson, Z. P., J. Lowe, V. Michopoulos, C. J. Moore, M. E. Wilson, and D. Toufexis. 2013. "Oestradiol differentially influences feeding behaviour depending on diet composition in female rhesus monkeys." *J Neuroendocrinol* 25 (8):729–741.

Jones, K. T., C. Woods, J. Zhen, T. Antonio, K. D. Carr, and M. E. Reith. 2017. "Effects of diet and insulin on dopamine transporter activity and expression in rat caudate-putamen, nucleus accumbens, and midbrain." *J Neurochem* 140 (5):728–740.

Joyce, J. N., R. L. Smith, and C. van Hartesveldt. 1982. "Estradiol suppresses then enhances intracaudate dopamine-induced contralateral deviation." *Eur J Pharmacol* 81 (1):117–122.

Kandiah, Jayanthi, Melissa Yake, James Jones, and Michaela Meyer. 2006. "Stress influences appetite and comfort food preferences in college women." *Nutr Res* 26 (3):118–123.

Kanter, Rebecca, and Benjamin Caballero. 2012. "Global gender disparities in obesity: a review." *Adv Nutr* 3 (4):491–498.

Kenny, P. J. 2011. "Common cellular and molecular mechanisms in obesity and drug addiction." *Nat Rev Neurosci* 12 (11):638–651.

Killgore, William D. S., and Deborah A. Yurgelun-Todd. 2010. "Sex differences in cerebral responses to images of high versus low calorie food." *Neuroreport* 21 (5):354–358.

Kinasz, Kathryn, Erin C. Accurso, Andrea E. Kass, and Daniel Le Grange. 2016. "Sex differences in the clinical presentation of eating disorders in youth." *J Adolesc Health* 58 (4):410–416.

Klenotich, S. J., and S. C. Dulawa. 2012. "The activity-based anorexia mouse model." *Methods Mol Biol* 829:377–393.

Klump, K. L., K. M. Culbert, J. D. Slane, S. A. Burt, C. L. Sisk, and J. T. Nigg. 2012. "The effects of puberty on genetic risk for disordered eating: evidence for a sex difference." *Psychol Med* 42 (3):627–637.

Klump, Kelly L., Sarah Racine, Britny Hildebrandt, and Cheryl L. Sisk. 2013. "Sex differences in binge eating patterns in male and female adult rats." *Int J Eat Disord* 46 (7):729–736.

Klump, Kelly L., Jessica L. Suisman, Kristen M. Culbert, Deborah A. Kashy, and Cheryl L. Sisk. 2011. "Binge eating proneness emerges during puberty in female rats: A longitudinal study." *J Abnorm Psychol* 120 (4):948–955.

Könner, A. Christine, Ruth Janoschek, Leona Plum, Sabine D. Jordan, Eva Rother, Xiaosong Ma, Chun Xu, Pablo Enriori, Brigitte Hampel, Gregory S. Barsh, et al. 2007. "Insulin Action in AgRP-Expressing Neurons Is Required for Suppression of Hepatic Glucose Production." *Cell Metab* 5 (6):438–449.

Kowalska, Irina, Monika Karczewska-Kupczewska, and Marek Strączkowski. 2011. "Adipocytokines, gut hormones and growth factors in anorexia nervosa." *Clin Chim Acta* 412 (19):1702–1711.

Lam, Brian Y. H., Irene Cimino, Joseph Polex-Wolf, Sara Nicole Kohnke, Debra Rimmington, Valentine Iyemere, Nicholas Heeley, Chiara Cossetti, Reiner Schulte, Luis R. Saraiva, et al. 2017. "Heterogeneity of hypothalamic pro-opiomelanocortin-expressing neurons revealed by single-cell RNA sequencing." *Mol Metab* 6 (5):383–392.

Lammers, Claas-Hinrich, Ursula D'Souza, Zheng-Hong Qin, Sang-Hyeon Lee, Shunsuke Yajima, and M. Maral Mouradian. 1999. "Regulation of striatal dopamine receptors by estrogen." *Synapse* 34 (3):222–227.

Ledikwe, Jenny H., Heidi M. Blanck, Laura Kettel Khan, Mary K. Serdula, Jennifer D. Seymour, Beth C. Tohill, and Barbara J. Rolls. 2005. "Dietary energy density determined by eight calculation methods in a nationally representative United States population." *J Nutr* 135 (2):273–278.

Leech, Rebecca M., Anthony Worsley, Anna Timperio, and Sarah A. McNaughton. 2015. "Understanding meal patterns: definitions, methodology and impact on nutrient intake and diet quality." *Nutr Res Rev* 28 (1):1–21.

Legrand, R., N. Lucas, J. Breton, P. Déchelotte, and S. O. Fetissov. 2015. "Dopamine release in the lateral hypothalamus is stimulated by α-MSH in both the anticipatory and consummatory phases of feeding." *Psychoneuroendocrinol* 56:79–87.

Leigh, Sarah-Jane, and Margaret J. Morris. 2018. "The role of reward circuitry and food addiction in the obesity epidemic: an update." *Biol Psychol* 131:31–42.

Leinninger, Gina M., Young-Hwan Jo, Rebecca L. Leshan, Gwendolyn W. Louis, Hongyan Yang, Jason G. Barrera, Hilary Wilson, Darren M. Opland, Miro A. Faouzi, Yusong Gong, et al. 2009. "Leptin acts via leptin receptor-expressing lateral hypothalamic neurons to modulate the mesolimbic dopamine system and suppress feeding." *Cell Metab* 10 (2):89–98.

Leranth, Csaba, Robert H. Roth, John D. Elsworth, Frederick Naftolin, Tamas L. Horvath, and D. Eugene Redmond. 2000. "Estrogen is essential for maintaining nigrostriatal dopamine neurons in primates: implications for Parkinson's disease and memory." *J Neurosci* 20 (23):8604.

Liu, C. M., E. A. Davis, A. N. Suarez, R. I. Wood, E. E. Noble, and S. E. Kanoski. 2019. "Sex differences and estrous influences on oxytocin control of food intake." *Neuroscience*

Liu, Clarissa M., and Scott E. Kanoski. 2018. "Homeostatic and non-homeostatic controls of feeding behavior: Distinct vs. common neural systems." *Physiol Behav.*

London, T. D., J. A. Licholai, I. Szczot, M. A. Ali, K. H. LeBlanc, W. C. Fobbs, and A. V. Kravitz. 2018. "Coordinated ramping of dorsal striatal paathways preceding food approach and consumption." *J Neurosci* 38 (14):3547–3558.

Lovejoy, J. C., A. Sainsbury, and Group the Stock Conference Working. 2009. "Sex differences in obesity and the regulation of energy homeostasis." *Obes Rev* 10 (2):154–167.

de Luca, Carl, Timothy J. Kowalski, Yiying Zhang, Joel K. Elmquist, Charlotte Lee, Manfred W. Kilimann, Thomas Ludwig, Shun-Mei Liu, and Streamson C. Chua. 2005. "Complete rescue of obesity, diabetes, and infertility in db/db mice by neuron-specific LEPR-B transgenes." *J Clin Invest* 115 (12):3484–3493.

Margules, D. L., and J. Olds. 1962. "Identical "feeding" and "rewarding" systems in the lateral hypothalamus of rats." *Science* 135 (3501):374–375.

Martin, Laura E., Laura M. Holsen, Rebecca J. Chambers, Amanda S. Bruce, William M. Brooks, Jennifer R. Zarcone, Merlin G. Butler, and Cary R. Savage. 2010. "Neural mechanisms associated with food motivation in obese and healthy weight adults." *Obesity* 18 (2):254–260.

Mauvais-Jarvis, Franck. 2015. "Sex differences in metabolic homeostasis, diabetes and obesity.", *Biol Sex Differ* 6:14.

McCutcheon, J. E., J. A. Beeler, and M. F. Roitman. 2012. "Sucrose-predictive cues evoke greater phasic dopamine release than saccharin-predictive cues." *Synapse* 66 (4):346–351.

McCutcheon, J. E., S. R. Ebner, A. L. Loriaux, and M. F. Roitman. 2012. "Encoding of aversion by dopamine and the nucleus accumbens." *Front Neurosci* 6:137.

McGinnis, Marilyn Y., John H. Gordon, and Roger A. Gorski. 1980. "Influence of γ-aminobutyric acid on lordosis behavior and dopamine activity in estrogen primed spayed female rats." *Brain Res* 184 (1):179–191.

McVay, Megan Apperson, Amy L. Copeland, Hannah S. Newman, and Paula J. Geiselman. 2012. "Food cravings and food cue responding across the menstrual cycle in a non-eating disordered sample." *Appetite* 59 (2):591–600.

Mebel, Dmitry. M., Jovi. C. Y. Wong, Yifei. J. Dong, and Stephanie. L. Borgland. 2012. "Insulin in the ventral tegmental area reduces hedonic feeding and suppresses dopamine concentration via increased reuptake." *Eur J Neurosci* 36 (3):2336–2346.

Meli, Rosaria, Maria Pacilio, Giuseppina Mattace Raso, Emanuela Esposito, Anna Coppola, Anna Nasti, Costantino Di Carlo, Carmine Nappi, and Raffaele Di Carlo. 2004. "Estrogen and raloxifene modulate leptin and its receptor in hypothalamus and adipose tissue from ovariectomized rats." *Endocrinology* 145 (7):3115–3121.

Meneses, Alfredo, and Gustavo Liy-Salmeron. 2012. "Serotonin and emotion, learning and memory." *Rev Neurosci* 23 (5–6):543–553.

Meule, Adrian, and Claus Vögele. 2013. "The psychology of eating." *Front Psychol* 4 (215).

Milner, T. A., L. I. Thompson, G. Wang, J. A. Kievits, E. Martin, P. Zhou, B. S. McEwen, D. W. Pfaff, and E. M. Waters. 2010. "Distribution of estrogen receptor β containing cells in the brains of bacterial artificial chromosome transgenic mice." *Brain Res* 1351:74–96.

Misra, Madhusmita, and Anne Klibanski. 2014. "Endocrine consequences of anorexia nervosa." *Lancet Diabetes Endocrinol* 2 (7):581–592.

Monteleone, Palmiero, and Mario Maj. 2013. "Dysfunctions of leptin, ghrelin, BDNF and endocannabinoids in eating disorders: beyond the homeostatic control of food intake." *Psychoneuroendocrinol* 38 (3):312–330.

Morel, Gustavo R., Rubén W. Carón, Gloria M. Cónsole, Marta Soaje, Yolanda E. Sosa, Silvia S. Rodríguez, Graciela A. Jahn, and Rodolfo G. Goya. 2009. "Estrogen inhibits tuberoinfundibular dopaminergic neurons but does not cause irreversible damage." *Brain Res Bull* 80 (6):347–352.

Morissette, M., and T. Di Paolo. 1993. "Effect of chronic estradiol and progesterone treatments of ovariectomized rats on brain dopamine uptake sites." *J Neurochem* 60 (5):1876–1883.

Morton, G. J., D. E. Cummings, D. G. Baskin, G. S. Barsh, and M. W. Schwartz. 2006. "Central nervous system control of food intake and body weight." *Nature* 443 (7109):289–295.

Nohara, Kazunari, Yan Zhang, Rizwana S. Waraich, Amanda Laque, Joseph P. Tiano, Jenny Tong, Heike Münzberg, and Franck Mauvais-Jarvis. 2011. "Early-life exposure to testosterone programs the hypothalamic melanocortin system." *Endocrinology* 152 (4):1661–1669.

Norgren, R., A. Hajnal, and S. S. Mungarndee. 2006. "Gustatory reward and the nucleus accumbens." *Physiol Behav* 89 (4):531–535.

Opland, Darren M., Gina M. Leinninger, and Martin G. Myers. 2010. "Modulation of the mesolimbic dopamine system by leptin." *Brain Res* 1350:65–70.

Padilla, Stephanie L., Jill S. Carmody, and Lori M. Zeltser. 2010. "Pomc-expressing progenitors give rise to antagonistic neuronal populations in hypothalamic feeding circuits." *Nat Med* 16 (4):403–405.

Palmer, B. F., and D. J. Clegg. 2015. "The sexual dimorphism of obesity." *Mol Cell Endocrinol* 402:113–119.

Palmiter, R. D. 2008. "Dopamine signaling in the dorsal striatum is essential for motivated behaviors: lessons from dopamine-deficient mice." *Ann N Y Acad Sci* 1129:35–46.

Del Parigi, Angelo, Kewei Chen, Jean-François Gautier, Arline D. Salbe, Richard E. Pratley, Eric Ravussin, Eric M. Reiman, and P. Antonio Tataranni. 2002. "Sex differences in the human brain's response to hunger and satiation." *Am J Clin Nutr* 75 (6):1017–1022.

Piech, Richard M., Jade Lewis, Caroline H. Parkinson, Adrian M. Owen, Angela C. Roberts, Paul E. Downing, and John A. Parkinson. 2009. "Neural correlates of appetite and hunger-related evaluative judgments." *PLoS One* 4 (8):e6581.

Plum, Leona, Bengt F. Belgardt, and Jens C. Brüning. 2006. "Central insulin action in energy and glucose homeostasis." *J Clin Invest* 116 (7):1761–1766.

Pochon, Jean-Baptiste, Richard Levy, Jean-Baptiste Poline, Sophie Crozier, Stéphane Lehéricy, Bernard Pillon, Bernard Deweer, Denis Le Bihan, and Bruno Dubois. 2001. "The role of dorsolateral prefrontal cortex in the preparation of forthcoming actions: an fMRI study." *Cereb Cortex* 11 (3):260–266.

Prättälä, R., L. Paalanen, D. Grinberga, V. Helasoja, A. Kasmel, and J. Petkeviciene. 2007. "Gender differences in the consumption of meat, fruit and vegetables are similar in Finland and the Baltic countries." *Eur J Public Health* 17 (5):520–525.

Proaño, S. B., H. J. Morris, L. M. Kunz, D. M. Dorris, and J. Meitzen. 2018. "Estrous cycle-induced sex differences in medium spiny neuron excitatory synaptic transmission and intrinsic excitability in adult rat nucleus accumbens core." *J Neurophysiol* 120 (3):1356–1373.

Qu, Na, Yanlin He, Chunmei Wang, Pingwen Xu, Yongjie Yang, Xing Cai, Hesong Liu, Kaifan Yu, Zhou Pei, Ilirjana Hyseni, et al. 2020. "A POMC-originated circuit regulates stress-induced hypophagia, depression, and anhedonia." *Mol Psychiatry* 25 (5):1006–1021.

Ramirez, V. D., and J. Zheng. 1996. "Membrane sex-steroid receptors in the brain." *Front Neuroendocrinol* 17 (4):402–439.

Rehavi, Moshe, Miri Goldin, Netta Roz, and Abraham Weizman. 1998. "Regulation of rat brain vesicular monoamine transporter by chronic treatment with ovarian hormones." *Brain Res Mol Brain Res* 57 (1):31–37.

Richard, Jennifer E., Lorena López-Ferreras, Rozita H. Anderberg, Kajsa Olandersson, and Karolina P. Skibicka. 2017. "Estradiol is a critical regulator of food-reward behavior." *Psychoneuroendocrinol* 78:193–202.

Rocha, Milagros, Chen Bing, Gareth Williams, and Marisa Puerta. 2004. "Physiologic estradiol levels enhance hypothalamic expression of the long form of the leptin receptor in intact rats." *J Nutr Biochem* 15 (6):328–334.

Rolls, Barbara J., Ingrid C. Fedoroff, and Joanne F. Guthrie. 1991. "Gender differences in eating behavior and body weight regulation." *Health Psychol* 10 (2):133–142.

Rolls, E. T. 2012. "Taste, olfactory and food texture reward processing in the brain and the control of appetite." *Proc Nutr Soc* 71 (4):488–501.

Rossi, Mark A., and Garret D. Stuber. 2018. "Overlapping brain circuits for homeostatic and hedonic feeding." *Cell Metab* 27 (1):42–56.

Russo, S. J., E. D. Festa, S. J. Fabian, F. M. Gazi, M. Kraish, S. Jenab, and V. Quiñones-Jenab. 2003. "Gonadal hormones differentially modulate cocaine-induced conditioned place preference in male and female rats." *Neuroscience* 120 (2):523–533.

Rybakowski, Filip, Agnieszka Slopien, and Marta Tyszkiewicz-Nwafor. 2014. "Inverse relationship between leptin increase and improvement in depressive symptoms in anorexia nervosa." *Neuro Endocrinol Lett* 35:64–67.

Sackett, Deirdre A., Michael P. Saddoris, and Regina M. Carelli. 2017. "Nucleus accumbens shell dopamine preferentially tracks information related to outcome value of reward." *eNeuro* 4 (3):ENEURO.0058-17.2017.

Schalla, Martha A., and Andreas Stengel. 2019. "Activity based anorexia as an animal model for anorexia nervosa - a systematic review." *Front Nutr* 6 (69).

Schwartz MW, Woods SC, Porte D, Seeley RJ, Baskin DG. Central nervous system control of food intake. *Nature*. 2000;404(6778):661–671. doi: 10.1038/35007534

Sclafani, Anthony, and Karen Ackroff. 2012. "Role of gut nutrient sensing in stimulating appetite and conditioning food preferences." *Am J Physiol Regul Integr Comp Physiol* 302 (10):R1119–R1133.

Scott, Hayley M., J. Ian Mason, and Richard M. Sharpe. 2009. "Steroidogenesis in the fetal testis and its susceptibility to disruption by exogenous compounds." *Endocr Rev* 30 (7):883–925.

Segal-Lieberman, Gabriella, Richard L. Bradley, Efi Kokkotou, Michael Carlson, Daniel J. Trombly, Xiaomei Wang, Sarah Bates, Martin G. Myers, Jeffrey S. Flier, and Eleftheria Maratos-Flier. 2003. "Melanin-concentrating hormone is a critical mediator of the leptin–deficient phenotype." *Proc Natl Acad Sci U S A* 100 (17):10085–10090.

Shi, Haifei, Randy J. Seeley, and Deborah J. Clegg. 2009. "Sexual differences in the control of energy homeostasis." *Front Neuroendocrinol* 30 (3):396–404.

Shi, Haifei, April D. Strader, Stephen C. Woods, and Randy J. Seeley. 2007. "Sexually dimorphic responses to fat loss after caloric restriction or surgical lipectomy." *Am J Physiol Endocrinol Metab* 293 (1):E316–E326.

Shiferaw, Beletshachew, Linda Verrill, Hillary Booth, Shelley M. Zansky, Dawn M. Norton, Stacy Crim, and Olga L. Henao. 2012. "Sex-based differences in food consumption: Foodborne Diseases Active Surveillance Network (FoodNet) Population Survey, 2006-2007." *Clin Infect Dis* 54 (suppl_5):S453–S457.

Shimizu, Hiroyuki, and George A. Bray. 1993. "Effects of castration, estrogen replacement and estrus cycle on monoamine metabolism in the nucleus accumbens, measured by microdialysis." *Brain Res* 621 (2):200–206.

Sinclair, Elaine B., Britny A. Hildebrandt, Kristen M. Culbert, Kelly L. Klump, and Cheryl L. Sisk. 2017. "Preliminary evidence of sex differences in behavioral and neural responses to palatable food reward in rats." *Physiol Behav* 176:165–173.

Smeets, Paul A. M., Cees de Graaf, Annette Stafleu, Matthias J. P. van Osch, Rutger A. J. Nievelstein, and Jeroen van der Grond. 2006. "Effect of satiety on brain activation during chocolate tasting in men and women." *Am J Clin Nutr* 83 (6):1297–1305.

Soriano-Guillén, L., L. Ortega, P. Navarro, P. Riestra, T. Gavela-Pérez, and C. Garcés. 2016. "Sex-related differences in the association of ghrelin levels with obesity in adolescents." *Clin Chem Lab Med* 54 (8):1371–1376.

Stice, Eric, Sonja Yokum, Kyle S. Burger, Leonard H. Epstein, and Dana M. Small. 2011. "Youth at risk for obesity show greater activation of striatal and somatosensory regions to food." *J Neurosci* 31 (12):4360–4366.

Stoeckel, Luke E., Rosalyn E. Weller, Edwin W. Cook, Donald B. Twieg, Robert C. Knowlton, and James E. Cox. 2008. "Widespread reward-system activation in obese women in response to pictures of high-calorie foods." *NeuroImage* 41 (2):636–647.

Striegel-Moore, Ruth H., Francine Rosselli, Nancy Perrin, Lynn DeBar, G. Terence Wilson, Alexis May, and Helena C. Kraemer. 2009. "Gender difference in the prevalence of eating disorder symptoms." *Int J Eat Disord* 42 (5):471–474.

Strubbe, Jan H., and Stephen C. Woods. 2004. "The timing of meals." *Psychol Rev* 111 (1):128–141.

Stuber, Garret D., and Roy A. Wise. 2016. "Lateral hypothalamic circuits for feeding and reward." *Nat Neurosci* 19:198.

Swanson, S. A., S. J. Crow, D. Le Grange, J. Swendsen, and K. R. Merikangas. 2011. "Prevalence and correlates of eating disorders in adolescents: Results from the national comorbidity survey replication adolescent supplement." *Arch Gen Psychiatry* 68 (7):714–723.

Thammacharoen, Sumpun, Nori Geary, Thomas A. Lutz, Sonoko Ogawa, and Lori Asarian. 2009. "Divergent effects of estradiol and the estrogen receptor-[alpha] agonist PPT on eating and activation of PVN CRH neurons in ovariectomized rats and mice." *Brain Res* 1268:88–96.

Thammacharoen, Sumpun, Thomas A. Lutz, Nori Geary, and Lori Asarian. 2008. "Hindbrain administration of estradiol inhibits feeding and activates estrogen receptor-alpha-expressing cells in the nucleus tractus solitarius of ovariectomized rats." *Endocrinology* 149 (4):1609–1617.

Thompson, T. L., S. R. Bridges, and W. J. Weirs. 2001. "Alteration of dopamine transport in the striatum and nucleus accumbens of ovariectomized and estrogen-primed rats following N-(p-isothiocyanatophenethyl) spiperone (NIPS) treatment." *Brain Res Bull* 54 (6):631–638.

Thompson, Tina L., and Robert L. Moss. 1994. "Estrogen regulation of dopamine release in the nucleus accumbens: genomic- and nongenomic-mediated effects." *J Neurochem* 62 (5):1750–1756.

Ulrich-Lai, Yvonne M., Stephanie Fulton, Mark Wilson, Gorica Petrovich, and Linda Rinaman. 2015. "Stress exposure, food intake and emotional state." *Stress* 18 (4):381–399.

Valle, A., A. Catala-Niell, B. Colom, F. J. Garcia-Palmer, J. Oliver, and P. Roca. 2005. "Sex-related differences in energy balance in response to caloric restriction." *Am J Physiol Endocrinol Metab* 289 (1):E15–E22.

Van Vugt, D.A. , and R.L. Reid. 2014. "Neuroimaging menstrual cycle associated changes in appetite." In *Handbook of diet and nutrition in the menstrual cycle, periconception and fertility*, edited by Caroline Hollins-Martin, Olga van den Akker, Colin Martin and Victor R Preedy, 169–188.

van Zessen, R., G. van der Plasse, and R. A. H. Adan. 2012. "Contribution of the mesolimbic dopamine system in mediating the effects of leptin and ghrelin on feeding." *Proc Nutr Soc* 71 (4):435–445.

Volkow, N. D., G. J. Wang, J. S. Fowler, J. Logan, M. Jayne, D. Franceschi, C. Wong, S. J. Gatley, A. N. Gifford, Y. S. Ding, et al. 2002. ""Nonhedonic" food motivation in humans involves dopamine in the dorsal striatum and methylphenidate amplifies this effect." *Synapse* 44 (3):175–180.

Volkow, Nora D., Roy A. Wise, and Ruben Baler. 2017. "The dopamine motive system: implications for drug and food addiction." *Nat Rev Neurosci* 18:741.

Wang, G. J., A. Geliebter, N. D. Volkow, F. W. Telang, J. Logan, M. C. Jayne, K. Galanti, P. A. Selig, H. Han, W. Zhu, et al. 2011. "Enhanced striatal dopamine release during food stimulation in binge eating disorder." *Obesity (Silver Spring)* 19 (8):1601–1608.

Wang, Gene-Jack, Nora D. Volkow, Jean Logan, Naoml R. Pappas, Christopher T. Wong, Wel Zhu, Noelwah Netusll, and Joanna S. Fowler. 2001. "Brain dopamine and obesity." *Lancet* 357 (9253):354–357.

Wansink, Brian, Matthew M. Cheney, and Nina Chan. 2003. "Exploring comfort food preferences across age and gender." *Physiol Behav* 79 (4):739–747.

Wardle, Jane, Anne M. Haase, Andrew Steptoe, Maream Nillapun, Kiriboon Jonwutiwes, and France Bellisle. 2004. "Gender differences in food choice: the contribution of health beliefs and dieting." *Ann Behav Med* 27 (2):107–116.

West, E. A., and R. M. Carelli. 2016. "Nucleus accumbens core and shell differentially encode reward-associated cues after reinforcer devaluation." *J Neurosci* 36 (4):1128–1139.

Williams, Kevin W., Lisandra O. Margatho, Charlotte E. Lee, Michelle Choi, Syann Lee, Michael M. Scott, Carol F. Elias, and Joel K. Elmquist. 2010. "Segregation of acute leptin and insulin effects in distinct populations of arcuate proopiomelanocortin neurons." *J Neurosci* 30 (7):2472–2479.

Woods, Stephen C. 2009. "The control of food intake: behavioral versus molecular perspectives." *Cell Metab* 9 (6):489–498.

Wurtman, Judith J., and Michael J. Baum. 1980. "Estrogen reduces total food and carbohydrate intake, but not protein intake, in female rats." *Physiol Behav* 24 (5):823–827.

Xu, Yong, and Miguel López. 2018. "Central regulation of energy metabolism by estrogens." *Mol Metab* 15:104–115.

Yamanaka, Akihiro, Carsten T. Beuckmann, Jon T. Willie, Junko Hara, Natsuko Tsujino, Michihiro Mieda, Makoto Tominaga, Ken-ichi Yagami, Fumihiro Sugiyama, Katsutoshi Goto, et al. 2003. "Hypothalamic orexin neurons regulate arousal according to energy balance in mice." *Neuron* 38 (5):701–713.

Yilmaz, Zeynep, Allan S. Kaplan, Arun K. Tiwari, Robert D. Levitan, Sara Piran, Andrew W. Bergen, Walter H. Kaye, Hakon Hakonarson, Kai Wang, Wade H. Berrettini, et al. 2014. "The role of leptin, melanocortin, and neurotrophin system genes on body weight in anorexia nervosa and bulimia nervosa." *J Psychiatr Res* 55:77–86.

Yoest, Katie E., Jennifer A. Cummings, and Jill B. Becker. 2014. "Estradiol, dopamine and motivation." *Cent Nerv Syst Agents Med Chem* 14 (2):83–89.

Zandian, Modjtaba, Ioannis Ioakimidis, Cecilia Bergh, Michael Leon, and Per Södersten. 2011. "A sex difference in the response to fasting." *Physiol Behav* 103 (5):530–534.

Zellner, Debra A., Susan Loaiza, Zuleyma Gonzalez, Jaclyn Pita, Janira Morales, Deanna Pecora, and Amanda Wolf. 2006. "Food selection changes under stress." *Physiol Behav* 87 (4):789–793.

Zellner, Debra A., Shin Saito, and Johanie Gonzalez. 2007. "The effect of stress on men's food selection." *Appetite* 49 (3):696–699.

Zhang, D., S. Yang, C. Yang, G. Jin, and X. Zhen. 2008. "Estrogen regulates responses of dopamine neurons in the ventral tegmental area to cocaine." *Psychopharmacology (Berl)* 199 (4):625–635. doi: 10.1007/s00213-008-1188-6.

Zheng, Huiyuan, Laurel M. Patterson, and Hans-Rudolf Berthoud. 2007. "Orexin signaling in the ventral tegmental area is required for high-fat appetite induced by opioid stimulation of the nucleus accumbens." *J Neurosci* 27 (41):11075.

Zhou, Wenxia, Kathryn A. Cunningham, and Mary L. Thomas. 2002. "Estrogen regulation of gene expression in the brain: a possible mechanism altering the response to psychostimulants in female rats." *Brain Res Mol Brain Res* 100 (1):75–83.

Zigman, Jeffrey M., Juli E. Jones, Charlotte E. Lee, Clifford B. Saper, and Joel K. Elmquist. 2006. "Expression of ghrelin receptor mRNA in the rat and the mouse brain." *J Comp Neurol* 494 (3):528–548.

13 High-Throughput Evaluation of Metabolic Activities Using Reverse Phase Protein Array Technology

Hsin-Yi Lu

Baylor College of Medicine, USA,

Jian Xiong

The University of Texas Health Science Center at Houston, USA,

Dimuthu Nuwan Perera

Baylor College of Medicine, USA,

Kimal Rajapakshe

Baylor College of Medicine, USA,

Xuan Wang

Baylor College of Medicine, USA,

Myra Costello

Baylor College of Medicine, USA,

Kimberly R. Holloway

Baylor College of Medicine, USA,

Carlos Ramos

Baylor College of Medicine, USA,

Sandra L. Grimm

Baylor College of Medicine, USA,

Julia Wulfkuhle

George Mason University, USA,

Cristian Coarfa

Baylor College of Medicine, USA

The University of Texas Health Science Center at Houston, USA,

Dean P. Edwards

Baylor College of Medicine, USA

The University of Texas Health Science Center at Houston, USA,

Michael X. Zhu

The University of Texas Health Science Center at Houston, USA and

Shixia Huang

Baylor College of Medicine, USA

The University of Texas Health Science Center at Houston, USA

Contents

13.1 INTRODUCTION

Many markers that play significant roles in biological functions are proteins with very low expression in clinical samples and display large variations among individuals; measuring them accurately requires a large sample number and incurs a tremendous challenge on workload. Reverse phase protein array (RPPA) (Grubb Iii et al., 2009; Mueller et al., 2010; Creighton and Huang, 2015) is a high-throughput antibody-based protein analysis technology that can profile low abundance proteins on a large scale. RPPA analyzes nanoliter amounts of samples for hundreds of proteins on thousands of samples simultaneously. The samples can be tissue or cell lysates, serum, plasma, or other body fluids (Mueller et al., 2010). The measurement assesses not only the total levels of protein expression but also phosphorylation of some of the proteins (Grubb Iii et al., 2009). To achieve the high throughput, protein samples are arrayed as microspots on nitrocellulose-coated glass slides and probed with highly specific antibodies that have been validated for RPPA. Since each microspot contains the whole proteome repertoire of the original protein sample, this approach enables the determination of the proteomic profile in large collections of tissue or cell samples.

The Baylor College of Medicine (BCM) Antibody-based Proteomics Core currently has an inventory of 230+ validated antibodies that cover multiple total and phosphoproteins in the following protein pathways or functional protein groups: epithelial-mesenchymal transition (EMT), stem cells, apoptosis, DNA damage, autophagy, proliferation and cell cycle, growth factor receptors, cytokines/STATs, and nuclear receptors/transcriptional and chromatin regulatory proteins. The core continuously works with investigators to build RPPA assays for new protein pathways of interest and to validate the required antibodies. The RPPA platform can be applied to various sample types including cell/tissue lysates, small numbers of isolated stem cells (Chang et al., 2015; Creighton and Huang, 2015; Bu et al., 2019), as well as isolated protein complexes (Acharya et al., 2017) and has proven to be a robust platform for discovery research in cancer biology (Holdman et al., 2015; Elsarraj et al., 2020; Sharma et al., 2020). The core has also developed in-house normalization and statistical analysis algorithms for the RPPA results (Chang et al., 2015) and has been developing an informatics pipeline for data processing and integration (Coarfa et al., forthcoming).

This chapter describes detailed protocols on how to use RPPA for protein profiling. An example is provided for cultured mouse embryonic fibroblasts (MEF) maintained under normal (fed) conditions or subject to serum and amino acid deprivation for one hour (starved). The dramatic changes detected in the total and phosphoproteins involved in autophagy from the MEF cell lysates validate the utility of the RPPA assay. In addition, we compared the responses to starvation of wild type (WT) and mutant MEF cells with ablation of two-pore channel (TPC) 1 and 2 genes and observed differential changes. TPC1 and TPC2 are endolysosomal ion channels permeable to Na^+ and Ca^{2+} (Calcraft et al., 2009; Wang et al., 2012). Recent studies have implicated the role of TPCs in autophagy regulation (Cang et al., 2013; Lin et al., 2015; Xiong and Zhu, 2016). Therefore, the RPPA analysis offers important new clues as to which proteins and signaling pathways are regulated by TPCs and how they contribute to autophagy signaling and cellular response to starvation.

13.2 MATERIALS

13.2.1 Antibodies Used in RPPA

See the following weblink for vendors and related information of the 230+ antibodies we have validated and routinely used in our core: https://www.bcm.edu/academic-centers/dan-l-duncan-comprehensive-cancer-center/research/cancer-shared-resources/reverse-phase-protein-array/antibodies-list

13.2.2 Instrumentation and Small Equipment

1. Aushon 2470 arrayer (Aushion Biosystem/Quanterix, Billerica, MA, USA).
2. Autostainer Link 48 (Dako/Agilent, Santa Clara, CA, USA)
3. GenePix 4400A Microarray Scanner (Molecular Devices, San Jose, CA, USA)
4. GenePix SL50 Slide Loader (Molecular Devices)
5. GenePix Pro 7.2 Microarray Acquisition & Analysis Software (Molecular Devices)
6. TissueLyser II (Qiagen, Germantown, MD, USA)
7. Spectramax 340PC Microplate Reader (Molecular Devices)

8. Rocking Platform Model 100 (VWR, Radnor, PA, USA)

13.2.3 Cell Culture

1. WT and TPC double knockout (dKO) MEF cells were prepared from WT C57BL/6 and *Tpcn*1/2 double knockout mice (Ruas et al., 2014) (gift from Drs. Antony Galione and John Parrington, Oxford University) using the established protocol (Jozefczuk et al., 2012).
2. Dulbecco's Modified Eagle's Medium (DMEM) culture medium (MilliporeSigma, Burlington, MA, USA)
3. Amino acid-free DMEM medium (US Biological, Salem, MA, USA)
4. Fetal Bovine Serum (FBS) (GenDepot, Katy, TX, USA)
5. Phosphate-buffered saline (PBS, 137 mM NaCl, 8 mM Na_2HPO_4, 2.7 mM KCl, 1.47 mM KH_2PO_4, pH 7.4)
6. Cell lifter (Corning, Glendale, AZ, USA)

13.2.4 Sample Preparation

1. Novex™ Tris-Glycine SDS Sample Buffer (2X) (Invitrogen, Carlsbad, CA, USA)
2. 2-Mercaptoethanol (MilliporeSigma)
3. 1.5-mL Microcentrifuge tubes (Fisher Scientific, Fair Lawn, NJ, USA)
4. 5-mm stainless steel beads (Qiagen)
5. 2-mL sample tubes RB (Qiagen)
6. RPPA Lysis buffer (30 mL): 27 mL T-PER™ Tissue Protein Extraction Reagent (Pierce Biotechnology, Waltham, MA, USA) and 3 mL 5 M NaCl (Invitrogen). Store at 4°C.
7. 5X Protease inhibitors (10 mL): 5 Protease inhibitor tablets (Roche, Mannheim, Germany) and 10 mL T-PER Reagent. Make 1 mL aliquots. Store at –20°C. Expires in three months.
8. 5X Phosphatase inhibitors (10 mL): 5 Phosphatase inhibitor tablets (Roche, Mannheim, Germany) and 10 mL T-PER Reagent. Make 1 mL aliquots. Store at –20°C. Expires in six months.
9. RPPA Working Solution (5 mL): 3 mL RPPA Lysis buffer, 1 mL 5X Protease inhibitors and 1 mL 5X Phosphatase inhibitors. Prepare fresh.
10. Bovine serum albumin (BSA) (Cell Signaling Technology, Danvers, MA, USA)
11. BCA protein assay kit (Pierce Biotechnology)

13.2.5 Reverse Phase Protein Array (RPPA) Sample Printing

1. 384-well Microarray plates with lid (Genetix/Molecular Devices)
2. Viewseal sealer plate cover (Greiner Bio-One, Monroe, NC, USA)
3. Grace Bio-Labs ONCYTE® AVID™ nitrocellulose film slides (Grace Bio-Labs, Bend, OR, USA).

13.2.6 Total Protein Staining

1. Sypro Ruby Protein Fixative Solution: 7% v/v acetic acid (Fisher Scientific) and 10% v/v methanol (Fisher Scientific) in deionized water
2. Sypro Ruby Protein Blot stain (Molecular Probes, Eugene, OR, USA)
3. Microscope slide staining dish set (Fisher Scientific)

13.2.7 Reverse Phase Protein Array Immunostaining

1. Autostainer Link 48 (Agilent)
2. 5 mL, 25 mL, 50 mL reagent vials (Agilent)
3. Milli-Q® Advantage A10 Water Purification System (MilliporeSigma)
4. Tris-buffered saline with Tween (Agilent)
5. 10X Re-Blot Plus Strong Antibody Stripping Solution (MilliporeSigma): Dilute 10X Re-Blot to 1X Re-Blot with Milli-Q water.
6. I-Block™ Protein-Based Blocking Reagent (Applied Biosystems): Dissolve 2 g I-Block in 1 L PBS on a hot plate at 70°C with constant stirring until all the particles are dissolved. DO NOT BOIL. The solution will remain slightly gloomy. Add 2 mL Tween-20 (Fisher Scientific) after solution has cooled down to room temperature. The solution can be stored at 4°C for one week.
7. Avidin/Biotin blocking system (Agilent)
8. 3% hydrogen peroxide (Fisher Scientific)
9. Avidin/Biotin blocking system (Agilent)
10. Protein block (Agilent)
11. Primary and secondary antibodies: All antibodies were diluted with antibody diluent (Agilent).
12. Secondary antibodies (goat anti-rabbit biotinylated H + L, BA1000) or (goat anti-mouse biotinylated H + L, BA9200) (Vector Laboratories, Burlingame, CA, USA)
13. VECTASTAIN® Elite ABC-HRP Kit, Peroxidase (Vector Laboratories): Mix 400 μL reagent A and 400 μL reagent B in 20 mL 0.1% BSA solution. (0.1 % BSA solution: dissolve 1 g BSA (MilliporeSigma) in 1 L PBS.)
14. TSA plus biotin kit (Perkin Elmer, Waltham, MA, USA): Dissolve the Biotin Amplification Reagent with 300 μL DMSO and transfer 80 μL of the DMSO solution into 20 mL 1X Plus Amplification Diluent.
15. LiCor IR dye solution (20 mL): Add 400 μL LiCor IR dye 680RD Streptavidin (LI-COR, Lincoln, Nebraska, USA) in 20 mL 1% BSA PBS solution. (1 % BSA solution: dissolve 10 g BSA in 1 L PBS.)

13.3 METHODS

RPPA workflow: RPPA platform starts from (1) validating a set of antibodies by Western blotting (WB) and setting up the RPPA platform through (2) sample preparation, (3) slide printing, (4) antibody labeling and signal amplification, and total protein labeling, (5) array scanning and image analyses, (6) data normalization, QC, and data processing, and (7) statistical analyses (Figure 13.1.).

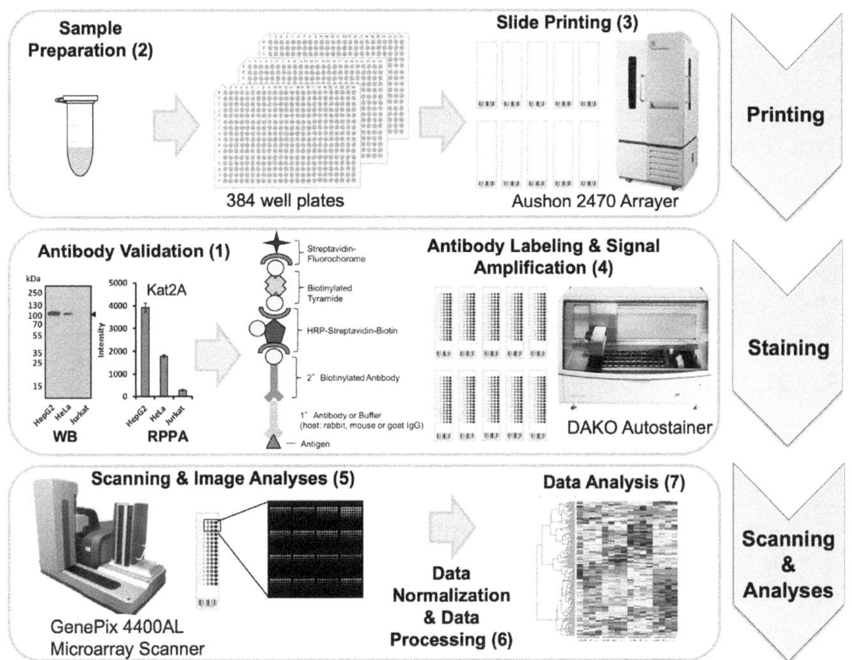

FIGURE 13.1. RPPA workflow: (1) antibody validation by Western blotting (WB) and RPPA, (2) sample preparation, (3) slide printing, (4) antibody labeling and signal amplification, and total protein labeling, (5) array scanning and image analyses, (6) data normalization, QC, and data processing, and (7) data/statistical analyses.

13.3.1 Antibody Validation

Antibody quality, specificity, and reactivity determine experimental reproducibility and reliability.

Antibody validation is carried out in four steps:

1. Identification of commercially available antibodies to targets of interest.
2. In-house validation by Western blotting.
3. In-house validation by RPPA and optimization of antibody dilution.
4. Correlation of RPPA and Western blotting results.

Since RPPA technology is highly dependent on the quality of the antibodies, a key feature is rigorous antibody validation for specificity and selectivity. Our criteria for antibody validation include an immunoblot assay (Western blotting) that results in a single protein band (or specific multiple bands for protein isoforms) of correct molecular size expected with known positive and negative control cells/tissues and an equivalent performance under RPPA assay conditions (Figure 13.1.). Most of the validated antibodies are from commercial vendors. Initial selection of commercial antibodies is based on vendor data demonstrating immunoblot detection of endogenous proteins as a predominant single band of the correct molecular mass in a known positive cell line or tissue. This is the minimal vendor data required. Additionally, a lack of immunoblot signal or substantial reduction of such a signal in a known negative cell/tissue type or sample after genetic knockdown or knockout is also required. We subsequently do our own in-house testing and validation. Because of well-known potential variations between antibody batches, we also test replacement batches in our inventory by RPPA and WB. We have built an inventory of 230+ validated antibodies. The antibodies detect key regulatory proteins of major signaling pathways and cellular processes with ~1/3 of them recognizing phosphorylation at specific sites of proteins to indicate functional states. An example of validation with antibody to Kat2A by both RPPA and WB is shown in Figure 13.1.

13.3.2 Cell Culture

1. MEF cells are routinely cultured in DMEM supplemented with 10% FBS, 100 units/mL of penicillin, and 100 μg/mL of streptomycin in a humidified incubator at 37°C, 5% CO_2. On the day before the experiment, seed MEF cells on 6-cm cell culture dishes at a density of ~50%. Cell density should reach ~80% the next morning. Use four dishes for each condition.
2. On the day of the experiment, replace the medium with fresh DMEM culture medium containing 10% FBS and incubate the cells for one hour.
3. For control cells, replace the medium with a free DMEM culture medium containing 10% FBS and incubate for one hour. For starvation, replace the medium with amino acid-free DMEM (without FBS) and incubate for one hour.

13.3.3 RPPA Sample Lysate Preparation

As in any high-throughput platforms, sample quality is the key to success. For tissue samples, snap-freezing in liquid nitrogen is recommended at the time of collection. The most critical steps for sample preparation include homogenizing tissues thoroughly, centrifuging multiple times to make sure that the protein extract is clear of debris or fat droplets, and keeping all lysates on ice and transferring to cold tubes during the processes. We recommend testing different lysis protocols and lysis buffers to achieve high quality samples. The detergent used in this protocol cannot be replaced by other detergent without rigorously testing the printing protocol. The homogenization method described below may be replaced by other traditional methods, as long as complete homogenization is ensured.

13.3.3.1 Protein Extraction (for Tissues)

1. Add an appropriate volume of RPPA Working Solution into Sample Tubes RB.
   a. Test tissue to volume ratio before doing large scale lysate preparation, since different tissues lyse differently. A starting point is 1:20 (w/v) for tissue weight (mg) over lysis buffer volume (μL).
   b. Tissue samples of 10–15 mg is usually lysed with 250 μL of RPPA Working Solution.
2. Lyse tissues using TissueLyzer (Qiagen).

a. Keep TissueLyzer and adapter in cold room all the time or precooled for at least one hour.
b. Add one piece of pre-cooled 5-mm stainless steel bead to each tube.
c. Check to make sure that the tubes are properly closed.
d. Homogenize tissues on the TissueLyzer using the following setting: two minutes at 23 Hz.
e. Take apart the adapter set and reverse the order of the tubes to ensure that all the tubes are evenly homogenized (samples on the inside of the adapter rack move more slowly than samples on the outside, merely rotating the adapter set is not sufficient).
f. Repeat TissueLyzer homogenization using the same setting as above.
g. Examine each tube after homogenization. Repeat homogenization if tissue debris are still visible.

3. Centrifuge samples at 14,000 rpm for 15 min at 4°C to remove any remaining insoluble material. Transfer the supernatant containing soluble proteins to a new tube. Repeat centrifugation at 14,000 rpm for 15 min at 4°C for two more times, each time transfer the supernatant to a fresh tube. Supernatant should be clear. If the supernatant is still cloudy, repeat centrifugation for one or two more times.
4. Perform Bicinchoninic assay (BCA) or Bradford assay to determine protein concentrations for individual samples. Use RPPA Working Solution as a blank when measuring protein concentrations.
5. The desired protein concentration is 1.1–3 μg/μL.

13.3.3.2 Protein extraction (for Cultured Cells)

1. Remove media from viable cell cultures.
2. Wash cells three times with cold PBS. Be sure to remove any excess liquid as this will dilute the lysate.
3. Add appropriate volume of RPPA Working Solution. For 5 x 10^6 cells, add 300 μL of the RPPA Working Solution. For smaller cell counts, e.g. 2 x 10^6 cells, add 100 μL of the RPPA Working Solution. Scrape or pipette lysis buffer over cells. The cell count here is based on the results from a few breast cancer cell lines tested. For your specific cell line, use this as a guideline to test and determine the final volume.
4. Transfer cell suspension to a 1.5-mL tube, vortex for 15 sec and incubate on ice for 30 min, with vortexing every 10 min. Alternatively, the tubes can be placed on an end-over-end rotator for 30 min at 4°C.
5. Centrifuge samples at 14,000 rpm for 15 min at 4°C to remove any remaining insoluble material. Transfer the supernatant containing soluble proteins to a new tube. Repeat centrifugation at 14,000 rpm for 15 min at 4°C, then transfer the supernatant to a fresh tube. Supernatant should be clear. If supernatant is still cloudy, repeat the centrifugation step for a third time.
6. Perform Bicinchoninic assay (BCA) or Bradford assay to determine protein concentrations. Use the RPPA Working Solution as a blank.
7. The desired protein concentration is 1.1–3.0 μg/μL.

13.3.3.3 Preparation of RPPA Lysate Samples (Carried Out on the Same Day, Immediately Following the Above Lysis Preparation Procedure):

1. Dilute the lysate samples by adding SDS Sample Buffer, 2.5% β-mercaptoethanol, and RPPA Working Solution to obtain a final concentration of 0.5 μg/μL.
2. Heat samples for 8 min at 100°C.
3. Bring to room temperature, centrifuge at 14,000 rpm for 2 min and collect supernatant.
4. Aliquot into two tubes and store all samples at –80°C for subsequent RPPA slide printing.

13.3.4 Reverse Phase Protein Array Design and Layout

For each run, control lysates are printed for quality assessment. Lysates from over 100 cell lines were screened to identify positive control cell lines, and those exhibiting high levels of antigens for most antibodies are selected and routinely used as positive controls. This extensive testing led to the creation of a mixture of cell lysate control (Cellmix control lysate, see below) for all the antibodies and confirmed the use of calibrators based on published data (Federici et al., 2013). We also determined 0.5 μg/μL as the optimal concentration for experimental samples through initially diluting all samples into eight serial dilutions from 1 to 0.0078 μg/μL, for all antibodies with varying affinities.

13.3.4.1 Preparation of RPPA Controls

1. Cell lysate mix controls (Cellmix): a mixture of four cell lysates (MDA-MB-415 cells, T-47D cells, pervanadate-treated HeLa cells, and calyculin A-treated Jurkat cells) is used as positive controls. It contains the majority of the antigens to be assayed, and also serves as standards (range of concentrations) for quality assessment on antibodies and array process. The mixed control lysate is serially diluted over a range of 0.0078 to 1 μg/μL to test for the linear range of the antibody recognition.
2. Calibrators:
   a. Cell lysates of pervanadate-treated Hela cells (HP100) mixed with untreated Hela lysates at 0 to 100% for phospho-tyrosine antibodies.
   b. Cell lysates of calyculin A-treated Jurkat cells (JC100) mixed with untreated Hela lysate at 0–100% for phospho-serine/threonine antibodies. Calyculin A is a potent phosphatase inhibitor which enhances serine/threonine phosphorylation.
3. Other controls and references (all lysates described below are spotted at 0.5 μg/μL unless otherwise indicated):
   a. NCI 60 cancer cell lines: lysates of selected individual cells and an equal mix (NCImix) of lysates from all 60 cell lines (Federici et al., 2013).

b. Breast cancer ATCC 39 cell lines: lysates of selected individual cells and an equal mix of lysates from all 39 cell lines (BCCmix).
c. Mouse tissue mix (mTissuemix) as reference for mouse proteins: an equal mix of lysates from multiple mouse tissues (heart, brain, lung, intestine, gastrocnemius, kidney, mammary glands, ovary and uterus, quadriceps, brown adipose tissue). Mouse liver and spleen are excluded due to a high background signal from tissue IgG content.
d. IgG mix: rabbit, mouse, and goat IgG are mixed at 0.05 μg/μL and spotted at four corners of the slides as gridding and positive controls for secondary antibodies.
e. BSA: one or two different sources of BSA are spotted at a range of 0.0078 to 1 μg/μL as non-specific binding controls.
f. RPPA cell lysis buffer: blank lysis buffer controls.

13.3.4.2 Design of the Slide Layout

1. Make a map for the samples, noting the sample spot location on the slide. Spot the same-treated group in neighboring locations of the slide to avoid variations caused by uneven background staining. Spot control samples in the top and bottom regions of each slide for the best quality control.
2. Generate excel files for each 384-well microplate, with the identity and location of each sample in the microplate. If the sample is to be printed on more than 100 slides, we strongly suggest to fill only a quarter of the plate with lysate samples; the remaining wells should be filled with water to increase the humidity of the plate and also decrease the time the plate is open during printing.
3. Generate GenePix Array List (.gal) file: import the excel files into Aushon 2470 software and create/edit the Source Well Plates and design a layout of slide. Check the Well Content Definition by .gal file generation with the Aushon 2470 software. The .gal file details the locations of individual spots to be printed and identities of the spots are annotated in the array.

13.3.5 Protocol for Printing Array Slides

RPPA platform is designed as a dot-blot layout (Spurrier et al., 2008). The Aushon 2470 Arrayer with a 40 pin (185 μm) configuration is used to spot samples and control lysates onto nitrocellulose-coated slides using an array format of 960 lysates/slide (2,880 spots/slide). Each slide (array) is probed with a single primary antibody. We routinely print 250–300 slides per experiment with 40 μL of each lysate sample at 0.5 μg/μL. This volume is sufficient for printing 400 slides with optimal spot morphology (full and round). When attempting to print more than 400 slides, some sample spots may become irregular due to evaporation.

1. Each sample prints three technical replicates and two depositions per spot in order to increase the protein concentration at each spot.

2. Wash the pins in between samples by immersing the pins into flowing water for two seconds and then making five dips at the next dip position.
3. The humidity is set at 60% during printing.
4. Fill the water container for washing and the humidifier for humidity control with Milli-Q water.
5. Load slides into Source Plate Elevator. Write down the slides barcode and printing slide order. (Caution: always wear gloves when handling slides and do not touch or scratch the slide pad with any fingers.)
6. Load the 384-well plates into Substrate Elevator.
7. Before clicking "START DEPOSITION," verify all material and instrument preparation steps.
8. The use of an SDS sample buffer with bromophenol blue allows examination of the applied spots under microscope. After printing a few slides, check the quality of the spotted slides. Each spot should be equal sized and round. If not, check the cleanness of pins or the quality of the lysate samples. Low volume or stickiness of lysates may cause uneven printing.
9. It is recommended that after printing every 100 slides, pin cleaning should be performed by loading 30 µL 70% ethanol into the wells of a 384-well plate and one nitrocellulose-coated slide into the arrayer. Immerse the pins into flowing water for five seconds twice and perform ten dips to 70% ethanol. Repeat the process eight times to comprehensively clean the pins.
10. After batch printing, perform pin cleaning following Aushon instruction of Pin Installation and Extraction Procedure. Put all pins in pin storage box. Examine each pin under microscope to check for dirt and residue carry over. Gently wipe the dirty area by a cotton swap soaked with acetone. After all pins have been checked and cleaned, install the pins back to the instrument.
11. The spotted slides can be stored in a slide box at room temperature until staining. If the spotted slides are not to be used immediately, they can be placed in a sealed Ziploc bag and stored at –20°C.

13.3.6 Total Protein Staining and Antibody Labeling

13.3.6.1 SYPRO Ruby Total Protein Staining

Total protein content of each spotted lysate is measured by fluorescent staining with SYPRO Ruby Protein Blot Stain. SYPRO Ruby is a sensitive ruthenium-based fluorescent dye that, similar to silver stains, interacts with basic amino acids, including lysine, arginine, and histidine. It is a highly sensitive method for detecting proteins on nitrocellulose membranes. The detection sensitivity of this assay (0.25–1 ng protein/mm^2) provides over three orders of magnitude of linear quantification range. Therefore, the protein levels of individual lysates on the slide can be easily determined and used for normalization of protein loading. Typically, we determine the total protein for each spot by staining 1 in every 20 slides with SYPRO Ruby protein blot stain following the manufacturer's instructions. All washing and staining steps are performed by gentle agitation on a rocking platform at 2 rpm.

1. Fix slides by immersing in the fixative solution at room temperature for 15 minutes in a small, glass staining dish with glass lid.

2. Wash the slides in deionized water four times for five minutes each time.
3. Immerse slides in SYPRO Ruby Protein Blot Stain for 15 minutes at room temperature in the dark. Cover the container with aluminum foil to prevent photo bleaching by light.
4. De-stain the slides in deionized water six times for one minute each. Protect from light.
5. Air dry slides.

13.3.6.2 Antibody Labeling

Immunolabeling is performed on an automated slide stainer, Autostainer Link 48 (Agilent), at room temperature. Re-blot, I-block, Biotin/avidin block, and protein block are used to optimize the block condition. Each slide is incubated with a single primary antibody followed by a goat anti-rabbit or anti-mouse IgG with biotinylated secondary antibody. A negative control slide is incubated with antibody diluent instead of a primary antibody. A Catalyzed Signal Amplification System kit and fluorescent IRDye 680 Streptavidin are used as the detection system (Figure 13.1.).

The Autostainer Link 48 can accommodate a maximum of 29 antibody slides and one negative control slide. For 230+ antibodies, we routinely divide them into nine to ten batches.

1. Prepare all the reagents with optimal dilutions (Table 13.1) in desired volume per the manufacturer's directions; enter associated information to each reagent into the stainer.
2. Prepare staining protocol according to details listed in Table 13.1 and each RPPA slide is arranged to react with one primary antibody or antibody diluent as negative control. Have a table match the antibody with RPPA slide barcode, and check the slide order carefully to avoid errors.
3. At the end of staining, take slides out of the Autostainer and rinse them twice with deionized water to decrease the background. This step washes away any residual fluorescent dye on the edge and backside of the slide. Without washing, some slides may show high background fluorescent areas.
4. Air dry slides and protect them from light. The slides are ready to scan.

13.3.6.3 Control Slides for Data Normalization

1. Total protein by SYPRO Ruby staining. The middle slide in every 20 slides printed, as well as the first and last slides of the entire batch, is stained for total protein with SYPRO Ruby. For example, with a total of 240 slides, slides #1, #10, #30, #50 … #230, and #240 are stained with SYPRO Ruby. The antibody labeled slides #2–#19 are normalized by #10 total protein slide while slides #21–#39 by #30 total protein slide, and so forth.

2. Negative control slides per run include replacing primary antibody with antibody diluent. For every batch of antibody labeling, one or two negative control slides are included. After incubation with antibody diluent, the subsequent steps are exactly the same as antibody labeling slides, including the incubation with either anti-mouse or anti-rabbit secondary antibodies plus Streptavidin-IRDye-680.

TABLE 13.1
Protocol for slide pretreatment and immunostaining

Step	Reagent Name	Category	Incubation (minutes)
1	Buffer	Rinse	
2	Re-blot	Strip and Re-probe	15
3	Buffer	Rinse	
4	Buffer	Auxiliary	5
5	Buffer	Auxiliary	5
6	Buffer	Rinse	
7	I-Block	Protein Block 2g/L	15
8	I-Block	Protein Block 2g/L	15
9	Buffer	Rinse	
10	Buffer	Rinse	
11	H_2O_2	Endogenous Enzyme Block 3%	5
12	Buffer	Rinse	
13	Avidin	Avidin/Biotin Blocking System	10
14	Buffer	Rinse	
15	Biotin	Avidin/Biotin Blocking System	10
16	Buffer	Rinse	
17	Protein Block	Protein Block 0.25% casein	5
18	Buffer	Rinse	
19	Primary Antibody	Primary Antibody Optimized Dilution for Each Antibody*	30
20	Buffer	Rinse	
21	Buffer	Auxiliary	5
22	Buffer	Rinse	
23	Anti-Rabbit/Mouse IgG, Biotinylated	Secondary Antibody 1:10,000	15
24	Buffer	Rinse	
25	Buffer	Auxiliary	5
26	Buffer	Rinse	
27	Vectastain-ABC	Avidin-Biotin Complex 1:50	15
28	Buffer	Rinse	
29	Buffer	Auxiliary	5
30	Buffer	Rinse	
31	TSA-plus-Biotin	Tyramide Signal Amplification 1:250	15
32	Buffer	Rinse	
33	Buffer	Auxiliary	5
34	Buffer	Rinse	
35	Fluorescent IRDye 680 Streptavidin	Fluorophore-label 1:50	15
36	DI Water	Auxiliary	1
37	DI Water	Rinse	
38	DI Water	Rinse	

* Antibody dilution usually starts with 1:200 dilution for commercial antibodies, 1:5 for monoclonal antibody supernatant, and optimized further.

13.3.7 Slides Scanning and Image Analyses

Air-dried, fluorescence-labeled slides are scanned on a GenePix 4400 AL scanner, along with accompanying negative control slides at an appropriate PMT to obtain an optimal signal for various samples on the slides. RPPA slides are spotted with different type of samples for different projects, and different samples may have big differences in antibody reactivity. For example, one set of samples may have a very high signal for one antibody, but another set of samples may have a very low expression level. In order to obtain an optimal signal for both sets of samples, we design our workflow to scan each slide by 2–5 different PMT settings, starting with the highest setting to accommodate the low expression proteins, and lower PMT settings for high expression proteins. Negative control slides (react with antibody diluent instead of primary antibody) are also scanned at every PMT setting used for all the antibodies in the same staining run. Total protein stained (Sypro Ruby) slides are scanned with one PMT setting to generate quality spots. Because of the consistency of total levels of protein in each spot, image quality is optimal from a single PMT scan setting.

The images are analyzed by GenePix Pro 7.2 software. A local background subtraction method was used by the software. Briefly, the local background is calculated using a circular region that is centered on the spot. This region has a diameter that is three times the diameter of the spot. All of the pixels within this area are used to compute the background except the spotted area and a two pixel wide ring around the spot. The median background value is used. For each spot on the slide, signal intensity (SI) is determined by median fluorescent intensity (median FI) minus background fluorescent intensity (background FI).

13.3.7.1 Slide Scanning

1. Launch the GenePix Pro 7.2.29 software and warm up the laser for at least 20 minutes.
2. Load the slides into the GenePix AL4400 scanner with the barcode faced down. Check for proper loading; set the correct scan area to cover the whole slide including the barcode.
3. Select manual scan and run a single preview scan to determine the scan setting. For the SYPRO Ruby protein stains, select excitement wavelength 532 nm, 100% laser power, emission filter 550–600 nm coupled with a neutral density filter to block light transmittance by 90%. For antibody LiCoR dye stains, select excitement wavelength 635 nm, 100% laser power, emission filter 655–695 nm coupled with a neutral density filter to block light transmittance by 90%.
4. Define optimized PMT setting: start with a high PMT and lower it until no spot saturation is observed. Note: the PMT setting should be in the linear range of the scanner (350–550 PMT).
5. Determine the scan setting and save the hardware setting as a .gps file.
6. Scan all slides at two PMT settings by Batch scan: one optimized (low) PMT applicable to most samples without any saturated spots; one high PMT useful for some very low signal spots. Review all images and rescan the slides that have saturated spots at the low PMT setting.
7. Rename each scanned image with barcode, date, PMT setting, and antibody name.

For the 230+ antibodies and associated negative control and total protein slides, scanning process generates ~1,000 images. Each image is evaluated for quality through manual inspection of spots and background uniformity. Antibody labeled spot images that fail the quality inspection are either repeated at the end of the staining runs or removed before data reporting.

13.3.7.2 Image Analysis

1. Manual single slide image analysis to generate a setting file: Open a scanned image (.tif file) and load the array list (.gal file generated from Aushon 2470 arrayer). Manually align the array list to all spots as close as possible. Set up the alignment factor: resize feature (60–150% diameter); limit feature movement (maximum translation: 50 μm) during alignment. Select "Align the features in all block" to automatically align all the spots. Check that each spot has been aligned properly. If not, manually adjust the spot size to make sure that all the signals are included in the spot circle. Save this well alignment setting as a modified .gps file for batch analyses.
2. Batch image analyses and data file generation: Add all the scanned images (.tif files) to do "batch analyses" and select the modified .gps files to align all the images. Perform the analysis to generate a result file (.gpr file) at the same time. Check gridding for each image. If gridding is not accurate, realign and repeat image analysis for the particular image. Sixty images can be analyzed within 20 minutes by batch analyses.
3. Batch image analyses are carried out for all the slides, including antibody slides, negative control slides, and total protein slides. When batch image analyses are finished, four files are automatically saved for each slide: two ".jpg" files, one analysis setting file ".gps" file, and one data file ".gpr" file. The data file (.gpr file) contains all the numeric data for individual spots, from spot coordination, spot size, signal intensity, background intensity, signal subtracted background intensity, quality, etc.
4. Quality assessment for image analyses:

The quality of aligned images is manually inspected after batch analyses. Misaligned images are realigned and data files are regenerated. Each data file (.gpr) is checked by an informatics program to ensure proper format for subsequent normalization and data processing.

13.3.8 Data Normalization and Data Processing

13.3.8.1 RPPA Data Normalization

All the ~1,000 data files are subject to data normalization. Every antibody data file is matched with a corresponding negative control file scanned at the same PMT scanning setting. The antibody and negative control slides were labeled at the same batch. Each antibody data file is also matched with a total protein data file based on the order of the slide printed (see Section 12.3.6.3 control slides for data normalization).

A group-based normalization approach is applied to the RPPA data as described (Chang et al., 2015). The antibody signal intensity (SI) of each spot (defined as median FI – background FI in data file after image analyses) is subtracted by the corresponding SI of negative control and then normalized to the corresponding SI of total protein (median FI – background FI) within the same group, which consists of all the spots from the same experiment (or any other conditions as defined by the investigators). The normalized antibody SI (N) is expressed as:

$$N = (A - C) * M / T$$

where A is the antibody SI, C is the negative control SI, M is the median SI of total protein of the spots within the same group, and T is the SI of total protein. If the antibody SI is lower than or equal to the negative control SI, the normalized SI is set to 1; if the antibody SI, negative control SI, or total protein SI has a flag indicating the SI to be problematic, the normalized antibody SI is set to NA (not analyzed).

13.3.8.2 Data Processing and Final Data Output

After data normalization and QC by both manual inspection and informatics program, a final data report is generated to include four excel spreadsheets for human samples or seven excel spreadsheets for mouse samples in one single excel file for each project. When mouse tissue samples are profiled by RPPA, some may have high mouse IgG content which binds to secondary antibody anti-mouse IgG thus producing a high non-specific signal. Separating data obtained from mouse tissues from antibodies allows researchers and statisticians to pay closer attention to the background of those samples, and decide whether to eliminate them from further analyses. We noticed that different mouse tissues have different levels of background signals, and some tissue types from different laboratories may also have different levels of background signals. Established cell lines from mice usually have a comparable low background signal for mouse and rabbit antibodies. To generate optimizing data output, one scanning setting is selected per antibody by the data processing program for each project. The selection criterion is that the saturated spot signal cannot be more than six spots, or two samples in triplicates in the entire project, thus ensuring a linear range of the protein signal for the project. Our project design recommends four biological replicates in each treatment group, ensuring a minimal three replicate samples per treatment group for data analysis, even after eliminating a potential technical outlier or a sample with high signal variation among technical replicates (see Section 13.3.9). As indicated in the previous section, we have pre-tested all antibodies and determined the optimal antibody dilution to achieve the highest possible signal without saturation of our control samples and experimental samples.

The worksheets for human samples are:

(1) Legend of final report, including explanation of antibody name, sample name, and printing ID.
(2) Normalized data for all antibodies, including the three replicate spots for each sample.
(3) Quality index data for all antibodies: this spreadsheet includes mean, medium, maximum of slide, RPPA controls, and calibrators (Cellmix, NCImix, BCCmix, mTissuemix, HP100, JC100, RPPA cell lysis buffer).

(4) Raw data for all antibodies: this worksheet includes the three replicate spots for each sample, negative control (without primary antibody but incubated with the same secondary antibody) signal at the same antibody scanning setting, total protein control signal. From this worksheet, all the raw data in the optimal setting of the antibody is included, and it could be used for renormalization if necessary.

For mouse samples:

(1)–(4) The same as human samples but only for antibodies from rabbit or goat.
(5) Normalized data for all the mouse antibodies.
(6) Quality index data for all the mouse antibodies.
(7) Raw data for all the mouse antibodies.

13.3.9 Statistical Analyses

After the final data report is generated for each project, the normalized data are used for statistical analyses. First, technical replicates for each sample from the normalized data are combined by using the median value. Then, antibodies displaying low expression or no expression signals across all the samples in the study are filtered out. We usually start by filtering out antibodies with normalized signal intensity <200 across all the samples (this cut-off value may be adjusted for antibodies/samples with higher background in some studies). The next step is to examine the coefficient of variant (CV) of technical replicates and expression levels of each protein across all the samples. Proteins with CV $\geq 25\%$ for the three technical replicates are marked with NA. If there are more than two NAs in any treatment group, the antibody is excluded from further analyses. Since there are typically four biological replicates per treatment group, eliminating two samples in a group makes the statistical analysis unreliable.

Principal component analysis (PCA) is a useful technique for data exploration and visualization (Hilsenbeck et al., 1999; Raychaudhuri et al., 1999). In RPPA analysis, proteins are treated as variables and PCA creates a set of protein-based principal components to examine and explain the observed variance among samples. PCA is performed on the median of each sample. If a sample is an outlier within the treatment group by PCA, closer attention is paid to that sample, including examining technical notes for sample preparation and data generation processes and reviewing background signals of this sample in comparison to other samples, to determine the source of this variation. If the outlier is found to result from technical problems such as sample treatment error or due to high mouse IgG content (high background signal), then it is eliminated from further analyses. If no obvious technical issues are found with the outlier, then all the samples will be kept for further analyses. The remaining data are then subject to further statistical analyses: analysis of variance (ANOVA) for multiple group comparison and t-test for two-group comparison. The orders of the above workflow may also be switched to evaluate data quality for RPPA projects.

13.4 RESULTS AND DISCUSSION: AN EXAMPLE

13.4.1 Background

mTORC1 (mechanistic target of rapamycin complex 1) is a master regulator of cell metabolism (Condon and Sabatini, 2019). When nutrients are abundant, mTORC1 activates the synthetic pathways and suppresses autophagy to promote anabolism. During nutrient shortage, the inhibition of autophagy by mTORC1 is lifted so that cells can regenerate essential building blocks to sustain basic cellular functions (Hosokawa et al., 2009). mTORC1 is localized to lysosomes under nutrient-rich conditions, but becomes dissociated from the lysosome in response to nutrient deprivation (Zoncu et al., 2011). A critical step of mTORC1 reactivation, which also terminates autophagy, is for mTORC1 to reassociate with the lysosome, a complex process that involves multiple sensing mechanisms for not only the status of growth factor stimulation but also the abundance of ATP, amino acids, and lipids both outside and inside the lysosomes (Kim and Guan, 2019).

TPCs are endolysosomal channels regulated by mTORC1 (Cang et al., 2013). Genetic knockout of the lysosome-localized TPC2 in mice led to a defect in autophagy termination in skeletal muscle cells, causing muscle atrophy (Lin et al., 2015). It has been proposed that TPCs may facilitate mTORC1 reactivation by preventing lysosomal export of amino acids generated from protein degradation through depleting Na^+ from the lysosomal lumen; this will allow the luminal sensing machinery to know whether enough amino acids have been produced by autophagy to support new synthesis (Xiong and Zhu, 2016). However, it remains unknown how TPC deficiency affects the overall metabolic activities and other cellular functions, and how it alters the cellular responses to serum and amino acid starvation. To understand the role of TPCs in cell signaling and metabolism, we isolated primary MEF cells from WT and TPC1/TPC2 dKO mice and utilized RPPA to profile the panoramic signaling in these cells under fed and starved conditions.

13.4.2 Changes in WT and TPC dKO MEF Cells in Response to Short-term Starvation

To learn how TPCs regulate cellular metabolism, we prepared lysates from WT and TPC dKO MEF cells either grown in the normal culture conditions (fed) or deprived of serum and amino acids (starved) for one hour and subjected them to RPPA analysis. Of the 210 antibodies included in the RPPA assay, 68 (32%) are phosphorylation site specific antibodies. Therefore, this assay is not only useful for analyzing alterations in protein expression but also particularly suitable for detecting changes in the activities of certain proteins and signaling pathways. Given that it takes some time for the transcriptionally regulated proteins to express, assessing phosphoprotein levels is particularly suited for the experiments designed here that focus on protein activity changes in response to short-term (one hour) starvation.

To evaluate the data quality for the entire array, we started our analysis workflow by performing PCA for all the proteins first, and then examined the CV for technical triplicates, followed by filtering out low intensity and high variation samples before

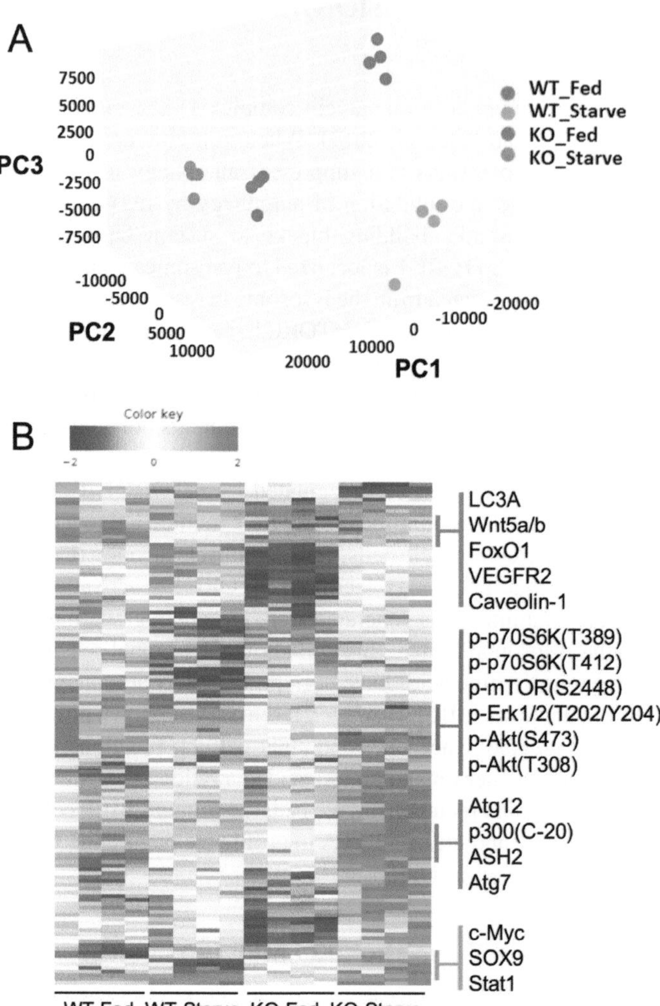

FIGURE 13.2. RPPA data analyses for metabolic activities and other cellular functions of embryonic fibroblasts. (**A**) Principal component analysis (PCA) of the RPPA data for all the proteins analyzed (***n*** = 210). X, y, and z axes represent three major principal components. (**B**) Heatmap of proteins (***n*** = 133) differentially expressed by one-way analysis of variance (ANOVA) among the four groups of samples subjected to supervised hierarchical clustering (p-value < 0.05). Selected proteins in four clusters representing changes in various treatment groups: decreased in KO but not affected by starvation (red); starvation-related in both WT and KO (blue); insensitive to starvation in WT but sensitive to starvation in KO (magenta); and increased in KO with opposite response to starvation (green).

statistical analyses. PCA of the RPPA data for all the proteins and phosphoproteins analyzed ($n = 210$) (the taken median of the normalized triplicate spots in each sample) clearly indicates that the four groups (WT-Fed, WT-Starved, KO-Fed, KO-Starved) are separated from each other without sample outliers in any group

(Figure 13.2.A). In addition, PCA shows that WT and TPC dKO cells respond differently to the short-term starvation (Figure 13.2.A).

Among the 210 antibodies, a total of 10,080 spot data points were generated for the four groups, representing 3,360 measurements for the 16 biological samples (quadruplicate samples printed in triplicates and labeled for each antibody). The technical variations of the triplicate spots of individual samples were examined and yielded CV ≤ 10%, 15%, 20%, and 25%, respectively, for 82%, 91%, 94%, and 97% of the 3,360 samples/antibodies measured. This indicates a high consistency of the RPPA data on technical triplicates. Only ~3% of the sample data had CV ≥ 25%, and all these were from the 24 antibodies that displayed a very low to low expression signal, with the maximal normalized signal intensity ≤316. Among them, 11 antibodies showed CV ≥ 25% in two or more samples in just one of the four treatment groups, again indicating the highly consistent data quality even in low expression samples. Next, we reviewed antibodies with low or no expression level. Since the negative control signal for samples in this study is around 200 or lower, we chose to filter out antibodies with normalized signal intensity ≤200 across all the samples: 57 antibodies met this criterion, including the ten above-mentioned antibodies with CV ≥ 25%. Thus, a total of 58 antibodies were eliminated based on the CV or low signal intensity cutoffs, leaving 152 proteins and phosphoproteins for further statistical analyses. Out of the 152 proteins, one-way ANOVA identified 133 to have significant difference among the four groups with $p < 0.05$ (Figure 13.2.B).

Consistent with a reduced anabolism, serum and amino acid deprivation of WT MEF cells led to changes in the levels of many phosphoproteins, as seen in the middle section of Figure 13.2.B. Among them, p-Erk1/2 (T202/Y204), p-p70S6K (T389), p-p70S6K (T412), p-Akt (S473), p-mTOR (S2448), and p-Akt (T308) levels were, on average, dramatically decreased by 62.5, 19.9, 19.0, 8.3, 2.7, and 2.6-fold, respectively, in the starved cells as compared to the fed ones (Figure 13.2.B, indicated by blue vertical lines). These proteins are well known to be the early responders of starvation with decreases in their activities, i.e. phosphorylation levels (Condon and Sabatini, 2019; Kim and Guan, 2019). Interestingly, these proteins also showed partially decreased phosphorylation in fed TPC dKO cells as compared to fed WT MEF cells, at 2.0, 1.9, 1.6, 1.6, 1.4, and 1.3-fold for p-Erk1/2 (T202/Y204), p-Akt (S473), p-p70S6K (T389), p-p70S6K (T412), p-mTOR (S2448), and p-Akt (T308), respectively. This would agree with the increased autophagy flux and therefore decreased mTORC1 signaling found in TPC2-deficient skeletal muscle cells (Lin et al., 2015). Despite these lower levels, TPC dKO MEF cells still responded to serum and amino acid starvation with decreases in p-Erk1/2 (T202/Y204), p-p70S6K (T412), p-p70S6K (T389), p-Akt (S473), p-Akt (T308), and p-mTOR (S2448) levels by 23.0, 9.9, 9.7, 6.0, 3.0, and 1.8-fold, respectively. These data indicate that both the genetic ablation of TPC1 and TPC2 and starvation dramatically affect metabolism and other cellular functions.

13.4.3 Homeostatic Alterations of Signaling Molecules between WT and TPC dKO MEF Cells

The RPPA data indicate not only rather widespread homeostatic changes in the TPC dKO MEF cells in the expression and function of many signaling molecules involved in metabolism, cell cycle regulation, and proliferation but also their differential responses to serum and amino acid deprivation as compared to the WT cells. The heatmap in Figure 13.2.B clearly shows several clusters of proteins with differential changes caused by the gene deletion and starvation. One of them, indicated by the red lines in Figure 13.2.B, includes proteins that are decreased in the TPC dKO MEF cells but are typically not affected by starvation at the level of expression. These include VEGFR2, caveolin-1, LC3A, Wnt5a/b, and FoxO1, which were decreased by 2.4, 2.8, 4.9, 2.8, and 3.8-fold, respectively, in fed TPC dKO cells as compared to the fed WT MEF cells. Interestingly, all of them have been reported to play certain roles in autophagy regulation, although usually not as negative regulators (Zhao et al., 2010; Bai et al., 2012; Shi et al., 2015; Liu et al., 2017; Jati et al., 2018). Their decreases in TPC dKO cells might reflect compensatory changes to dampen the enhanced basal autophagic flux in these cells.

Of the other two clusters indicated by the magenta and green lines in Figure 13.2.B, one represents proteins that are relatively insensitive to starvation in the WT cells, but become sensitive to starvation in the TPC dKO (magenta); and the other represents those that responded to short-term starvation with decreases in the WT cells but increases in the TPC dKO cells (green). Among them, Atg7 and Atg12 are members of the ubiquitin-like conjugation systems involved in autophagy (Reggiori and Klionsky, 2013). p300, ASH2, c-Myc, SOX9, and Stat1 have also been shown to play roles in autophagy regulation (Wysocka et al., 2003; Fielhaber et al., 2009; Wu et al., 2015; Goldberg et al., 2017; Mateo et al., 2017; Wan et al., 2017; Iezaki et al., 2018). The approximately four-fold increases in the levels of SOX9 and Stat1 in the TPC dKO as compared to the WT MEF cells under fed conditions also indicate that these proteins are important for the survival of TPC dKO cells. Their further increases, along with the other proteins shown in these two clusters, in response to short-term starvation, instead of no change or decreases as found in the WT cells, suggest that these proteins may be uniquely involved in overcoming the detrimental effect of TPC loss under fed and starved conditions.

Collectively, these data indicate that the loss of TPCs not only led to changes in the activities of metabolic proteins that reflect persistently increased autophagic flux, due to the impairment in mTORC1 reactivation, as suggested by the previous study (Lin et al., 2015), but also other homeostatic changes that are either secondary to the enhanced autophagic flux and/or reduced mTORC1 signaling, or necessary for cell survival under conditions of TPC deficiency. Further exploration of the mechanistic underpinning of these changes will improve our understanding of metabolic regulation and TPC functions and shed lights on new strategies to treat metabolic diseases.

ACKNOWLEDGMENTS

We thank Drs. Antony Galione and John Parrington for providing the *Tpcn1*$^{-/-}$/*Tpcn2*$^{-/-}$ mouse line used to prepare MEF cells, Dr. Xinghua Feng for preparing the MEF cells. We thank Eric Li for assistance on sorting ANOVA analyzed data and the heat-map protein list for cluster interpretation. This work was supported in part by the Cancer Prevention & Research Institute of Texas Proteomics & Metabolomics Core Facility Support Award (RP170005, DPE), NCI Cancer Center Support Grant

(P30CA125123, DPE) to Antibody-based Proteomics Core/Shared Resource (SH), and NIH grants (R01NS092377 and R01NS102452, to MXZ), as well as NIEHS grants P30 ES030285 (CC) and P42 ES027725 (DPE, CC).

REFERENCES

Acharya, K.D., Nettles, S.A., Sellers, K.J., Im, D.D., Harling, M., Pattanayak, C., Vardar-Ulu, D., Lichti, C.F., Huang, S., and Edwards, D.P. (2017). The progestin receptor interactome in the female mouse hypothalamus: Interactions with synaptic proteins are isoform specific and ligand dependent. *Eneuro* 4(5), doi: ENEURO.0272-17.2017.

Bai, H., Inoue, J., Kawano, T., and Inazawa, J. (2012). A transcriptional variant of the LC3A gene is involved in autophagy and frequently inactivated in human cancers. *Oncogene* 31, 4397–4408.

Bu, W., Liu, Z., Jiang, W., Nagi, C., Huang, S., Edwards, D.P., Jo, E., Mo, Q., Creighton, C.J., and Hilsenbeck, S.G. (2019). Mammary precancerous stem and non-stem cells evolve into cancers of distinct subtypes. *Cancer Research* 79, 61–71.

Calcraft, P.J., Ruas, M., Pan, Z., Cheng, X., Arredouani, A., Hao, X., Tang, J., Rietdorf, K., Teboul, L., and Chuang, K.-T. (2009). NAADP mobilizes calcium from acidic organelles through two-pore channels. *Nature* 459, 596–600.

Cang, C., Zhou, Y., Navarro, B., Seo, Y.-J., Aranda, K., Shi, L., Battaglia-Hsu, S., Nissim, I., Clapham, D.E., and Ren, D. (2013). mTOR regulates lysosomal ATP-sensitive two-pore Na+ channels to adapt to metabolic state. *Cell* 152, 778–790.

Chang, C.-H., Zhang, M., Rajapakshe, K., Coarfa, C., Edwards, D., Huang, S., and Rosen, J.M. (2015). Mammary stem cells and tumor-initiating cells are more resistant to apoptosis and exhibit increased DNA repair activity in response to DNA damage. *Stem Cell Reports* 5, 378–391.

Condon, K.J., and Sabatini, D.M. (2019). Nutrient regulation of mTORC1 at a glance. *Journal of Cell Science* 132 jcs222570.

Coarfa C, Grimm, SL, Rajapakshe K, Perera D, Lu HY, Wang X, Christensen KR, Mo Q, Edwards DP, Huang S. (forthcoming). Reverse Phase Protein Array (RPPA): Technology, Application, Data Processing & Integration. *Journal of Biomolecular Techniques* 32, 2

Creighton, C.J., and Huang, S. (2015). Reverse phase protein arrays in signaling pathways: a data integration perspective. *Drug Design, Development and Therapy* 9, 3519.

Elsarraj, H.S., Hong, Y., Limback, D., Zhao, R., Berger, J., Bishop, S.C., Sabbagh, A., Oppenheimer, L., Harper, H.E., and Tsimelzon, A. (2020). BCL9/STAT3 regulation of transcriptional enhancer networks promote DCIS progression. *NPJ Breast Cancer* 6, 1–14.

Federici, G., Gao, X., Slawek, J., Arodz, T., Shitaye, A., Wulfkuhle, J.D., De Maria, R., Liotta, L.A., and Petricoin, E.F. (2013). Systems analysis of the NCI-60 cancer cell lines by alignment of protein pathway activation modules with "-OMIC" data fields and therapeutic response signatures. *Molecular Cancer Research* 11, 676–685.

Fielhaber, J.A., Han, Y.-S., Tan, J., Xing, S., Biggs, C.M., Joung, K.-B., and Kristof, A.S. (2009). Inactivation of mammalian target of rapamycin increases STAT1 nuclear content and transcriptional activity in α4-and protein phosphatase 2A-dependent fashion. *Journal of Biological Chemistry* 284, 24341–24353.

Goldberg, A.A., Nkengfac, B., Sanchez, A.M.J., Moroz, N., Qureshi, S.T., Koromilas, A.E., Wang, S., Burelle, Y., Hussain, S.N., and Kristof, A.S. (2017). Regulation of ULK1 Expression and Autophagy by STAT1. *Journal of Biological Chemistry* 292, 1899–1909.

Grubb Iii, R.L., Deng, J., Pinto, P.A., Mohler, J.L., Chinnaiyan, A., Rubin, M., Linehan, W.M., Liotta, L.A., Petricoin Iii, E.F., and Wulfkuhle, J.D. (2009). Pathway biomarker profiling of localized and metastatic human prostate cancer reveal metastatic and prognostic signatures. *Journal of Proteome Research* 8, 3044–3054.

Hilsenbeck, S.G., Friedrichs, W.E., Schiff, R., O'connell, P., Hansen, R.K., Osborne, C.K., and Fuqua, S.a.W. (1999). Statistical analysis of array expression data as applied to the problem of tamoxifen resistance. *Journal of the National Cancer Institute* 91, 453–459.

Holdman, X.B., Welte, T., Rajapakshe, K., Pond, A., Coarfa, C., Mo, Q., Huang, S., Hilsenbeck, S.G., Edwards, D.P., and Zhang, X. (2015). Upregulation of EGFR signaling is correlated with tumor stroma remodeling and tumor recurrence in FGFR1-driven breast cancer. *Breast Cancer Research* 17, 141.

Hosokawa, N., Hara, T., Kaizuka, T., Kishi, C., Takamura, A., Miura, Y., Iemura, S.-I., Natsume, T., Takehana, K., and Yamada, N. (2009). Nutrient-dependent mTORC1 association with the ULK1–Atg13–FIP200 complex required for autophagy. *Molecular Biology of the Cell* 20, 1981–1991.

Iezaki, T., Horie, T., Fukasawa, K., Kitabatake, M., Nakamura, Y., Park, G., Onishi, Y., Ozaki, K., Kanayama, T., and Hiraiwa, M. (2018). Translational control of Sox9 RNA by mTORC1 contributes to skeletogenesis. *Stem Cell Reports* 11, 228–241.

Jati, S., Kundu, S., Chakraborty, A., Mahata, S.K., Nizet, V., and Sen, M. (2018). Wnt5A signaling promotes defense against bacterial pathogens by activating a host autophagy circuit. *Frontiers in Immunology* 9, 679.

Jozefczuk, J., Drews, K., and Adjaye, J. (2012). Preparation of mouse embryonic fibroblast cells suitable for culturing human embryonic and induced pluripotent stem cells. *JoVE (Journal of Visualized Experiments)*, 64, e3854.

Kim, J., and Guan, K.-L. (2019). mTOR as a central hub of nutrient signalling and cell growth. *Nature Cell Biology* 21, 63–71.

Lin, P.-H., Duann, P., Komazaki, S., Park, K.H., Li, H., Sun, M., Sermersheim, M., Gumpper, K., Parrington, J., and Galione, A. (2015). Lysosomal two-pore channel subtype 2 (TPC2) regulates skeletal muscle autophagic signaling. *Journal of Biological Chemistry* 290, 3377–3389.

Liu, K., Ren, T., Huang, Y., Sun, K., Bao, X., Wang, S., Zheng, B., and Guo, W. (2017). Apatinib promotes autophagy and apoptosis through VEGFR2/STAT3/BCL-2 signaling in osteosarcoma. *Cell Death & Disease* 8, e3015.

Mateo, F., Arenas, E.J., Aguilar, H., Serra-Musach, J., De Garibay, G.R., Boni, J., Maicas, M., Du, S., Iorio, F., and Herranz-Ors, C. (2017). Stem cell-like transcriptional reprogramming mediates metastatic resistance to mTOR inhibition. *Oncogene* 36, 2737–2749.

Mueller, C., Liotta, L.A., and Espina, V. (2010). Reverse phase protein microarrays advance to use in clinical trials. *Molecular Oncology* 4, 461–481.

Raychaudhuri, S., Stuart, J.M., and Altman, R.B. (1999). "Principal components analysis to summarize microarray experiments: application to sporulation time series," in *Biocomputing 2000*. World Scientific), 455–466.

Reggiori, F., and Klionsky, D.J. (2013). Autophagic processes in yeast: mechanism, machinery and regulation. *Genetics* 194, 341–361.

Ruas, M., Chuang, K.-T., Davis, L.C., Al-Douri, A., Tynan, P.W., Tunn, R., Teboul, L., Galione, A., and Parrington, J. (2014). TPC1 has two variant isoforms, and their removal has different effects on endo-lysosomal functions compared to loss of TPC2. *Molecular and Cellular Biology* 34, 3981–3992.

Sharma, M., Khong, H., Fa'ak, F., Bentebibel, S.-E., Janssen, L.M.E., Chesson, B.C., Creasy, C.A., Forget, M.-A., Kahn, L.M.S., and Pazdrak, B. (2020). Bempegaldesleukin selectively depletes intratumoral Tregs and potentiates T cell-mediated cancer therapy. *Nature Communications* 11, 1–11.

Shi, Y., Tan, S.-H., Ng, S., Zhou, J., Yang, N.-D., Koo, G.-B., Mcmahon, K.-A., Parton, R.G., Hill, M.M., and Del Pozo, M.A. (2015). Critical role of CAV1/caveolin-1 in cell stress responses in human breast cancer cells via modulation of lysosomal function and autophagy. *Autophagy* 11, 769–784.

Spurrier, B., Ramalingam, S., and Nishizuka, S. (2008). Reverse-phase protein lysate microarrays for cell signaling analysis. *Nature Protocols* 3, 1796.

Wan, W., You, Z., Xu, Y., Zhou, L., Guan, Z., Peng, C., Wong, C.C.L., Su, H., Zhou, T., and Xia, H. (2017). mTORC1 phosphorylates acetyltransferase p300 to regulate autophagy and lipogenesis. *Molecular Cell* 68, 323–335.

Wang, X., Zhang, X., Dong, X.-P., Samie, M., Li, X., Cheng, X., Goschka, A., Shen, D., Zhou, Y., and Harlow, J. (2012). TPC proteins are phosphoinositide-activated sodium-selective ion channels in endosomes and lysosomes. *Cell* 151, 372–383.

Wu, Y., Li, Y., Zhang, H., Huang, Y., Zhao, P., Tang, Y., Qiu, X., Ying, Y., Li, W., and Ni, S. (2015). Autophagy and mTORC1 regulate the stochastic phase of somatic cell reprogramming. *Nature Cell Biology* 17, 715–725.

Wysocka, J., Myers, M.P., Laherty, C.D., Eisenman, R.N., and Herr, W. (2003). Human Sin3 deacetylase and trithorax-related Set1/Ash2 histone H3-K4 methyltransferase are tethered together selectively by the cell-proliferation factor HCF-1. *Genes & Development* 17, 896–911.

Xiong, J., and Zhu, M.X. (2016). Regulation of lysosomal ion homeostasis by channels and transporters. *Science China. Life Sciences* 59, 777–791.

Zhao, Y., Yang, J., Liao, W., Liu, X., Zhang, H., Wang, S., Wang, D., Feng, J., Yu, L., and Zhu, W.-G. (2010). Cytosolic FoxO1 is essential for the induction of autophagy and tumour suppressor activity. *Nature Cell Biology* 12, 665–675.

Zoncu, R., Bar-Peled, L., Efeyan, A., Wang, S., Sancak, Y., and Sabatini, D.M. (2011). mTORC1 senses lysosomal amino acids through an inside-out mechanism that requires the vacuolar H+-ATPase. *Science* 334, 678–683.

Index

Page numbers in *Italics* refers figures; **bold** refers table

X

Y

Z

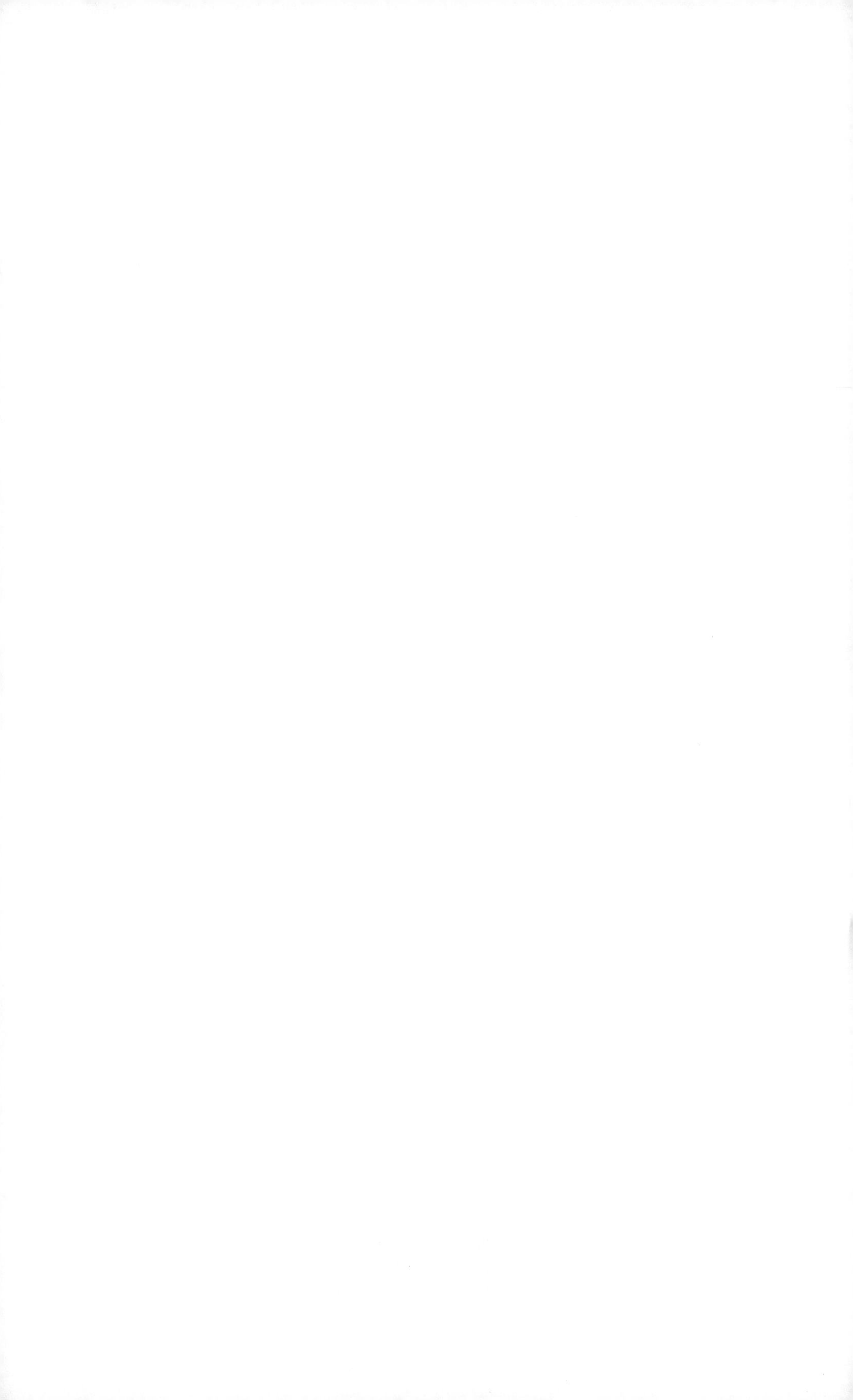

T - #0040 - 171024 - C84 - 234/156/16 - PB - 9780367744663 - Gloss Lamination